*By Variorum Publications:*

**Neoplatonism and Early Christian Thought**
**Essays in honour of A. H. Armstrong**
edited by H. J. Blumenthal & R. A. Markus

*By Variorum Reprints — Collected Studies Series:*

**DAVID C. LINDBERG**
Studies in the History of Medieval Optics

**EDWARD GRANT**
Studies in Medieval Science and Natural Philosophy

**CHARLES B. SCHMITT**
Studies in Renaissance Philosophy and Science

**CHARLES B. SCHMITT**
The Aristotelian Tradition and Renaissance Universities

**D. P. WALKER**
Music, Spirit and Language in the Renaissance

**FRANCIS OAKLEY**
Natural Law, Conciliarism and Consent in the Late Middle Ages

**WILLIAM J. COURTENAY**
Covenant and Causality in Medieval Thought

**YVES CONGAR**
Thomas d'Aquin. Sa vision de théologie et de l'Eglise

**JAN PINBORG**
Medieval Semantics
Selected Studies on Medieval Logic and Grammar

**ROBERT M. KINGDON**
Church and Society in Reformation Europe

**JOHN W. O'MALLEY**
Rome and the Renaissance: Studies in Culture and Religion

**PAUL GRENDLER**
Culture and Censorship in Late Renaissance Italy and France

**S. M. STERN**
Medieval Arabic and Hebrew Thought

**MAX MEYERHOF**
Studies in Medieval Arabic Medicine

# Religion and Neoplatonism in Renaissance Medicine

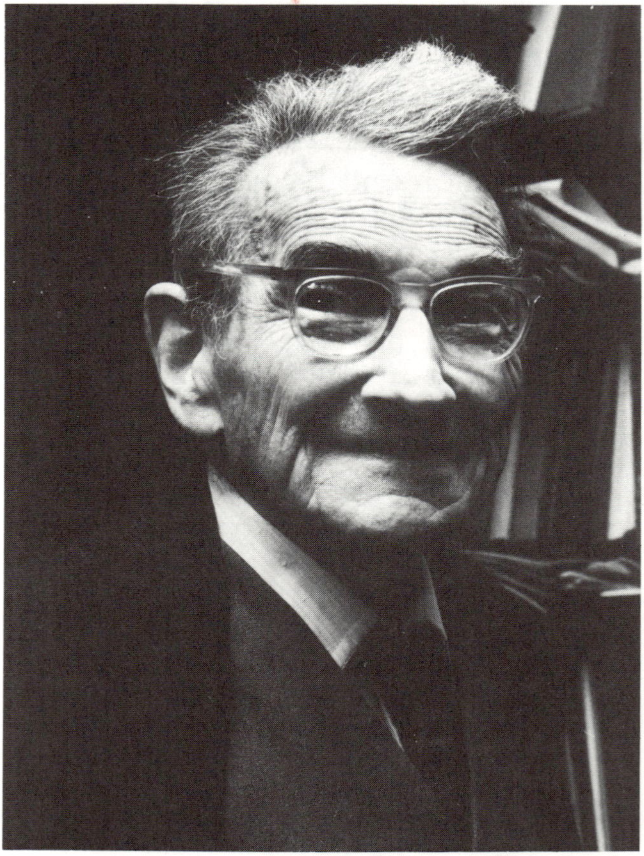

*Wellcome Institute Library, London*

Walter Pagel (1898–1983)

Walter Pagel

# Religion and Neoplatonism in Renaissance Medicine

Edited by Marianne Winder

VARIORUM REPRINTS
London 1985

*British Library CIP data*

Pagel, Walter
Religion and Neoplatonism in Renaissance medicine. — (Collected studies series; CS226)
1. Medicine — History
I. Title II. Winder, Marianne
610′.9′031 R145

ISBN 0–86078–174–7



*Published in Great Britain by* Variorum Reprints
20 Pembridge Mews London W11 3EQ

*Printed in Great Britain by* Galliard (Printers) Ltd
Great Yarmouth Norfolk

VARIORUM REPRINT CS226

## CONTENTS

This volume contains a total of 346 pages.

# PREFACE

The philosophical background to Renaissance Medicine and its close connection with religious ideas and with the Neoplatonism and Gnosticism of the past were some of the many subjects Walter Pagel was preoccupied with in his writings on medical history.

Walter Pagel (12.11.1898 — 25.3.1983) was born in Berlin and became a physician, like his father Julius Leopold Pagel before him, also an eminent historian who had published an authoritative history of medicine and was Professor in that subject at Berlin University. Walter Pagel, after obtaining a Berlin M.D. degree in 1922, worked at the Tuberculosis Hospital, Berlin, 1928–1930, and taught at Heidelberg University (1930–1933). Being Jewish, he emigrated first to Paris where he worked at the Pasteur Institute (1933) and then to Cambridge where he worked at the Papworth Hospital (1933–1939). From 1939 to 1956 he was Consultant Pathologist at the Central Middlesex Hospital, London, and from 1956 at the Clare Hall Hospital where he remained Honorary Consultant Pathologist after 1965, when he retired to devote himself entirely to the study of the history of medicine. At that time he lived in Mill Hill with his wife Magda, who sustained him, body and spirit, with her care and love through years of ill health and exile. The many visitors from all over the world who made the 'pilgrimage' there remember the inspiration, stimulation and encouragement they invariably received in their own particular subject of research.

More details about Walter Pagel's life and development can be found in his autobiographical sketch, 'Erinnerungen und Forschungen' in *Wege zur Wissenschaftsgeschichte* II, ed. K. Mauel, Wiesbaden, F. Steiner, 1982, pp. 45–66, and in English in the Obituaries in *The Times*, 4.4.1983, the *Daily Telegraph*, 5.4.1983, the *British Medical Journal*, 23.4.1983, the *Lancet*, 16.4.1983, and *Medical History*, vol. 27, July 1983. A complete list of his writings up to 1971, comprising over 200 items, is contained in a bibliography in the two volumes of Essays published in his honour in 1972 under the title, *Science, Medicine and Society in the Renaissance*, edited by Allen G. Debus, New York, Neale Watson Academic Publications, Inc. But the last eleven years of Walter Pagel's life saw many more books, reviews and articles three of which are contained in the present volume. Two more from that period will be published by Variorum Reprints in 1986 in another volume of studies by Walter Pagel, devoted to Renaissance science and medicine.

Even a cursory glance through the bibliography will show that up to around 1960 pathology and particularly that of tuberculosis were the chief subjects of Walter Pagel's publications. Nevertheless, already in 1930 he had published a monograph on J. B. Van Helmont not from the biographical and descriptive point of view as was the custom at the time but training his searchlight on the philosophical background from which Helmont's ideas emerged.

I, 'The vindication of "rubbish"', has been included because it represents a turning point in the historiography of medicine and science. Originally it was the response to a request from students for a light-hearted contribution to the *Middlesex Hospital Journal*. Here, for the first time, it was demanded that a scientist or medical man of the past should not be measured against the requirements of today but against the intellectual background of his own time, however incongruous it would seem today. Nowadays, the view that theories unacceptable to us have to be included in a historical work has become a commonplace, due in no small measure to the impetus and constant reminders of Walter Pagel. Again, the subject of II, the view that religious motives have been often the main springs of scientific and medical discoveries and inventions has been taken up by cultural historians since. But even fifty years after its first appearance this study commands attention and will provide new insights to those who read it for the first time. The theme of III can be summarised in the sentence on p. 13: 'We can now understand why the scientist (Van Helmont) who used the balance, who designed scientific instruments, who expressed his results so admirably in quantitative and chemical terms, who founded Biochemistry and Pathology on experimental knowledge, — why this man deprecated "Ratio", accepted magic effects and miracles as genuine natural phenomena and never completely concealed his ultimate doubts in the possibility of full human knowledge.'

IV leads to Paracelsus on whom Walter Pagel has written two different books, one in English (1958), and one in German (1962). Paracelsus, who has been regarded as an early representative of modern medicine because he introduced chemical remedies into a pharmacopoeia hitherto chiefly herbal and because of his contempt for Scholastic Medicine, also drew on mediaeval, Gnostic and

Neoplatonic sources, partly literary like Konrad von Megenberg's *Buch der Natur* and partly from folk tradition. Various groups of people have adopted him as their protagonist — Roman Catholics, Protestants and even the German National Socialists. The latter supported their view by pointing out the anti-Semitic utterances of Paracelsus of which there are indeed quite a number. On the other hand, there is the praise of the Jew Techellus and of the 'revelations granted by God to the Israelites' mentioned in the Paracelsian corpus, with which V is concerned. The passages may well be spurious. But in genuine works Paracelsus does praise the Kabbalah. VII deals with an important concept in alchemy and the Hermetic philosophy: prime matter. VI, VIII, IX and X discuss the probable sources of Paracelsus and the origin of many of his ideas. IX has also one of the more immediate sources as a subject, namely his contemporary Georgius Venetus. Finally, XI tells of Paracelsus' belief in a Messianic alchemist who will be capable of transmuting base metal into gold.

Considering the depth and breadth of Walter Pagel's vision it is no wonder that he was honoured with the Dexter Award in the History of Chemistry in 1969, the Sarton Medal in 1970, the Julius Pagel Medal in 1971, the Robert Koch Medal in 1973, the William H. Welch Medal in 1976, the Fellowship of the British Academy in 1976, and the Paracelsus ring of the city of Villach in 1978.

MARIANNE WINDER

*The Wellcome Institute*
*for the History of Medicine, London*
*March 1985*

## PUBLISHER'S NOTE

The articles in this volume, as in all others in the Collected Studies Series, have not been given a new, continuous pagination. In order to avoid confusion, and to facilitate their use where these same studies have been referred to elsewhere, the original pagination has been maintained wherever possible.

Each article has been given a Roman number in order of appearance, as listed in the Contents. This number is repeated on each page and quoted in the index entries.

# I

## The Vindication of "Rubbish"

THE Medical Historian selects and simplifies. The material at his disposal is overwhelming. He chooses from it what he thinks relevant to his particular task—Medical Biography; History of Discovery in Anatomy; Physiology; Pharmacology; Theories of Pathology; and the changes which diseases have undergone throughout the ages, as the case may be. He endeavours to trace the stepping-stones leading to the modern point of view; he sketches a line of steady progress taking us to a climax—present-day medicine and science. All these tasks involve processes of selection and simplification guided by the modern point of view —that of the historian himself and his contemporaries. His is the extraction of "correct" and "still valuable" facts from their original setting, which may appear to him quite "useless" and unscientific.

It is well known that the discovery of the flow of blood from the right heart through the pulmonary artery and the lungs into the left heart (as against passing through fictitious pores in the ventricular septum)[1] occurs in a religious tract. This tract sets out a Unitarian point of view, and is entitled "Restitution of Christianity" (1553). The historian does not dare to waste time, or try his reader's patience with its actual contents. Those who afford the patience of perusing them will see that Servetus was a fundamentalist intent on proving the literal truth of the scriptural idea that the blood is the seat of the soul, and not the heart, as Aristotle believed. With this aim in mind Servetus found that the blood must acquire a fundamental change in the lungs which in his opinion enabled it to act as the vector of the soul. Three hundred years before Servetus, the author of this tract, an Arab, Nafis, anticipated his discovery ; perhaps legitimately—that is, by anatomical observation and induction from factual evidence. About this, we are not quite clear ; but the record of his discovery is embedded amidst lengthy arguments on the correct interpretation of certain passages of Galen, whose voluminous works formed the " Bible " of medieval medicine. Here again, the setting is unscientific, and apparently devoid of interest for the modern observer. Finally, we may recall the famous case, in the history of science, of Kepler's laws, to be found in two books—" The Mystery of the Kosmos " (1596), and the " Harmony of the World " (1619). Kepler, a Platonic theologian and metaphysician believing in " Planet-Souls," desired to trace the progress and rationale of divine creation. Both titles and contents of these works amply demonstrate this desire. He achieves this largely through scientific observation, and, in particular, mathematical reasoning. The results only, not the work as a whole, attract the historian's attention, with his audience of scientists.

Yet it remains to be seen how far the true historian can afford to ignore the original setting in which the discoverer presented new knowledge. The foremost concern of the historian is truth. It is taken for granted that his facts must be correct. Only a few realise, however, that the usual construction of a line of progress, based on the selection of material from the modern point of view, may endanger the presentation of historical truth. The work of historical appreciation, comparisons of past short-comings and present achievements, the distribution of prizes among the *dramatis personæ* of Medical History, however legitimate and valuable in themselves, are, in my submission, not the main tasks of the historian. For it is difficult to maintain a straight-line view of progress, when discoveries and theories of the past are taken from their original background to be judged alongside modern scientific and medical entities.

Modern Physiology may be said to begin with Harvey's discovery of the blood circulation, published 1628. Harvey proved his point scientifically; that is, by observation and induction, presenting it in terms of quantitative consideration, as does the modern physiologist.[2] Yet blood circulation was only *one* idea which Harvey cherished, as an Aristotelian thinker and natural philosopher. It is *the* idea which made him immortal; but by that very fact—that it had its place in a natural philosophy—it is essentially different from any modern discovery.

In Harvey's time, a strong opposition grew up to Aristotle's philosophy. This had governed the oriental and occidental mind for many centuries; yet was felt to be inimical to scientific progress, as it tended to subordinate observation to reasoning, and insisted on fitting it into the narrow framework of logical theories and categories. It is this feeling which actuated Sir Francis Bacon, when he formulated his principles, to pave the way for the establishment of "inductive science." But the school of Padua, to which Harvey belonged, upheld the Aristotelian tradition. In Aristotle's world it was the heart which was the centre of the living being, and therefore deserved the main attention of the philosopher.

Now it is hardly an accident that the great masters of cardiovascular anatomy, Realdo Colombo (1516-59), and Fabricius of Aquapendente (1537-1619), were typical exponents of the Aristotelian school of Padua and the immediate predecessors of Harvey. Cesalpino (1519-1603), who came even nearer it than did Colombo,[3] was the latter's pupil, and one of the greatest Aristotelian thinkers of his time. His correct estimation of the pulmonary artery as a " public," and not a " private " vessel merely destined for the nutrition of the lung parenchyma ; his knowledge of the blood content of the left auricle and of the flow of the blood from the heart through the lungs back to the heart, and his insight into the centripetal direction of the flow in the veins towards the heart and its centrifugal direction (towards the tissues) in the arteries*—all these corrections of the wrong, but then ruling, opinions of Galen—corrections foreshadowing Harvey's work, are to be found in his " Questions concerning Peripatetic (*Aristotelian*) Philosophy " (1571). More-

---

* This is an important point in judging Cesalpino's merits and shortcomings which are not always given with the desirable clarity. I therefore quote what he says : " . . . rien ne peut faire craindre que l'échange se fasse des artères vers le cœur : la chaleur entraînant l'aliment, le mouvement se fait des veines au cœur, et en même temps, du cœur aux artères, parce que le chemin ne s'ouvre que dans ce sens, étant donnée la position des membranes ; le même mouvement ouvre de part et d'autre les orifices, de la vein vers le cœur, du cœur vers les artères. Or, les membranes ont reçu cette disposition pour que jamais il ne se produisît un mouvement contraire, ce qui eût pu se faire dans les émotions violentes de l'âme, ou par d'autres causes qui ramèneraient le sang au cœur ; les membranes s'opposent a ce mouvement. Si elles n'avaient été disposées ainsi, le feu du cœur s'éteindrait pour la plus petite cause. Si en effet un mouvement contraire se faisait, tous se passerait comme quand on rabat de force une flamme sur du combustible : qu'il soit préparé en quantité insuffisante, ou trop abondante, on étouffe le feu . . ." (Questions Péripatéticiennes. French Translation by Maurice Dorolle. Paris Alcan, 1929. Book V, question 4 ; p. 219ff). Cesalpino's correct arguments are part and parcel of his defence of Aristotelian doctrines versus Galen and partly based on correct observation. It is a " mixture of tradition and experience, a mixture of rationalism and observation " which he presents (Dorolle loc. cit., p. 87). It is thus that he still believes in nutritive " spirits " conveyed by the arteries to the tissues and in the openings of the veins by which the tissues draw substances necessary for their growth, and remains ignorant of the fact that *all* the blood passes through veins and arteries in the direction which he had described correctly, in other words that it circulates. What Max Neuburger has shown with regard to Servetus and Colombo (loc. cit., footnote 1), applies therefore to Cesalpino too.

over, Haller (1708-77), the great physiologist, said of Cesalpino, that it was his concentration on the heart and abandonment of the liver as a "central organ" which enabled him to achieve what he did; that is, his progress was due to adherence to Aristotelian doctrines rather than those of Galen.

For Aristotle not only made the heart the origin and "principle" of the heart and vessels, but devoted much to the logical demonstration that circular movement is the noblest of all forms of movement; and that the circular motion of the heavens forms the pattern to which motions of "sublunary bodies," especially the microcosm of living organisms, aspire. Aristotle said that circular movement is "perfect," since "there is no other form of motion opposed as contrary to it" (as upward and downward movement are contraries to each other); "it is the only motion which is continuous; and it is a great marvel in that it is made up of contraries which are present together, namely motion and rest, the concave and convex, and its moving simultaneously to a forward and backward position."

No such speculations can be found in Harvey's works. Nevertheless Harvey's adherence to Aristotle and Aristotelian ways of thinking and observing are easy to recognise, particularly in his work on Embryology (1651), and in the comparative anatomical methods which he employed. Aristotle may rightly be called the founder of Scientific Embryology and Comparative Anatomy, and Harvey's master Fabricius a worthy follower of Aristotle on these lines. Harvey made no secret of his leanings towards Aristotelian principles. Harvey felt he had proved the main Aristotelian tenets —the sovereignty of the heart, its independence of the brain in sense and motion, its supremacy in being the first part which exists, in its containing blood, life, sensation, motion, before either the brain or the liver were in being.[4]

Harvey concludes : " The heart like a prince in a kingdom, in whose hands lie the chief and highest authority, rules over all ; it is the original and the foundation from which all power is derived, on which all power depends in the animal body."[5] The stroke of genius by which Harvey welded the multitude of his observations into the concept of blood circulation, he describes as follows : " I began to think whether there might not be *a motion as it were in a circle*. Now this I afterwards found to be true . . . which motion we may be allowed to call circular, in the same way as Aristotle says that the air and rain emulate the circular motion of the superior bodies ; for the moist earth, warmed by the sun, evaporates ; the vapours drawn upwards are condensed, and descending in the form of rain, moisten the earth again ; and by this arrangement, are generations of living things produced ; and in like manner, too, are tempests and meteors engendered by the circular motion, by the approach and recession of the sun. And so in all likelihood, does it come to pass in the body, through the motion of the blood ; the various parts are nourished, cherished, quickened by the warmer, more perfect, vaporous, spirituous, and as I may say, alimentive blood ; which, on the contrary, in contact with these parts becomes cooled, coagulated, and, so to speak, effete ; whence it returns to its sovereign the heart as if to its source, or to the inmost home of the body, there to recover its state of excellence or perfection. Here it resumes its due fluidity and receives an infusion of natural heat—powerful, fervid, a kind of treasury of life, and is impregnated with spirits, and, it might be said, with balsam ; and thence it is again dispersed ; and all this depends on the motion and action of the heart. The heart, consequently, is the beginning of life ; the sun of the microcosm, even as the sun in his turn might well be designated as the heart of the world ; for it is the heart . . . which is indeed the foundation of life, the source of all action."[6]

Here, the circulation of the blood is visualised as the microcosmic copy of a general cosmological pattern and principle. It no longer remains a discovery of scientific detail, but obtains a position in a view of the world which complies with two of the main Aristotelian tenets : the excellence of circular motion ; and the parallelism of the microcosm and the macrocosm—that is, the living organism and the universe. We need not be surprised, therefore, that the mystic Robert Fludd (1574-1637) was the first to recognise Harvey's discovery, calling him, " his friend, colleague, and compatriot, well-versed, not only in Anatomy, but also in the deepest mysteries of Philosophy," and saying that his theory was a demonstration that the spirit of life retains an impression of both the planetary system and the zodiac.[7] In other words, he regarded the essential requisite of Harvey's work to be the genuine Aristotelian idea of the " fountain of life " in the living body imitating the circular movement of the " common parent and producer " in the bigger world, namely the sun. It should be borne in mind that at this time Harvey was widely disbelieved and attacked by the exponents of " scientific " and professional medicine, as then understood.

Boyle tells us that Harvey was led to his discovery by the reflection that " so provident a cause as nature had not placed so many valves without design." This is a consideration of final causes in the true Aristotelian sense—for it was Aristotle who had said that : " Nature like mind always does whatever it does for the sake of something, which something is its end."

But to Harvey adherence to Aristotelian philosophy did not mean subjection of empiricism to reasoning, for he refers to Aristotle's advice : " Faith is to be given to reason if the matters demonstrated agree with those that are perceived by the senses ; when all things have been thoroughly scrutinised, then are the senses to be trusted rather than the reason." Moreover, he said against those who attacked him for refuting the authority of Galen : " The facts cognisable by the senses wait upon no opinions, and the works of nature bow to no antiquity ; for, indeed, there is nothing either more ancient or of higher authority than nature."[8]

I am not concerned with the question whether Harvey's general attitude was " reactionary " or " progressive,"[9] for the tremendous progress achieved by his discoveries in physiology, as well as in embryology, needs no discussion. But I have tried to show that only a process of abstraction from a world of seventeenth-century ideas will take his discoveries to the level of modern research, and that this abstraction endangers the historical understanding of the chapter which Harvey's work constitutes in the History of Medicine. By " historical understanding " I mean an attempt to develop a medical theory or discovery from the world of ideas cherished by its author and characteristic of his period, disregarding their scientific or non-scientific value ; so that ultimately one tries to explain why each discovery was typical of the period which begot it.

I feel, then, it is necessary first, to look at Harvey as a whole, not separating the scientist from the philosopher, but trying to discover the influence of the various aspects of his personality on one another ; and secondly, to study the general background, including Aristotelian philosophy, being responsible for the cardiovascular bias of the school of Padua, and the spirit of the seventeenth century in general—the " Baroque " period. This dissolved the strictly finite and linear forms, of the " static " attitude of the Renaissance, into the perspective of things infinitely movable or " dynamic." It is the period which interested itself far more in " coming into being " than in " being " itself. All this is obvious in Art, but the concepts " Renaissance " and " Baroque " cover a much wider field ; they indicate a world of ideas which create, and penetrate into, all branches of culture, such as literature, music, politics, fashion—and science. As Sigerist[10] has shown, Anatomy, the knowledge of the " static " forms, is consequently a typical offspring of the Renaissance period ; while Physiology owes its existence to the Baroque spirit of which Harvey is a typical example. Without an understanding of Baroque culture, an understanding of Harvey is impossible.

Let us turn to another naturalist and philosopher of this period, an example even more obvious than Harvey. John Baptista van Helmont (1579-1644) discovered " Gas." This, in itself, is *true* ; he did distinguish air and water vapour, on the one hand, from " gas "—notably carbon dioxide and the other " gases " which he had isolated, on the other. But this is not the *whole truth*. The whole truth is that the discovery of gas as a physico-chemical, or scientific entity, is a by-product of some quite unscientific ideas. Van Helmont was trying to detect the divine spark implanted in things when created, their " time-table " of development towards a destined end—something " spiritual," yet of finest corporality, which could not be apprehended unless its coarse material cover was removed. The " spagyric " art of chemistry, the " Philosophy by Fire " (the employment of combustion), seemed to van Helmont the most promising method to attain his end. He found that charcoal heated in a closed vessel never substantially disappears, but is almost completely transformed into a " wild spirit "—called " wild " because it cannot be held in an open vessel and solidified. Van Helmont felt that this was a new entity, for which he had to coin a new term—" gas." He argued that each organised body in nature (everything that is not insipid water, or air) contains its gas, a spirit, under normal conditions " concrete " or " coagulated," like a solid body, and thereby kept dormant.

The whole body may, however, become volatile—reveal its gaseous nature, when it has combined with an appropriate "ferment," such as seen in fermenting grapes left lying about with their skins damaged. If the skin is intact, however, and the ferment thus prevented from access, they simply dry up without liberation of "their gas." Gas is, to van Helmont, unlike water vapour and air, no common volatile medium of which all things partake, but something specific; it is the material vector of specificity, such as the "life-spirit" in our blood, a vital principle in all things, in organic beings more easily perceptible than in inorganic objects. Van Helmont set out to search for the divine spark in beings, and discovered a scientific, a chemical entity. It is difficult to understand the circumstances of his discovery—why van Helmont was responsible for it, why it was discovered in his time, and what it originally meant—unless the "dark" chapters of van Helmont's work, his religious philosophy and cosmology, his leanings towards Alchemy—briefly the "rubbish"—are subjected to as close a scrutiny as the "scientific light" which he has seen.[11]

Before we conclude let us meet two objections—first of all, am I not exaggerating? Was the "rubbish" really meant as seriously as I try to make you believe? Are we not dealing with mere figures of speech, with poetical arabesques, meant to adorn a dry scientific text or an old-fashioned clumsy language, a cloak in which the ancient author had to present knowledge in a then customary way? I do not think so. Harvey's small book on the circulation is famous for its conciseness, for its clear language, for its logical structure in which fact follows upon fact, argument on argument, proof on proof. Yet Harvey himself cannot have deemed the pages of his book too precious to be devoted to bits of Aristotelian philosophy as outlined above. In van Helmont's case there is so much philosophy and religion interwoven in the scientific detail, and so intimately blended with it, that it must be regarded as an integral part of all his treatises. It is not merely an odd mode of expression, or the clumsiness of an obsolete language, which creates a religious or philosophical impression in his work, since there are other seventeenth-century scientific works in which the contemporary style of expression has no trace of philosophy or religion—such as the treatises of Galileo and Santorio.

Secondly, who cares about the religious or philosophical views of present-day, or nineteenth-century, scientists ? Pasteur (1822-95) and Schwann (1810-82) were firm Catholics—we forget this in relation to their work ; does it really matter what Harvey's views were ? Now it is not unlikely that present-day scientists do not escape the bias of faith and philosophy when speculating about general problems, as the nature of life, or the mysterious universe ; yet the actual work in the laboratory, the approach to scientific problems will be unaffected by outside considerations. But nineteenth- and twentieth-century scientists were, and are, in a situation quite different from that which confronted earlier scientists, notably those of the seventeenth century who saw the creation of modern science. Then there were no university departments, no laboratories, in which professors and their staff of specially trained assistants devoted time and public means to specialised and well-defined tasks. Science then was in the hands of individuals, wealthy noblemen such as van Helmont and Boyle ; of adventurers, men like Paracelsus (1493-1541) and his followers, mostly vagrant doctors and alchemists ; or of clergymen such as formed the nucleus of the early Royal Society —with the result that "Philosophia Naturalis," Nature in her entirety, cosmology in its widest sense—that is, a mixture of Science, Theology and Metaphysics—formed the subject of the studies of early scientists. This is recognisable not only in the two examples given, but in many others too, of whom Robert Boyle (1626-1691), Francis Glisson (1597-1677) and John Ray (1628-1705) may be cited.

Thus our aim in Medical Historiography is to outline spheres of ideas, centred round men, with peculiar and contemporary motives, around trends of thought, scientific and non-scientific, and around economic and political factors ; in other words to understand the facts of medical history as the outward expression of their time. Then we shall be able to see why problems and discoveries at certain times are " in the air," why certain facts are forgotten and rediscovered in quick succession ; to quote only two examples : the insight into the cellular structure of man and animals, Dutrochet-Schwann ; or the causation of fermentation by organisms, and the proof that " spontaneous generation " does not exist, Schwann-Pasteur.[12] It will then appear that not only certain standards of technical equipment made discoveries possible, but that these can be seen also as the offspring of certain non-scientific ideas and of a particular cultural background. Finally, we learn from Harvey and van Helmont that philosophical insight and metaphysical views were not always detrimental to scientific work and discovery.

The history of Medicine will then appear much more complicated than it does in the usual perspective of straight lines of progress. Yet we will have to embark on the cumbersome task of reconstructing ancient thought if we wish to write history—and not best-sellers.

## REFERENCES

[1] Max Neuburger (of the Wellcome Historical Medical Museum) conclusively showed in 1930 that

we have no right to call this " the discovery of the lesser circulation." The early pre-Harveian anatomists demonstrated the correct anatomical pathways for the blood's passage through the lungs, but did not recognise that it is the whole blood that passes through in the unit of time. Without a knowledge of the greater, there was no knowledge of the lesser circulation; so Harvey remains discoverer of both.

[2] For the detail, *cf.* Singer, C., " The Discovery of the Circulation of the Blood," London, 1928; Sir H. Rolleston, " Harvey's Predecessors and Contemporaries"; *Annals of Medicine*, 1928, X, 323; Sir M. Foster, " Lectures on the History of Physiology," Cambridge, 1901; Willis, R., " Wm. Harvey," London, 1878.

[3] Foster, loc. cit., p. 35.

[4] " Anatomical Disquisition on the Motion of the Heart and Blood in Animals," cap. XVII. In " Works," transl. by R. Willis, London Sydenham Society, 1847, p. 83; also Second Disquis., p. 136.

[5] Loc. cit., " Motion of Heart," p. 83.

[6] " Motion of the Heart and Blood," cap. VIII, transl. by R. Willis, loc. cit., p. 46; on the supreme role played by the sun as " common parent and producer, or at all events, immediate and universal instrument of the Creator in the work of reproduction " and his agreement with the Aristotelian pattern of this doctrine, *see* Harvey, " On Generation," Exercise L, transl. Willis, loc. cit., p. 367.

[7] Pagel, W., " Religious Motives in Seventeenth-Century Medical Biology: *Bulletin Johns Hopkins Institute of the History of Medicine*, 1935, iii, 97-312, partic. p. 277.

I



[8] Harvey, Second Disquis to J. Riolan, jun., in "Works" transl. by Willis, loc. cit., p. 123.

[9] *See* Needham, J., "History of Embryology," Cambridge, 1934, p. 128.

[10] Sigerist, H. E., "Harvey's Position in the History of European Thought": *Arch. f. Kulturgesch.*, 1928, xix, 158; Man and Medicine, New York, 1932.

[11] Pagel, W., "Van Helmont's Science and Medicine," Supplem. Bullet. History of Medicine, No. 2, Baltimore, 1944; *Nature*, 1944, cliii, 675; *Brit. Med. J.*, 1945, i, 59.

[12] *Cf.* A. R. Rich's ingenious paper, "The Place of R. J. H. Dutrochet in the Development of the Cell Theory," *Bull. Johns Hopkins Hospital*, 1926, xxxix, 330.

# II

# RELIGIOUS MOTIVES IN THE MEDICAL BIOLOGY OF THE XVIITH CENTURY

INDEX

I. General religious motives leading to empiricism in medical biology during the XVIIth century.

Piety as the source of the scepticism and the fundamental doctrines of Paracelsus.

Comparison of the writings of Paracelsus with

(a) the medical literature of his time (Fracastoro)

(b) medieval authors (Arnald of Villanova, Roger Bacon).

II. The pious scepticism of Hieronymus Hirnhaim as the philosophical basis of " idealistic " biology and pathology.

Comparison with Agrippa of Nettesheym's pious scepticism.

III. The pious conception of Nature and Magic in the writings of the alchemists of the XVIIth century (" Themis aurea," Mich. Maier, Suchten, Croll, Quercetanus). Their adversaries.

IV. The speculative embryology of Marcus Marci and his application of the metaphysics of light to the explanation of life according to the principles of optics.

V. The " Medicina catholica " of Robert Fludd. Metaphysics as the source of a mechanistic explanation of life. Similarity of Fludd's conceptions with those of the " Romantic natural philosophy " during the early XIXth century. The fundamental differences.

---

* This paper is dedicated to Mrs. Elisabeth Gundolf. I wish to express my deepest gratitude to Mrs. Jeanette Stott, without whose aid the paper could not have been produced.

VI. Dissentient trends of thought during the XVIth century and the process of dissociation in mystical natural philosophy.
The non-religious scepticism of Sanchez.
The rationalism of Mersenne.
" Inductive " natural philosophy of Francis Bacon.
Robert Boyle and the theory of corpuscles as scientific explanation of the " mystery " of " specificity," " forms " and " final causes."

In modern medical biology the connection between reason and empiricism is obvious. An historical survey of the evolution of that science, however, will scarcely fail to suggest that in the past this union has not always been regarded as indispensable. Even as late as in the XVIIth century, a period of decisive importance in the development of modern natural science, there is evidence of a significant tendency to discriminate between reason and experiment, and from this differentiation medical biology derived notable inspiration. An increasing opposition to the deliberations of formal logic was the stimulus which gave impulse to a desire for experimental investigation. The limitations of formal logic being realized, its general application since antiquity to the solution of the problems of natural research and medicine was found to be an error in method resulting in fallacies. It became apparent that reason had not made any contribution whatsoever to the cause of natural science. Logic is " inutilis " [1] for the purpose of natural research, for at all times it explains its own statements only, without adding anything new. Its truth is ever opposed to reality. But reality is the aim of the new science. Aspiring inquiry feels capable of grasping the things themselves. They seem to be delivered into her hands.

In this case ratiocination and intellectual analysis are useless. Everything must be apprehended in its entirety and regarded as an aspect of the whole. Elements of the divine creation — how shall human understanding presume to penetrate its mystery?

By divine grace alone may the virtuous acquire knowledge, either in sleep or in visionary ecstasy; or by bold incursion into the garden of nature, by means of unprejudiced experiment inspired by divine revelation, may the adept attain his end.

Thus, knowledge is a divine favour, science and research divine

[1] See van Helmont's treatise " Logica inutilis " and Fr. Bacon, *Nov. Organum*, I, 11 . . . " Logica . . . inutilis est ad inventionem scientiarum."

service, the connecting link with divinity. Grace from above meets human aspiration for knowledge from below. Natural research is the search for God. Knowledge in nature is rather the result of the experiences of the individual soul than of rational deliberation which is generally incontestable and objectively constraining. ("Zwingendes Wissen.")

Hence we find religious motives leading to natural research and to experiment.

The pious naturalist regards the world in its unity as the independent creation of God, its laws as the manifestations of the divine freedom. The laws of nature are the instruments by means of which the Deity coördinates the manifold diversities of his creatures. This Creator is omnipotent. He is the God of the Bible to whom all things are possible — not the demiurge of antiquity who is bound by the laws of nature, in accordance with which he may work his will. Mind and matter, things spiritual and things corporeal, emanations of the will of the Creator, according to this conception of the world, are in all stages connected, and finally identical. There is a general law, a general "reason," a soul in all things of the world, in "Nature," a belief which has been foreshadowed in the philosophy of the stoics.[2] The world is made up of corporeal units, graduated according to the kind and amount of divine force with which they are endowed during creation. This sovereign influence of the divine power must be discovered in the living creature in its entirety as well as in its organs and in the most elementary parts of the organs. This is the seed in all things, the gauge of their development, which constructs their forms and gives direction to their functions until they arrive at their destined end. By virtue of this seed all things live.

In this sense Paracelsus regarded the world as constructed monadically. The "Logos" in things has the same action on their substance as human imagination on the corporeal world. It is the mediator between spirit and matter as was once and for ever Christ. Everything is predetermined. The world does not consist of ever constant matter in a state of continual transformation, due to the

[2] See the note on the importance of stoicism for the philosophy of the Renaissance: Dilthey, *Weltanschauung und Analyse der Menschen seit Renaissance und Reformation*, 3. Aufl., Gesamm. Schriften., II (Leipzig, Teubner, 1923), p. 17 ff.

displacement of the fundamental elements, as the ancients believed. It is rather a mosaic of individual units, each performing its own task. They may unite in various ways, one may even take possession of another, but "never can anything develop from what is not in itself."[3] An important source of this doctrine is St. Augustine, who taught that matter alone cannot be the origin of life unless there are present the implanted seeds of the organisms. Like a mother with child the world is pregnant with the causes of being. The world resembles a grain of seed. All beings have been preformed during the Creation, which, although the result of a single act, is unfolded gradually according to the laws of nature.[4]

Paracelsus was the enemy of all learned science. His source of knowledge was the experience of the common people. By analogies he grasped the obvious. Thus he started from the parallelism between the world as the macrocosm and man as the microcosm.[5] The

[3] Paracelsus, *Op. Paramirum,* III, 1; I, 7 etc.

[4] Compare: Augustinus, *de trinit.*, III, 9, 6; and Meyer, H., *Geschichte der Lehre von den Keimkräften von der Stoa bis zum Ausgange der Patristik* (Bonn, 1914).

[5] An early English expression of the macro-microcosmos doctrine in the sense of Paracelsus is given by the dedication of the English edition of Croll's "Discovering the great and deep mysteries of nature" and Paracelsus' "Philosophy to the Athenians" ("Discovering the wonderful mysteries of the creation") by H. Pinnell under the title Philosophy reformed and improved in 4 profound tractates, London 1657:

"What is above is likewise here below
as this anatomy of man does show.
The man in all the parts of him consists
of what the macrocosme composed is.
The world itselfe's a man though great and big
and man himselfe's a world; do but here dig,
A treasure will appear more worth than all
by which he may be ransom'd from his fall
. . . .
Nature, grace, physick and divinity
so returning to their first unity.
. . . .
Sure, Paracelsus has obtained the skill
through permission of the holy will
To ensee the secrets of each thing
and so of it to mortal's tydings bring.
Praise too the attempt of him that made him speak
in English and the sealed ark to break
That so his treasure might in common be
to the great wonder of posterity."

human organs correspond to the celestial bodies, e. g. the heart to the sun, diseases to natural occurrences, for example, dropsy to rain, phthisis to drought. But beyond this obvious sense there is a deeper meaning.[5a]

The heavens are the example of the harmonic coöperation of the parts in the whole. As the stars follow their own laws of movement, the organs of men fulfil the functions defined by their peculiar structures; and this existence as a microcosm endowed with definite purpose is the power in men. According to the constellation of the organs and impelled by its innate energy, the function of the whole organism proceeds without regard to external influence.

The constellation of the organs varies like the constellation of the stars. Each peculiar constellation defines the characteristics of the individual organism, its temper, which is therefore determined by the relation between the organs and not, as the ancients believed, by those existing between the humours.

According to the ancient views the physical world was the result of a process of constant change in matter, the aggregation and dissipation of the elements. Similarly, the constitution of man was regarded as solely dependent upon the harmonious mixture of the humours and innate heat, i. e. nothing more than a certain arrangement of matter. Humoralism governed ancient biology and pathology. The humoral theory was rejected by Paracelsus,[5b] who argued that if man, like other things, has been developed from a peculiar seed created by God, he must be a peculiar entity. He can not be the result of a mixture of humours, quantitatively varying with the individual.[6] There must be something qualitatively new in him, producing his personality. This makes him live and saves him from decay. It is the immortal in him, his "*mummy.*" The mixture of humours is something secondary, a later occurrence, as

[5a] Vol. *Paramirum,* III, 1.

[5b] *Opus Paramirum,* I, 4.

[6] See Alexander Ross, the adversary of Francis Bacon, *Arcana microcosmi,* 2nd edition (London, 1652): "The whole composition cannot be transformed into another composition nor the form to another specificall form nor the matter into another matter . . . for generation is not the changing of one composition into another, but an introduction of a new form into the matter. . . . Transmutation then of species is impossible to nature, not to chemists who think to transform silver into gold, not to the Roman church which holds a transubstantiation of bread into Christ's body . . ."

far as the humours really exist. Paracelsus imagined each living being as having a centre or "Archeus." Everything in the world is living insofar as it contains an archeus, which ensures the fulfilment of its peculiar purposes. The archeus of Paracelsus corresponds to the Entelechia of Aristotle. This is the purpose of a thing, and therefore the cause of its development; thus it is identical with our conception of a thing. But the life process, according to Paracelsus, is seen rather in movement. In his conception the things are realities. Therefore in their cause and purpose they are not the result of our thought.

Paracelsus' belief in God, his piety, is the basis of all these assumptions. God has arranged the world. As well as life, He has created death and disease. In His wisdom, however, He has made plants containing remedies to grow in the garden of nature. These remedies are specific, their virtue is beneficial to certain organs and antidotal to certain diseases. Their specificity originates in the general sympathy and antipathy by which all things are attracted and repelled. The knowledge of their specific virtue can only be achieved by the godfearing. Experiment and experience must be employed rather than such logical deductions as are contained in the tables of remedies drawn up by Galen.

Paracelsus' doctrine of sympathy and antipathy is the basis of the modern theories of immunity. Even at this period it was suggested that the blood of convalescents had a curative virtue in cases of the same disease and that poison in small doses had the effect of an antidote or prophylactic.

I am inclined to believe that his experience in the mines had a profound influence on the mental attitude of Paracelsus. There is no doubt that it was the origin of his predilection for chemistry, which resulted in the introduction of inorganic substances as remedies, and especially of those of metallic origin.[7] It may also have affected his whole view of biology and pathology. Like everything else in the world the various ores in the mines appeared to be constituted of substance and properties. Their growth seemed to signify

[7] See Paracelsus' achievements in chemistry in the remarkable work of E. Darmstädter, "Arznei und Alchemie. Studien zu Paracelsus," *Studien z. Geschichte der Medizin*, XX (Leipzig, Barth, 1932), founded on an *imitation* of *Paracelsus'* experiments.

a unique process of life, i. e. the pursuit of certain aims by means of the natural operations of motion, alimentation and generation. Thus, even a stone has a peculiar individuality, a peculiar ens, which is not merely the result of an accidental mixture of the elements common to all things. A living individual is never the sum of his parts. Therefore everything has a kind of soul which is revealed by its structure, function and virtue. When absorbed by another body a substance, such as a remedy or food, is not destroyed entirely; its active essence unites with the active essence of the absorbing body with a result which varies according to its ability to penetrate that body.[7a]

These are not merely physical processes. Any influence exerted by one thing on another is primarily something spiritual, just as imagination produces physical effects, e. g., when a pregnant woman is frightened by the sight of some monstrosity, deformity of the child is caused. The bite of a mad dog transfers the imagination of this animal to the person bitten, causing him to behave like a mad dog, to rage and bite other people. Pious contemplation of the suffering of Christ causes stigmatization, the development of haemorrhages in the parts corresponding to the wounds of Christ. These are examples of psychical causes of anatomical changes. They form the basis of the religious biology of Paracelsus. Things influence each other not by purely physical processes, like attraction and repulsion, rarefaction and condensation, but by the mutual influence of their dynamic principles, of the non-corporeal spark inherent in things, the Logos, connecting the General with the Particular, the One with the Many. Christ is the mediator who bestows on things their aim, on material possibility, realization.[7b]

As the magnet attracts iron by virtue of inherent properties which are not to be explained by intellectual analysis, the remedy develops its effects on the corresponding disease. In case of disease one can not simply give the remedy. It is always necessary to await the propitious constellation, a fact which is never accessible to causal analysis. The Christian awaits the inspiration for healing from God, the heathen tries to heal in each case and every time by means

[7a] *Op. Paramirum,* I, 7.

[7b] *Op. Paramirum,* IV, and "Fünf Bücher über unsichtbare Krankheiten," *passim.*

of his reason. Therapy belongs to the world of magic which is remote from reason, having existed before all reason and language. It is the world of the spirit. "Whatever lives according to reason, lives contrary to spirit." [8] This world of spirit is ever connected with the depth in men, the sphere of will, and thus it is connected with the influence of the stars.

Just as every being is a peculiar entity the essence of which can never be the result of a simple mixture of matter, every organ within this being has its peculiar form, function and life. If man were nothing more than a mixture of humours, what could explain his peculiar organization, the "anatomy" of his organs? In that case every organ should have a peculiar humour, because no organ can take the place of another.

Moreover, Paracelsus' reformation of *pathology* depends on the abolition of humoralism, as the consequence of his religious doctrine of seeds. To the Greek physician disease was a disturbance of the harmonious mixture of the humours affecting the organism as a whole. There was no idea of disease as an invading entity which attacks definite parts of the body. Thus there was only the conception of disease, never of diseases (H. E. Sigerist).[9] It was impossible to differentiate diseases either according to the organ involved or according to the causes of the morbid conditions. Paracelsus created the modern conception of disease by emphasizing the importance of its external causes and its seat in a particular organ. He was actually the first to teach that there are different diseases which can be classified, and that each disease is a peculiar reality, an Ens.

Since, according to Paracelsus, humours are only the constituents of the external appearance of man, they have no importance in disease. For the ancient humoral pathologists on the other hand illness was closely connected with the normal life of the individual, because if health is dependent upon the humours, the form and course of disease must vary according to the particular humours predominating in the individual in question. To Paracelsus, however, disease and

[8] Vol. *Paramirum*, Ens spirituale, ed. Achelis (Jena, Diederichs, 1928), p. 96.

[9] See the delightful and fundamental description of the ancient conception of "disease" in H. E. Sigerist, *Antike Heilkunde* (München, Heimeran, 1925); and *Einführung in die Medizin* (Leipzig, Thieme, 1931), p. 136.

normal life were as different as fire and water. Disease and life are opposed. Everything is an entity, men, metal, particles of dust. Even disease is an entity.[10] The essence of these entities does not consist in their substance, but in the spark of spirit or logos inherent in them. This spirit or essence is the cause of the disease. There is no doubt that the theory was inspired by his experience in the mines, for he observed that miners frequently contracted diseases which varied according to the vapors inhaled in the air. When he found it possible to differentiate diseases according to the metals present in the mines where they occurred, he naturally came to regard the various metals and ores or, rather, their "spiritual essence," as the causes of the corresponding diseases. Therefore, he imagined the cause of disease in general to be of finest corporality, a kind of spirit or germ which penetrates into the body, and, as male seed actively produces new living entities, the spiritual cause, in coöperation with the body, creates the disease as a new entity with a peculiar form, function, and life.

In antiquity there were as many diseases as patients. To Paracelsus there were as many diseases as causes. Humoral pathology disregarded the organs and their peculiarities in favour of the whole organism. Paracelsus pointed out that in each disease some particular organ is usually involved and that local events are of great importance. Each organ with its peculiar structure and function, has its own "alchemist," who attracts suitable food from the general supply. His function resembles that of a stomach or a kitchen attached to the organ, which governs its metabolism. Life is metabolism. The organ ingests, changes the food into the specific

[10] See *Op. Paramirum,* III, 1. *Krankheiten ex ingestis.* "Und wiewol die alten Skribenten und ihr Hauf die choleram, phlegma, melancholiam heftig zeihent in solchen Sachen, dieweil es aber unergruendt ist, was soll dann auf dasselbige gemercket werden. Sie betrachten nit, so sie von den Dingen schreiben, den grund philosophiae, also dass sie nit moegen mit ihren humoribus stat und platz haben. Denn bedencket am ersten, wie sies doch reimen wollen, dass auss der phlegmate, melancholia, sanguine, cholera solche generation moegen geboren werden, so doch solche naturae in inen nit seind. . . . Diese krankheiten sind Stein und Sand Leim und Letten. Nun saget mir von eueren humoribus, wie sie moegen zu steinen werden, zu Sand, zu Letten, zu Leim und das sie anfaenglich nicht seind? Soll ein Stein werden im Menschen oder ein Sand oder ein Letten oder ein Leim, so muss es sein in dem, darauss es wird, ist es nicht im selbigem, so wird es nit dasselbig geboren, das es nicht ist."

substance of the organ and gives off the waste. When the irritant of disease is united with this alchemist of the organ, the process of metabolism is disturbed, because the irritant influences the alchemist in the direction of its own purposes. Consequently the waste material is deposited instead of being excreted, with the result that anatomical changes are to be observed as the expression of the disturbance in the metabolism of the organ. Paracelsus compares this process with the deposit of " Tartarus " in wine vats. He calls those diseases during the course of which such waste material appears in the organs, tartaric diseases, e. g. calculus and other pathological conditions characterized by calcification, such as tuberculosis.[11]

Thus disease is a local process, the expression of which is to be found in anatomical changes. The difference of the organs involved and the differences in the anatomical changes — like their causes — permit a classification of diseases.

Hence it is to Paracelsus and his religious view that we owe the modern conception of disease in the establishment of three new doctrines:

(1) The external cause is the essense of disease.
(2) The organ involved and the anatomical changes decide the nature of disease.
(3) Disease consists of a complicated disturbance of organ-metabolism, which secondarily reflects on the whole system.

It is obvious that these principles must cause a new movement in *therapy*. Therapy is *now* directed towards the abolition of the external causes in order to restore the normal metabolism of the organ. God has created the physician, enabling him to cure diseases by means of remedies containing specific virtues against the cause and essence of the disease. Thus the hitherto incurable diseases appear to be curable by the physician installed by God. " He who does not know how to cure leprosy does not understand the power of medicine. He who does not make a lame leg straight is no

[11] *Op. Paramirum,* III, 1-4. Crit. edition by Sudhoff, IX, p. 150. See my I. B. van Helmont, *Einführung in die philosophische Medizin des Barock* (Berlin, Springer, 1930), p. 84 ff.

physician. He should know that God has not set up the physician in order to cure cold in the head and headache. They justify their lack of skill by saying, 'This disease is incurable,' demonstrating nothing but their own stupidity and mendacity, because God never caused a disease for which he has not created a remedy." [12]

Hence we may conclude from the doctrines of Paracelsus that the ideology of religious philosophy permeates the medical biology of the Renaissance period giving it inspiration and impulse. At the same time natural science is also closely connected with magic, a term embracing for the natural philosopher of this epoch, all natural events inaccessible to analysis and therefore classified as miracles or delusions of sorcery. As a matter of fact, this magic includes important phenomena which may be regarded as realities because they are to be produced by experiment. Karl Joel in his most delightful book on the " Birth of natural philosophy from the spirit of mysticism," [13] gives an account of the connection between mysticism and scientific thought during the epoch of the Renaissance.

But, with the exception of Paracelsus, in the *medical* literature of the period of the Renaissance *sensu strictiori*, no direct reference to the association of religion with biological experience can be found. Let us take Fracastoro as an example:

Although he begins his treatise on the causes of the critical days first by extolling the wonders of nature, especially as seen in the existence of organic beings, as the " Munus Dei optimi," and then by stressing the necessity of proving his results by experience, there is every reason to assume that the former expression is only a figure of speech, while the latter is designed to serve as an apology for his defection, in the matter of the influence of the stars on the critical days, from the teaching of Galen, whose opinions he held in high esteem. Fracastoro strictly adheres to the ancient doctrine of humoralism, pointing out that it is not the influence of the stars but an irritation of the humours which produces critical days, the most marked paroxysm being due to the rivalry of the humours.[14] The

[12] *Op. Paramirum,* I, 7-8.

[13] *Der Ursprung der Naturphilosophie aus dem Geiste der Mystik* (Jena, 1903), 2. Aufl., 1928.

[14] Fracastoro, Hieron., " Die causis criticorum dierum libell.," *Opp. omn.* (Venet., Junt., 1574), p. 48 ff. The influence of the stars: " . . . si enim per ea quae in

effect of the "Spiritualia," however, is fully acknowledged and its possibility discussed. The doctrine of the "Contagium," as a spiritual entity, is without doubt derived from this point of view, and it is to Fracastoro that we owe its elaboration in his recognition of the independence of the Contagium with regard to vapors, and the contagious nature of certain diseases. In all this, in spite of the prominence given to humoralism, are to be observed, in *individual points*, important resemblances to the doctrines of Paracelsus and van Helmont and to the "ontological" conception of disease. To this subject we shall return later.

There are, however, *fundamental differences.* There is no trace of religious motives in Fracastoro's scientific work. To him nature is not so much the great world system embracing macrocosm and microcosm, as the "Physis" of the individual body, which is removed in its activity both from the macrocosmic forces and from the stars. The influence of the latter is not theoretically denied, but is, as far as possible, restricted to give place to the theory of the simple reaction between the Galenic humours. Similarly, in research, he rejects the "Universalia" in favour of the immediate "Causae." He is acquainted with the general consensus of all things in the world, but explains it by the application of mechanical principles. Just as the movements of the atoms consist of expansion and contraction, the reactions of the soul and members of the animal body are constriction and dilatation.[15] Most emphatically does

nobis sunt, ratio omnis et causa criticorum dierum ostendi possit, bene erit, ab eo labore lunam et beata illa corpora liberare, quae cum alioqui multa penes nos faciant, tum et multa a nobis et a natura fieri sinunt." On the reliability of authorities and own results: "neque prius credi audirique volumus quam et re ipsa ac rerum (ut aiunt) magistra experientia fuerint comprobata, eiusmodi enim sunt, ut et rationibus credi et observationibus plane sperari possint." ". . . longa primum diligentique inquisitione comperta, mox et re ipsa observationibusque comprobata sic enim me excusare poterunt, si a parente medicinae Galeno, quem in reliquis ut deum veneramur et colimus hac una in re discedere ausus sum." Natura: ". . . Dei optimi munus cum tota quae aut oculis cernitur aut concipitur animo, admirationis multae plena est, tum maxime qua in animalibus viget." "Crisim atque expulsionem tentat natura quoniam stimulatur."

[15] De sympathia et antipathia rerum liber ad Alexandr. Farnesium card. ampl., a paper, "sine quo natura contagionum plane perquiri et monstrari posse non videbatur." "Nihil admirabilius, nihil scitu desideratum magis quam de latenti rerum consensu et dissensu." In chapter 2 the general consensus of things is acknowledged. "Primus autem communis rebus omnibus et admirandus est ipsius universi con-

Fracastoro state: "Universalissimis vero stare ignavi et rustici ingenii est, medias vero inquirere et ad proprias niti (quantum homini datur) philosophi certi est." In his opinion the whole doctrine of contagium is incomprehensible without the theory of sympathy and antipathy, but he definitely condemns the simple acceptance of such things as have been described by the catchword "Qualitates occultae," and those persons who, having nothing to say or to teach, explain problems by means of unknown things. On the other hand, there appear in Fracastoro's writings certain purely humoralistic doctrines which seek to trace the origin of the contagium to the establishment of peculiar mixtures of the humours occurring in addition to simple putrefaction. Once again we find the old theory that the frequent cases of contagious diseases among indolent young men are due to their warm and moist constitution which causes the opening of the pores.

"The latter generation had nothing to add to the sound doctrines of infection and therefore introduced the worthless "qualitates occultae" (Fracastoro).

The work of Paracelsus, on the other hand, both in its negatively critical and its constructive aspects, seems to me to derive peculiar importance from the association of the religious and the scientific conception of the world already described.

The new science of Paracelsus knows only a single infinite universe. Therefore it is dedicated to the perception of the Divine in the individual, of the One in the multiplicity of His manifestations.

sensus, in quo quae sunt corpora, ita omnia invicem connexa, ita haerentia esse volunt, ut nulla potentia sit, quae eorum extrema, quibus sese mutuo tangunt, seiungere prorsus possit atque ita separare, ut vacuus locus intercidat." Therefore the place of all things is determined, which preserves them from decay. Thus everything is harmonically arranged, there is no place for a "Contrarium," the latter being introduced by the development of the properties of the individual. Sound and movements originate in the changing condensation and rarefaction of the constituents, "more undarum." Simple attraction in inanimate nature is achieved by means of pores. The plant needs more than mere pores in order to attract food and to give off the waste. In animals and men the "spiritus" of the soul cause contraction and expansion of the material atoms and help to maintain the "consensus" of the parts.

It is interesting to note that certain followers of Paracelsus, like Fludd, accepted this doctrine of condensation and rarefaction of matter as the basis of natural philosophy. We shall discuss this conception later.

It leads to a new reality, to life. According to the doctrine of Paracelsus, this science begins here below with experiments, but it must be blessed by the Grace from above. Only thus does it acquire the power to penetrate to the source of life and therewith to the destiny of things.[16]

This is the basis of a mental attitude from which, a little later, proceed discoveries in experimental science and fundamental innovations in pathology. In both branches the theoretical and practical achievements of J. B. van Helmont are outstanding. His work belongs to the new natural science and stands in intellectual relationship to that of Kepler and Leibniz.[17] Helmont's " Rise of the science of medicine " (" Ortus medicinae ") appeared at the same time as Jacob Boehme's " Aurora."

Thus we may conclude: One of the spiritual tendencies leading to modern medical biology was mysticism, and one of the motives to experimental research in medical biology was religion.

But this religion was not that of the Middle Ages, when faith demanded intellect, and when experimental science was relegated to the realm of magic with the result that in a certain sense a development from magic to experimental science took place; compare the classical work of Lynn Thorndike.[18] Furthermore, the mysticism of the Middle Ages may be regarded as the native soil of a contempt for book-learning and scholarly wisdom. " The tree of science cheats many of the tree of life or exposes them to the severest pains of purgatory," threatens Bonaventura. " What is all science but a picture without life, a phantom without movement or feeling? ", complains Richard of St. Victor. " Instruction maketh men learned, but it is feeling which giveth wisdom. The sun doth not give warmth to all on whom he shineth. It is one thing to know of

[16] Compare the remarkable interpretation of Paracelsus, given by Strunz, " Mensch und Natur in der Weltanschauung des Paracelsus," *Acta Paracelsica* 1, 108, 1930.

[17] Pagel, W., " Helmont, Leibniz, Stahl," *Arch. Gesch. d. Med.*, XXIV, 1, 1931, p. 19-59, and *J. B. van Helmont* (Berlin, Springer, 1930). With special reference to Helmont's vitalism and its relation to contemporaneous religious trends of thought, compare the excellent introduction in two vitalistic treatises of Helmont edited by F. G. M. de Feyfer, " Helmont, Gaubius, Schroeder van Kolk on vitalism," *Opera Select. Medicor. Neerlandicorum* (Amsterdam, 1932).

[18] *A history of magic and experimental science during the first XIII centuries of our era* (London, 1923).

treasure and another to possess it" are the admonitions of St. Bernard. But Hugo of St. Victor expresses his pious contemplation rather than a real demand for natural research, when he declares that the wisdom of God is invisible unless it is revealed by his work: Nature, who speaks of her Creator and indicates the events of his creation to those who are able to understand.[18a]

The day of scholasticism is over when the "Liber naturae" is recommended as a source of knowledge and revelation by Raymundus de Sabunde[18b] and when Nicolaus de Ultricuria regards things themselves and not Aristotle and his interpreters as the aim of research.

Therefore it is in vain that we seek either in the scholasticism or in the mysticism of the Middle Ages that yearning for a knowledge of nature which inspired the work of Paracelsus.

In the medicine and natural science of the Middle Ages, in spite of the inevitable subordination of all learning to religion, the rational element preponderated in the sense of the formal logical deduction of diagnosis, pathology and therapy according to the authoritative humoralistic prescriptions and tables.[19] Science then ran parallel to dogmatic belief, to which it was adapted. As in the picture of a medieval town the Church occupies the most prominent position, and even science remains hidden by the shadow of her wings, both belief and science were governed by the same rules of formal logic and rationalism, I might even say, by the same juridical manner of thinking. Objectively, the spirit of the age may have checked the so-called progress of science; subjectively, this state of affairs

[18a] *De sacramentis christ. fid.*, I, 3.

[18b] *Theologia naturalis s. liber creaturarum,* 1436 (Francf., 1635). Compare Neuburger, M., *Geschichte der Medizin,* II, 1, 2, p. 418 (Stuttgart, 1911).

[19] Compare the striking remarks of Joseph Needham: "Science . . . never was an appeal to reason, but to the facts of empirical observation and experiment, as is seen . . . in Galileo, Sanctorius and Gilbert: the scholastics were the real rationalists." *The Sceptical Biologist* (London, 1929), p. 227. Compare further: Schiller, F. C. S., *Scientific discovery and logical proof.* Ch. Singer's *Studies in the History and Method of Science,* I, 235 (Oxford, 1917). — Whitehead, A. N., *Science and the modern world* (Cambridge, 1926), p. 12 with reference to Galileo ("mistake to conceive this historical revolt as an appeal to reason . . . it was through and through an anti-intellectualist movement . . . based on a recoil from the inflexible rationality of medieval thought").

ensured an eminent position for science and the learned professions, separating the wide field of their activities from that of practice, empiricism and technique.

" Reason," the effort to limit and to comprehend the illimitable, compressing it where possible into the framework of generally valid *tables* in which, according to the categories of logic, all combinations of chance were taken into account, was the highest aim and dream of the medieval scholars. In this sense even astrology could claim a peculiar importance. But this rational magic of the tables, which, from the sum of the causes and qualities arbitrarily assumed, or according to accepted authorities, logically deduced the effect, was fundamentally different from the mode of thought of Paracelsus and the mystic philosophers of the XVIIth century, with their religious empiricism and irrationalism, although if in the case of some, such as Fludd, the whole ancient mystery of tabulation was resurrected.

Even so independent a thinker as Arnaldus of Villanova manifests a strict adherence to the medieval ideal of power derived from a rational determination of properties and qualities and their logical deductions from tables. This is to be observed in his doctrine of the " Proprietas." His attention is particularly drawn to our ignorance of the properties of matter, especially of materials actively affecting the body's substance. Two things of the same composition may differ in action, whereas two things of different composition may be similar in action. We are well acquainted with the effect, but the " modus operandi " remains unknown, as it is derived from the " mirabilitas mistionis " (" forma ") which causes the peculiar changes in the things. Hence many physicians have called the proprietas a " virtus occulta." The possible combinations of things (" Forma mistionum ") are infinite according to the number of the constituents, and hence the knowledge of the " forma specifica," and therefore the explanation of the effects, to us is impossible, nor is a " rationabile experimentum " able to solve this problem. Without knowledge of the " proprietas " we cannot tell whether the remedy exercises its specific action on the solid parts, on the humours, or on the spirit. No reasoning can ever inform us that coral affects the stomach, only "experimentum casuale" or some manner of divine revelation gives us this information.[20]

These doubts on the capability of the human intellect, which led directly to a belief in the superiority of experiment, especially in the matter of the discovery of the right remedy, specific by virtue of its properties, foreshadowed the revolutionary ideas of Paracelsus.

Galen himself was conscious of the limitations of human knowledge, a fact to which the 13th of the Parabolae of Arnaldus refers.[21] Although the individual properties of remedies cannot be determined, the physician must be acquainted with them. Moreover, Galen declares: Although we can never exclude by reason the possibility that some particular substance may influence the course of hydrophobia, a condition so dangerous as that resulting from a dog's bite requires the immediate application of a known and tried remedy; for we must not endanger the life of the patient in order to try out a new cure.[22] Furthermore, in the case of renal calculus, when a remedy, which, according to either logical deduction or its known properties, should be effective, fails, perhaps because the body, by reason of some latent "proprietas" prohibits the action, we must then "descend" (*χωρεῖν*) to those things which operate by virtue of their inherent properties which, being inaccessible to rational analysis, have been discovered by trial and irrational practice (as dream, oracle, accident, etc.). Such remedies include sparrows' and goats' blood, that is to say, the known therapy of magic. Much of this is to be avoided as abomination and pure nonsense, and no great faith should be put in such things, since so far, we have been unable to discover by reason the manner of their efficacy.[23]

But it is also a "descent" according to Arnaldus, when the

[20] *Specul. introduct. medic.*, 18. Opera c. Taurelli adnot. (Basileae, 1585), 48g. Comp. *Parab.*, 16: "Proprietas incognita ratione vel syllogismo revelatione vel experimento iuvantium et nocentium innotescit," *Opp.*, p. 914.

[21] "Proprietates individuales corporum sanabilium licet scribi non valeant necesse est tamen ut operarius non ignoret." Galen 3, *de ingen. san.*, 3 u. 7; Avicenna 4, *physicor.*

[22] *De compos. medicam*, I, 16.

[23] Küehn XIX, 677 (*περὶ τῆς τῶν ἐν νεφροῖς παθῶν διαγνώσεως καὶ θεραπείας* *V* i. f.): "... *ἐπὶ τὰ τῶν παλαιῶν ἄρρητα καὶ καθ' ὅλην τὴν οὐσίαν ἐνεργοῦντα χωρεῖν, ἃ ἐκ πείρας καὶ ἀλόγου τριβῆς εὑρημένα εἰσί* ..." by "*τύχη, αὐτοσχέδιον, μιμητικόν, ὄνειρα, χρῆσμα, μάθησις* ... *ἐξ ὧν συνέστηκεν ἐμπειρική.*"

physician abandons the " via recta rationis," e. g. when a " vulgaris medicus " in a single case mixes together all the drugs he knows, so that one at least may be effective. By such a course of action we fail to make use even of our knowledge of the effects of the simple remedies. This knowledge appertains to the " ordinata mens " by which alone man resembles God, and for such wisdom he has to seek fervently, unmindful of the convenience of old customs.

The parabolae deprecate " omnis motus animi vel appetitus inordinatus " and the " vagus animus," for these distract the " mens " of the practitioner, from which, as from a clear mirror, he obtains guidance in his work " claro intuitu." He who knows the nature of the body, the kinds of diseases, the diversity of causes, the possibility of instruments, will treat his patients " cum ratione " and by his art give aid to the sick.[24]

The physician who acquires a knowledge of the occult proprietates, is " inter ceteros mirabilis." How may this knowledge be obtained? By means of speculative medicine and philosophy which instruct in the primary, secondary, tertiary and quaternary *qualities*,[25] to which latter, according to Hermes, only the " homines experti, iusti ponderis et valde elevati super alios " attain. For this purpose Arnaldus has drawn up *tables* of all forces and all practices in which the ingenious scholar can find by analysis whatever information he requires, thus ensuring that his work shall be " valde mirabile." Moreover, it is advisable that he keeps secret the wisdom of the tables.[26]

Such contradictions and his general attitude to magic[27] show

[24] Parabolae medicat. sec. instinctum veritatis aeternae., *Opera*, 914, VI, VII, X, XI, XII.

[25] See Galen, *loc. cit. de renum affectionib.* "Δεῖ δὲ τὸν μέλλοντα κατὰ λόγον πράττειν ἰατρόν κατὰ τὰς δραστικὰς ποιότητας, δυνάμεις τε καὶ ἐνεργείας σεμνύνεσθαι τὸ θαῤῥεῖν, ὡς εἰδότα διὰ τῆς μεθόδου τὴν δύναμιν θερμοῦ τε καὶ ψυχροῦ, ξηροῦ τε καὶ ὑγροῦ, τῶν τε στρυφνῶν, αὐστηρῶν, ὀξέων, γλυκέων . . . καὶ τῶν λοιπῶν κατὰ μέρος."

[26] *De simplicibus*, 81, opp. *2 c.* 376.

[27] On Arnald's position to magic, compare Diepgen, *Studien zu Arnald von Villanova* IV. Arnald's " Stellung zur Magie, Astrologie und Oneiromanthie," Sudhoff's *Archiv. Gesch. Med., 5,* 1912, p. 88; and III: " Arnald und die Alchemie," *ib. 3,* p. 369, 1910.

According to Diepgen, Arnald's position is not clear and uniform. There are

that the position of Arnald cannot be clearly defined. There is no doubt that, not only does the terminology he employed bear a certain resemblance to that of the writings of Paracelsus, but in substance the work of the two authors contain many similarities.[27a] The rational element, however, which greatly exceeds mystical revelation, irrationalism, and empiricism in importance and ultimately culminates in the Lullian ideal of a universal table, is the outstanding feature of Arnald's work. Hence we may conclude that, in spite of certain theories indicating a later mode of thought, Arnald should be placed among the exponents of scholasticism in science, although, in his case, this certainly does not exclude experimental research. But never does he undertake this on the grounds of conscious withdrawal from rational knowledge and the edifice of Galen. Moreover, the dependence of the "proprietas occulta" on the mixture, which he emphasizes, is an important principle in the system of Galen; there is also no mention in his work of the ontological idea of "seeds" in the sense of Paracelsus, who denies the whole doctrine of mixtures. The ideal of Arnaldus is the Galenic doctrine of qualities constructed to the last detail of the "proprietates."

"Halbheiten" and contradictions. Indeed he is deeply influenced by the official ecclesiastical trends of thought. Thus he believed in witchcraft. But on the other hand this belief in the reality of sorcery and magic is not incontestable. Like Roger Bacon, but with less resolution than this philosopher, Arnald tried to give natural explanations of magic phenomena by reducing them to the emanation of spirits and vapors from the sorcerer which are effective under certain constellations of the stars. Similar contradictions can be found in his refutation of magic remedies which are sometimes recommended and employed as such (e. g. against "Verrucae"), but, on the other hand are explained in their influence by the force of psychical imagination on the body; Diepgen, *loc. cit.*, p. 99. Similarly, according to Diepgen, Arnald is not original in his alchemy, where boasting and charlatanry are predominant. But, on the other hand, Arnald may have believed in his achievements in chemistry and indeed he worked industriously in empirical chemistry and endeavoured to attain to the aims of alchemy: the transmutation of the metals, their reduction to their source, mercury, in order to render them "perfect."

[27a] Compare Neuburger's appreciation of Arnald's yearning for empirical knowledge, *Geschichte der Medizin,* l. c. II, 1, 2, pp. 388, 395, 398. Arnald desires to describe, "quae expertus sum"; he learns from empiricists and uneducated women and rebukes those who disregard empiricism. With reference to his religious point of view: "Beatus igitur ille medicus, cui Deus dat scientiam (sc. naturas et potentias rerum simplicium et imaginativam fortem) et intelligentiam, quin est naturae socius" (Arnald, *De vinis*). Neuburger points out the contradictions in Arnald's rationalism and mysticism.

The position of Roger Bacon is similar, although, in many respects, perhaps it is clearer, for he approaches more nearly than Arnald to the ideas of the school of Paracelsus. Roger Bacon shows an aspiration for an impartial knowledge of reality, for liberalism, and science.

In Bacon's doctrine of sciences one criterion of the dignity of a science is its utility.[28] This conception is closely connected with a high estimation of experiment.

The "scientia experimentalis" is "perfectior omnibus," providing for them certainty in a miraculous manner. Experimental science is able to neglect the "argumenta," because these alone do not give any certainty, and even if they are very strong, they provide it only in connection with the "experientia."[29] "Sine experientia conclusionum nunquam fit scientia." Man does not rest until he sees his arguments confirmed by experiment. Thus it is not those well versed in book learning who obtain certainty and truth, but the experimental worker, who may learn from animals, women, slaves. Furthermore, experiment precedes reason and stimulates the investigation of causes. On the other hand, there is no doubt that reason must be employed in order to make mere empiricism a science. This is interwoven with all the other sciences, e. g., our knowledge of the virtue of a simple remedy depends upon our knowledge of animals and plants. Alchemy leads to a knowledge of simple remedies in inanimate nature.

By means of magic, man penetrates to the heart of the hidden processes of nature, and the knowledge obtained is only concealed by the useless ceremonies. He must make the processes so discovered profitable to the progress of mankind. Sympathy and antipathy, the attraction of animate and inanimate, is not to be invoked by incantations and characters nor by the orgies of sorcery. It is a state which exists "propter naturae conformitatem." There are emanations from animate beings which can have a strengthening

[28] "Ceterum ante omnia utilitas cuiuslibet rei consideranda est," *Op. tert.*, Cap. 5; Brewer, *Fr. Rogerii Baconis opera quaed. hacten. inedita*, Vol. I (London, 1859), p. 19.

[29] *Ib.*, p. 43 (12/13); *Op. maius*, VI, 1/2. — De retardatione accidentium senectutis cum aliis opusculis de rebus medicinalibus, ed. A. G. Little and E. Withington (Oxonii, 1928), p. 169.

or weakening influence (infectio) on other beings, not as the result of magic but of " spiritus " and " vapores," which, according to Galen, these beings exhale. It is only the uneducated who use the word " magic " to denote the secrets of nature. There is still much unknown and unexamined which in later centuries will be the common knowledge of every student. The ceremonies of the magician have suggestive power which perhaps the physician may use for the healing of the sick. On the other hand, it is the privilege and duty of the scholar not to expose his wisdom freely to the masses. He must conceal it so that it is only to be understood by those worthy to receive it.[30]

The neglect of experience and experiment is the reason why many things which are well known to the empiricist are unknown to official medicine, e. g., the art of prolonging life. It is the empiricist who gives the sciences orders, just as the sailor gives the carpenter the order to build a ship. The alchemist, on finding out the ways to prolong life, commissions alchemy to produce a substance which is " aequalis complexionis " with long-living or regenerating animals.[31] Thus it is its utility which elevates alchemy above all the other sciences. By its practical results alchemy justifies the employment of speculative natural philosophy and theoretical medicine, for not only does it make possible the prolongation of the life of the indi-

[30] *Epistolae fratris Rogerii Baconis de secretis operibus artis et naturae et de nullitate magiae.* Ed. Joh. Dee (Hamburg, Froben, 1618) ; Von den geheimen Wirkungen der Kunst und Natur und Nichtigkeit der Magie mit Joh. Dee und eines Ungenannten Anmerkungen a. d. Latein. uebers. nebst Raimundus Lullus Clavicula. Hof. Vierling. 1776. — Brewer, pp. 393-519. See *Op. tert.*, Brewer, 46-47, Little, 1912, 46. — About John Dee, the pretended editor, see: A. E. Waite, *Lives of alchemystical philosophers* (London, 1888) and the same: *The Brotherhood of the Rosy Cross* (London, 1924) ; Smith, Ch., *John Dee* (London, 1909), a novel. Dee lived from 1555-1608. He is said to have made gold by means of the " tincture " of a vagabond alchemist Kelly. During his journey with Kelly to the court of Maximilian II in Prague his property in England was confiscated. He returned 1589 to England, where he was rehabilitated, while, on account of his failure to make gold, Kelly was detained a prisoner in Vienna for many years until his death.

[31] *Op. tert.*, Brewer, p. 43 (12) : " Sed experimentator fidelis consideravit aquilam et cervum et serpentem et phoenicem et multa prolongare vitam et renovare iuventutem et scit quod haec dantur brutis ad instructionem hominis, propter quod excogitavit vias nobiles ad hoc et iussit alkimiae practicae praeparare ei corpus aequalis complexionis, ut hic experimentator uteretur eo."

vidual, but it also provides treasure for the state. Very few, however, possess the wisdom of practical alchemy in its correct form.[32] This explains the ignorance and errors in pharmacology.[33] Humoralism demonstrates fundamental contradictions. The same drug is said to influence contrary humours. In composite remedies the mutual abolition or attenuation of the different constituents is generally unrecognized.

Neither the *quantity* nor the weight of the constituents determines the effect of a substance or a mixture of substances, but the " proprietas et operatio, quae est in re." The recognition of this property in a remedy, however, requires exact rational knowledge (" Ratiocinatio ") of the simple constituents, for it is only thus that harm may be avoided.[34]

Now all these remedies which assist in the prolongation of life and the restitution of youth are occult. They are " Secreta magna," because they are concealed in the ancient writings, which cannot be interpreted correctly by the official science. The books of the Chaldeans, Arabs, and Greeks are full of such " secreta," hidden by analogies and symbols. Roger Bacon learned from their study that there is in plants, animals, words, and stones a strange virtue, the knowledge of which has illuminated the spirit of ancient philosophers, but remained unknown to the rest of mankind. This spirit is the inventor of the sciences, the salvation of the soul, the judge of the right and the wrong, the discoverer of the virtues, and it leads to the revelation of the truth in the occult writings.[35]

These quotations from the works of Bacon show many features typical of the conceptions of Paracelsus: the refutation of the predominance of reason and argument in favour of experience and experimental science; the estimation of magic as a source of genuine knowledge of nature, and its importance for the benefit of mankind; the criticism of contemporaneous humoralism, as contained in the

[32] *Ib.*, 40 (12).

[33] *De errorib. medicor.*, Little-Withington, p. 150 ff.

[34] *Capit. antidot.*, Little-Withington, p. 115: " Multi compositores compositarum medicinarum fuerunt decepti credentes quod pondus faceret operationem et non proprietas . . . nec credas laudibus compositarum medicinarum nisi examinaveris medicinam per ratiocinationem."

[35] *Expositio epistolae de retardat. accident. senect.*, Little-Withington, p. 84.

emphasis laid upon the specific " proprietas " of a substance instead of upon the quantitative relations between the qualities imagined by ancient humoralism.

On the other hand the ideal of Roger Bacon is that of a universal knowledge and a science leading to truth and reality, but religious motives *sensu strictiore* cannot be recognized in his new scientific views, neither in his refutation of reason nor in his estimation of experimental science, in spite of the fact that he charges the Church with the task of superintending science and the power derived from it, and of saving mankind from all deceptions of demons and the antichrist. Thus Bacon's ideal is that of science and not that of faith,[36] and is far removed from Paracelsus' search for God by means of research in nature.

Finally, the rôle of religion in Bacon's scientific doctrines may be more important than it appears (Carton),[37] (Liebeschuetz),[38] because he refers to the Bible as the chief source of the occult science as well as to a kind of divine wisdom revealed to the ancient heathen philosophers. Our knowledge is not the result of our work, but of divine grace and revelation. Hence, according to Roger Bacon also, only the sinless and believers attain to science. A contradiction between the view of infinity and the recommendation of simple sensual perception and experience as the ways leading to truth seems here to be dissolved by a kind of religious pragmatism,[39] just as we find it in the philosophy of Paracelsus, which combines the tendencies to search for God, research in nature, practical medicine and ethics.

In *conclusion:* The combination of religious irrationalism and vitalistic empiricism characteristic of the XVIIth century originated

[36] See Liebeschuetz, H., "Der Sinn des Wissens bei Roger Bacon," *Vortr. Biblioth. Warburg.*, IX, 1932, p. 53: ". . . trotz dieser Einfuegung der Wissenschaft in einen kirchlichen Rahmen und religioesen Endzweck ihr eigentlicher Gehalt . . . noch keine positive Formung durch religioese Antriebe zeigt." "Es ist der Sinn der Wissenschaft, Zwecke des Lebens zuverlaessig zu verwirklichen; religioes geistige Endzwecke beruehren das eigene Wesen der theoretischen Disziplinen jedenfalls nicht."

[37] *L'expérience physique chez R. Bacon* (Paris, 1924); *L'expérience mystique de l'illumination intérieure chez R. Bacon* (Paris, 1924).

[38] *Loc. cit.*, p. 56 ff. See also Thorndike, *loc. cit.*, II, p. 631.

[39] Liebeschuetz, *loc. cit.*, p. 59.

in Paracelsus, in his refutation of formal logic and reason as methods of natural research, his mysticism and his realism. In all fundamental points of his doctrine, religious motives can be recognized: in his employment of analogy like that of macrocosm and microcosm, in his theory of sympathy and antipathy, in his rejection of ancient humoralism in favour of his doctrine of seeds and created entities. To this last doctrine are due: his view of specificity and virtues, his belief in the importance of the solid organs and their metabolism, and his conception of the diseases as entities, varying according to their external causes and their seats. These religious fundamentals are obvious in the predominance of spirit and imagination as emanations of the universal logos in things based upon the assumption that they, like Christ, represent the mediator between the One and the Many.

In the medical literature of the Renaissance Paracelsus alone seems to give voice to these trends of thought, as the comparison with Fracastoro demonstrates.

The relation of empiricism in medical biology to religion and mysticism is quite different from that of medical science to religion during the Middle Ages. There are certain points of contact between Paracelsus and some independent medieval scholars such as Arnald of Villanova and Roger Bacon, but even here there are fundamental differences in the ideals and the final results.

## II

In order to illustrate religious motives in the development of modern medical biology the present investigation will bring into prominence some practically unknown witnesses of the XVIIth century. The fact that they are scarcely mentioned in the current histories of philosophy and science in no way militates against their importance as memorials of the spirit of the age. There are no particular scientific results achieved by their work, they play no definite part in the progress of discovery and invention, but the typical repetition of the same fundamental ideas in a considerable number of writings of this epoch exhibits their authors as representatives of important and almost imperceptible tendencies. They indicate the motive of the period quite as much as the brilliant figures, well known in the history of science.

Just as mystic theology begins with the rejection of all statements concerning God, because any statements inevitably limit His infinity, certain exponents of the view of the world, characteristic of the XVIIth century, even question the possibility of human participation in knowledge, because it is infinite.

A century earlier Agrippa of Nettesheym gave pointed expression to a contemporaneous wave of scepticism.[40] Like the medieval mystics we have mentioned, he contrasts the value of the arts and sciences with that of the life of man and the welfare of his soul. Not with rhetoric and superficial arguments will he defend his opinion, but he will test things accurately in their innermost essentials. He is not interested in rhetoric but in the truth, which has its seat in the heart and not on the tongue. His aim is happiness, which exists not in the knowledge of goodness but in goodness itself. It is not understanding which is important, but life in understanding. It is not understanding but the will to goodness which connects man with God. These ideas lead to a destructive analysis of contemporary therapy and medicine,[41] very similar in its negatively critical attitude to that of Paracelsus and van Helmont.[42] The uncertainty of medical knowledge is primarily revealed by the lack of unanimity among the investigators in quite fundamental matters, such as the process of development. There prevails the same jealousy among the schools as among the systems of philosophy. Hippocrates refers the causes of disease to the pneuma, Herophilus to the humours, Erasistratus to the arterial blood, Asclepiades to the pores, Alcmaeon ascribes them to the lack or excess of physical energy, Diocles to inequality of the elements composing the body and to the air, Strato to excess and indigestibility of food. Medical practice [43] is built upon absolutely erroneous experiments, and hence the patients frequently suffer more from the physician and remedy than from the disease itself. The best physician is he whom the

[40] *De incertitudine et vanitate scientiarum omnium et artium*, 1528. (Francof., et Lipsiae, Planer, 1714), p. 2: "Nil perniciosius, nil pestilentius hominum vitae, animarumque nostrarum saluti . . . quam ipsas artes ipsasque scientias. . . . Non intelligere sed in intellectu vivere, neque enim bona intelligentia sed bona voluntas coniungit homines deo."

[41] *Loc. cit.*, Cap. 82: *de medicina in genere*, p. 428.

[42] See in my "I. B. van Helmont," *loc. cit.*, pp. 14 ff., 47 f., 144, 146 ff.

[43] *Loc. cit.*, Cap. 83: *De medic. operatrice*, p. 435.

apothecary, who shares the fees, recommends. Magnificent garments, stained fingertips, a foreign origin or even only a difference of faith, a boldly lying tongue and the continual prescription of drugs create authority, renown, and confidence. The physician observes the patient with gravity, inspects the urine, feels the pulse, looks at the tongue, examines the chest, tests the excretions, asks questions concerning the customary diet and other intimate details, as though, by such means, he could weigh the elements and the humours of the body and bring them into equilibrium. Then, with great solemnity, he prescribes the medicine. Mild illnesses he protracts as long as possible, suggesting ridiculous measures which will be agreeable to the patient, such as water dripping into a basin as a cure for insomnia. If the illness is severe and the outlook doubtful or hopeless, he prescribes a special routine, orders unusual things, forbidding the usual, finds fault with whatever has been given to the patient, threatens death, promises life, and demands a high fee. If death occurs, it is the result of a pulmonary œdema or some other incurable condition,[44] or, no doubt, it is due to the disobedience of the patient or the carelessness of the nurses, or it may even be a colleague or the apothecary who is responsible. Aesculapius himself was a rogue, the offspring of an incestuous marriage. In fact, physicians are the greatest criminals, the most quarrelsome, envious, and deceitful of all men. One physician will never approve of the prescriptions of another. They are always dirty, because for the sake of gain they roam around privies and make their homes in the filth of men. Cato was right when he forbade all physicians to reside in Rome. They fall into three categories: The very learned who lose all their patients, the illiterate who cure them all, even those who have been given up, and a third class whose rich patients alone recover, while peasants and the common people either die or suffer greatly.

If physicians themselves knew all the virtues of the elements, of roots, plants, flowers, fruits, seeds, animals and stones, that is, all things created by nature, and if they put all this knowledge into practice, they would not be able to make men immortal or be sure

[44] Compare Helmont on morbid anatomy in my "I. B. van Helmont," *loc. cit.*, p. 113.

of curing even a slight illness. How often has the remedy, which should have been effective, failed? How often has that, which should have expelled, not expelled? How often must the patient return to the physician and finally die? What hope have we in the practice of medicine, when even the master Hippocrates has said: " Experience is deceptive "? If this be so, there is no other possibility than to return to the simple wisdom of experience applied before the age of science by primitive people, who thereby attained to great age. That is: the homely skill by which many an old wife has confounded the most learned doctors with all their expensive and carefully considered (" elaboratis ") prescriptions. A simple remedy, because its action is known and proved — *expertis viribus* — relieves even great suffering, while the complicated mixtures prescribed by the professional doctor perform a cure, if ever this occurs, by accident. These physicians acquire their knowledge from incorrect books and illustrated manuscripts, while the old wife searches wood and field for the individual plants, learning (" contemplata et edocta ") their colours, forms, taste, scent and species, and, according to her experience (" experta ") of their virtues, in cases of illness and accident, administers, free of charge, to everyone the surest remedy.

I have referred in detail to Agrippa's attitude towards medicine because the *religious impulse to criticism* and scepticism is pronounced, and this *leads* to the *recommendation of simple empiricism.*

During the period with which we are now dealing, Hieronymus Hirnhaim denies the validity of the scientific axioms which he, like Agrippa, examines individually.[45] But by Hirnhaim's time the doctrines of Paracelsus and Helmont have become more widely disseminated, and this explains why his recommendation of simple empiricism is combined with the important innovations in pathology

[45] See Barach, C. S., "Hieronymus Hirnhaim," *Beitrag z. Geschichte d. philos. theolog. Kultur im 17. Jahrhdt.* (Wien, 1864). H. was born in 1637 at Troppau, entered the order of Premonstratenses at Prague, was appointed Doctor of Divinity at St. Norbert's, then abbot, 1670, was adversary of the Jesuits especially during the quarrel about the foundation of the second chair of canon law, died 1676.

Besides the elder Sanchez, Daniel Pierre Huet (1637-1721) is contemporary of the sceptic Hirmhaim. Huet was adversary of Descartes. His scepticism was combined with unlimited religious faith and a high estimation of antiquity. See Barach, D. P. Huet (Wien. a. Leipzig, 1862).

derived from these authors. Agrippa, on the other hand, does nothing more than advise the application of the old wife's remedies.

Hirnhaim's book is dedicated to the "Typhus generis humani." [45a] The title page shows a ship in full sail on a calm sea, a building, and a tame bird on a man's hand, a picture representing the peace and prosperity following the Flood. Charitas has created this happy time, "charitas ædificat, nutri ædificantem." On the other side of the page is the ship capsizing in a storm and the building falling. Science has evoked the Flood, "inflat, exsuffla inflantem."

Science is dependent on the senses. These deceive. Even the axioms of science are uncertain, being called in question by the very existence of God and His Creation. This came from nothing thus controverting the atomistic axiom of the eternity of matter, that "out of nothing comes nothing." With God all things are possible. Hence a pious scepticism, similar to that of medieval mysticism, is the origin of the doubt in the possibility of science. The inner, immediate light alone reveals the truth, but even this is no source of science, since we cannot know whether we are following this light or our own deceptive understanding. "Diminutae sunt veritates a filiis hominum." True knowledge is the infinite problem insoluble by human intelligence. "Scientiam non dari," "Magna hominum ignorantia in explicandis naturae magnalibus, inter quae primo rerum sympathiae censentur," are characteristic chapter headings in the work of this author.

But this scepticism is not actuated by a desire to leave an absolute nothing in the knowledge of nature, the rational and scientific character of which it certainly denies. While rejecting the rationalistic explanation of natural phenomena this author admits the possibility of their simple perception, and, guided by the spirit of faith, he advises the employment of experiment. Sympathy and antipathy are "magnalia naturae" recognized by Hirnhaim as fundamental phenomena.[46] They are the basis of therapeutics. There existence is evident from the remedies for the various organs to be considered, "quae occulta quadam familiaritate certas corporis partes

[45a] Prague, 1676.

[46] Compare Bacon, Fr., *Hist. de ventis, loc. cit.*, p. 118. Sympathia et antipathia as "Magnalia naturae."

adiuvant." [47] The origin of diseases also follows the laws of sympathy and antipathy. Thus, diabetes insipidus occurs because the body magnetically attracts water from the air.[48] On account of antipathy appear signs of immunity, as in the case where two infants suckled by a plague-stricken nurse remain healthy.[49] "Nature" is reality. She is everywhere "continua" and tolerates no interruption of her ubiquity.[50] She can never exist "sine corpore." She avoids a vacuum, for, when this is imminent, the nearest body is attracted to the vacant space. This is sympathy appearing as a "magnale" of nature. If there is something acting as a soul in man, nature operates, as the soul of the cosmos. According to St. Augustine all is "ratione condita," a statement on which the important "doctrina idearum" was founded and elaborated by van Helmont and Marcus Marci.[51] The ideas are to be understood as the "rationes rerum omnium efficiendarum creandarumque," since they are decreed, eternally unchangeable and true in the "mens" of the Deity. The world is filled with them, they give movement and purpose to the things, endowing them with life and soul. This reminds us of Campanella's "sensus rerum." [52] Hirn-

[47] *Typh. gen. hum.*, p. 53 ff. Remedies operating by antipathy, Cap. 8, p. 85.

[48] Cap. VII, p. 73.

[49] According to *Camerarius.*

[50] Cap. XII, p. 145.

[51] Cap. XII, p. 146 H. In spite of the fact that Hirnhaim's doctrines are deeply influenced by those of Paracelsus and Helmont, these authors personally are not esteemed. By their moral deficiencies they are said to have suppressed the truth which they held in their hands. Many readers are deterred by the inordinately confused method, the barbaric expressions, the unnecessarily gruff polemics against scientific medicine, and the boastful style, particularly of van Helmont. With reference to the modest attitude of the latter: "Vereor ne omnibus maior esse voluerit." He was preceded by Theophrastus Paracelsus: "you may go through all his writings and yet you will remain unlearned as before, although satiated with execrations and futile significations" (Cap. XV). Accordingly, Helmont was better understood by the XVIIth century than Paracelsus, especially outside Germany.

Similarly, the author of the "Themis aurea" follows Paracelsus, not without blaming his general behaviour. P.'s polemics went too far. He wished to cure medicine rather than diseases. His claim for "monarchy" and so many calumnies are not in keeping with the virtues of a "homo rationalis." With reference to his regardless polemics: "Personae maneant intacte. Communis hostis est morbus eiusque causa et effectus symptoma . . . ," p. 95.

[52] Compare with Glisson, *Tract. de natura substantiae energetica*, 5: "Quamvis igitur perceptionem naturalem substantiis in genere assero, praecipue tamen scopus est hoc in rebus materialibus manifestare et probare."

haim was probably greatly influenced by the archei and "seeds" of Paracelsus and Helmont, who defined and limited everything qualitatively. Since each remedy benefits some particular organ in the body, according to the doctrine of ideas, the body is monadically divided. There are the "ideae singularum partium" whose existence is indispensable to life. Thus there is an "idea chyli" in the stomach, an "idea sanguinis" in the heart, in the liver. Every limb has its own idea which governs its nutrition and is therefore a force giving direction to the functions. Such a thing, independent by virtue of its own idea, is disease.

The new ontological theory of disease, foreshadowed by Paracelsus and founded by van Helmont, appears also in Hirnhaim's treatise as the result of the monadic conception of the world. The "idea morbi" is determined by the cause of the disease. This is the contagium [53] which is generally inhaled with the air. Being able to assimilate matter, it is also called ferment.

In the case of Fracastoro the study of the contagium led, rather as an afterthought and unconsciously, to ontological conceptions of disease. Here [54] indeed the virus is the representative of disease. It wanders "per partem post partem ad interna et demum ad precordia," e. g., in syphilis the contagium creeps through the blood until it becomes embedded in the mucus. The lighter parts are cast into the skin, where they condense to form the substance of the pustules, the heaviest of which reside about the nerves and ligaments. The course of the disease depends on the gradual change in the contagium. For, on account of its penetration into the body, this departs ever more markedly from its original form and grows old. Nevertheless, for Fracastoro, the essence of disease is always a lack

[53] ". . . morborum ideae, quae potissimum in peste aliisque morbis infectiosis et malignis deprehenduntur suntque ipsa morbi contagio et semen quoddam quod cum aere attractum in morbum sibi analogum progerminat et ideas vitae humanae abolet. . . . Dantur etiam similes ideae in ipsis mortalium corporibus in quarum suscitatione mira est vis humanae apprehensionis." P. 154.

[54] De contagione. Independent nature of the contagium: II 4, Migration of the virus in hydrophobia: II, 10, in syphilis II, 12. Compare, e. g. Sacheti, *Hieron. Aeliani, de podagricis et arthriticis morbis* (Brixiae, 1586). In men with current diseases there is a "Vis et natura quaedam" which stimulated from outside or inside, at a certain time "morbos sui generis tanquam fructus quosdam suis temporibus renascentes procreent." It is *not* the quantity of the *humours* but the reaction of this Ens, within the body which determines the time of maturity. Cap. 6.

of something, e. g., he distinguishes between the melancholics who have a positive disposition to depression, and the sick, who, on account of something lacking in the mixture of their humours, can no longer find joy in joyful things.[55]

In the theories of contagiums and ferments typical of the trends of thought described we have before us the origin of our modern conception of the living causes of disease, which we similarly represent as being combined through all transitions with inanimate matter. The etiological conception of today is the same as that of the XVIIth century, but then it was inseparably united with the view of the *world* in which it originated. Doubt in the existing science of humoralism inspired the search for the new reality of the contagium. As we have demonstrated, this new pathology with its bias towards etiology had, at the same time, a tendency to localize disease, and thus was interested in morbid anatomical changes.[56] But it did not develop on the lines of Morgagni's morbid anatomy wherein the organic changes were also regarded as the *causa morbi*.[57] This conception of Morgagni has perhaps been the source of the recognition of the anatomical basis of the morbid symptoms and therefore fruitful for the general development of modern medicine, yet the older ontological doctrine of the contagium of Paracelsus and Helmont was more important to the realization of the essence and the general understanding of disease. This doctrine also had a tendency to localize the disease and was concerned with the organic changes, as we have already shown with reference to Paracelsus' doctrine of " Tartarus."

Such theories originated in the tendency to subject matter to ideas, both as regards dignity and order of occurrence. The non-corporeal idea seeks its material and forms it (Contagium, Semen, Astrum). There is no " appetite for forms " inherent in matter, which was regarded as " principum individuationis " by Aristotle.

[55] *De sympath. et antipath.*, Cap. XVIII.

[56] Furthermore my " I. B. van Helmont," *loc. cit.*, p. 36 ff.; my " Helmont, Liebniz, Stahl," *loc. cit.*, p. 55; my *Virchow und die Grundlagen der Medizin des XIX. Jahrhunderts* (Jena, Fischer, 1931), p. 4.

[57] Naïvely the first pioneers of morbid anatomy derive properties of living men from anatomical changes in the body, e. g., Ant. Beniveni when he refers the vileness of a hanged criminal to his *cor villosum* found in his autopsy (De *abditis* et mirandis morborum *causis* (Basileae, 1529), Cap. 83, p. 284).

After van Helmont, Marcus Marci, also an authority quoted by Hirnhaim, worked out this doctrine of ideas. By combination with matter the idea suffers a diminution, insofar as it is subjected to extension and multiplication. When the idea is made concrete, it becomes "contracted." Therefore if the individual is destroyed, although the form itself is indestructible, its external features disappear.

It is in this sense that the preservation of form after the destruction of matter to ash is one of the points on which Sir Thomas Browne bases his "Religio medici." This preservation or resurrection of forms which can be seen by experiment, as in the ashes of a plant, is reality, and demonstrates from "the visible effects of nature" the reality of godliness. Just as many things in theology are true "which are not inducible by reason or confirmable by senses, many things in philosophy are confirmable by sense, yet not inducible by reason." [58]

Thus: the work of Hirnhaim indicates the continued existence in the XVIIth century of the negative theory of knowledge as the basis of the new biological and pathological science [59] which is closely connected (a) with the negatively critical reforms of Paracelsus (the result of his view of the world), and (b) with the work of van Helmont, which actually belongs to modern experimental science. The sceptical examination applied to all branches of science has left standing a natural philosophy which is accepted as reality, and which, on the basis of simple observation, in biology has led to knowledge of secular importance.

[58] *Religio medici*, ed. W. A. Greenhill (London, 1898), Sect. XLVIII.

[59] I cannot agree with Hirnhaim's biographer, Barach, in his denial that Hirnhaim's scepticism leaves room for knowledge and research in nature. According to Barach not even mystical revelation is appreciated by Hirnhaim — notwithstanding his reverence for St. Bernhard, — because mystical revelation includes faith in one's own internal experiences and is therefore illusory. But, as a matter of fact, Hirnhaim seems to me to justify his natural philosophy by his faith and by the doctrine of ideas and the soul of the world in the sense of Paracelsus, Helmont, and Marci. According to Hirnhaim, their natural research approached the truth. He was right to interpret these doctrines leading to induction and empirical knowledge—as having been derived from the religious conceptions and cosmology of these scholars.

## III

Against what type of reason and science is the new demand for empiricism directed? The answer to this question is supplied by one of the principal documents of the Order of the Rosicrucians, the "Themis aurea" of Michael Maier, physician to Rudolph II.[1] It is chiefly that type of reason which, like Galen, in his well known tables on the effects of remedies, desires to calculate and explain the properties and actions of substances from their qualities. The specific element of the remedy, that is, the unknown part which operates, the "proprietas" of Paracelsus, exercises its function directly ("immediate").[2] This function of the remedy is its form or idea and is identical with the ideas of all the other things

[1] See Craven, J. B., *Count Michael Maier, Doctor of Philosophy and Medicine, Alchemist, Rosicrucian, Mystic*, 1910 (quoted after Waite, A. E., *The Brotherhood of the Rosy Cross* (London, 1924). Mich. Maier lived from 1568-1622, the title of his paper is: "Themis aurea h. e. de legibus fraternitatis R. C. tractatus, quo earum cum rei veritate convenientia, utilitas publica et privata, nec non causa necessaria evolvuntur et demonstrantur" (Frankfurt, 1618).

[2] "Proprietas est quaedam virtus vel naturalis positio continens immediàte et inseparabiliter formam substantialem rei adductam super ipsam sub determinata proportione adiuvante coelesti influentia." V, p. 47. This conception of "Proprietas" is in many respects identical with that of the ὅλη οὐσία of Galenos, and it is from this doctrine that Haeser derives the medical belief in magic and supernatural forces (*Geschichte der Medizin*, 3. Edition, 1875, p. 357). On the other hand the practical value of this doctrine was not very high within the system of Galenos (compare his "de renum affectionibus," previously mentioned, further III, simpl. med. 12; *ibid.*, V, 18 — comparison of the proprietas with the virtue of the magnet — and particularly the treatises on "Theriac" in the XIVth volume of Kuehn's edition of Galen's *Opera omnia*. Avicenna repeats the comparison with the magnet ("Sicut est in magnete virtus attractiva ferri, quam nulla elementariarum virtutum invenitur habere." Canon, Tr. 2 de vir. corp. Venet. Junt. 1608, vol. II, p. 340). Accordingly Averroës recommends experiment rather than syllogism in order to find out the "Complexio medicinae" ("Sciuntur per rationes, sed verificantur experimenti." A "Compositum per rationem" should not be given to a noble patient unless it has been proved harmless in a peasant with strong constitution. Super Cantic. Avicennae. In the Edit. of the Colliget Venet. Junt. 1553, p. 104 and De theriaca. Venet. Junt. 1552, p. 141.

of the world, and likewise dependent on the influence of the stars. These are the shining signs of divine law, immutable and inaccessible to intellectual analysis, but apprehensible by means of experiment.

The true physician learns the properties of remedies by means of " ratio experimenti " alone.[3] Accordingly he selects " pauca probata infallibilia," mixes them deliberately (" iudicio "), not in order to give the impression of a longer prescription, but to ensure that they are actually suitable, and that his estimate of their action is correct. The " Proprietas " has nothing to do with the complexion, which was the sole object of investigation by the ancients. For things of different complexion can have the same effect. Rhubarb and tamarinds " a tota proprietate " attract black bile, but they are not of the same complexion. Whereas the complexion is deduced by rational calculation, the proprietas is obtained by experiment. Hence from the opposition to automatic reason results the preference for empiricism and experiment.

It is in this sense that Suchten[4] emphatically states that he will describe only that which he knows " exacte et certe," which his own eyes have seen, his own hands have touched, and experience confirms; but this is entirely for the benefit of the young who are not yet contaminated by doctrines and opinions, and not for the followers of Galen, because they pretend to discover more secrets in nature than ever existed, and not for the followers of Paracelsus, because they claim that the knowledge they have obtained from their master is greater than that of the author himself.

How is this experience to be achieved? The necessary work is done by chemistry, which separates the superfluous matter from the essential nucleus, thus creating medicines of greater purity than are otherwise to be obtained. Therefore there is already a new science appearing in place of the old.

True medicine is the gift of God, only to be obtained by the devout and worthy, whose human reason is illumined by God, while pride is allied with ignorance. The physician must be " born by the light of grace and nature, by the internal and invisible angel in man, in

[3] " Multa stant in experimento quae nunquam fuere nec de praesenti stant in ratione," p. 47.

[4] *De secretis antimonii,* 1570. Ed. Forberg latine (Basil, 1575).

the light of nature which instructs man like a true preceptor."[5] Thus, there develops a peculiar conception of nature. Nature is defined first of all by her relation to God to whom, as His workshop, she is subjected; and secondly by her relation to men to whom she appears as part and product of the Divine. Hence knowledge resulting from the investigation of nature is the beatitude of the present life. Theology is the natural and supernatural source of science.[6] Therefore the heathen writings on nature are almost always wrong; it is a waste of time and diligence to seek wisdom there.[6a] Authorities like Galen and Aristotle are not to be acknowledged. Every sect[7] is based on some element of truth. The physician who wishes to excel must therefore abstain from sectarian doctrines. Experience alone enables him to detect the errors of the ancients and to elucidate all that is occult, and thus to fulfil the ordinance of God. The knowledge of sympathy and antipathy as the results of divine providence, the signs of the macrocosm, chiromancy and physiognomy lead to a medical science which God has miraculously inscribed in the book of nature, i. e., in the heavens and in the earth. The human soul, by a mystic process of internal contemplation and reversion to itself, attains to "mens," and hence it approaches God, seeing all without need of external instruction, a mysterium incomprehensible by the "spiritus academicus."[8] This is the illumination of reason by the mens, a state which is due to the Divine Right, while the perception "per sensus" includes a removal from God. On the other hand, only the physician who prepares remedies with his own hands and not by "ratione" like the

[5] Crollii, Oswald, *Basilica chymica cum notis Hartmanni et praxi chymiatrica* (Marburg, 1611), pp. 6, 11, 13, 28.

[6] It is therefore described in the "Themis aurea" as characteristic of the Rosicrucians that they live for godliness, search the scriptures and practise mercy and holiness without thought of reward. But immediately after this there follows the statement that they investigate "omnem naturam," making the secrets of nature the basis of experiments ("eiusque arcana in experimenta ducunt"). They are in possession of many of these secrets in astronomy, physics, mechanics, medicine and chemistry, all fundamentally true, by means of which they work wonders. Finally, Nature allows her processes to take their course according to her own laws, in the operations of which only God in his providence can interfere.

[6a] Compare Roger Bacon's entirely different appreciation of the ancient authors in the I. chapter of this paper.

[7] According to Pico della Mirandola. Croll, *ibid.*, p. 65.

[8] P. 71.

" medicus rationalis " and who knows how to separate the remedy from the poison and to reduce composite substances to their " pure simplicity " [9] is the genuine physician.

But nature which we are investigating is " ministrans," that is, the servant of the independent Creator. She proceeds in her allotted task " fideliter et naturaliter." Her work can bring man good or evil, and under these headings come disease, healing and death. They are provided by God for every individual, and this providence of God changes nothing in the natural course of events, " sed cursum sinit naturae ordinatum." Nevertheless Divine Will in its absolute independence has also power to operate against the destined course of nature and to interrupt it sometimes " nunc in his, nunc in aliis emendando et derogando." [10] The evil to which a man is doomed " secundum naturae ordinem " is allowed to take its course as this man's punishment which binds him to the earth, to the causal, compulsory course of natural events.

The secrets of nature, to which the true divine medicine leads, represent the development (" explicatio ") of God and therefore accomplish what is known as " ars magica." [11] Magic, in this sense, is the highest, the most perfect and the richest knowledge of " philosophia naturalis." It is assisted in its wondrous works by profound experience and the occult virtues of things, which, applied to a suitable substratum, perform miracles in the natural course of events (" rerum natura ").[12] Thus the magician is a particularly

[9] Pp. 77, 4.

[10] Compare the well known doctrine of St. Augustine (De gen. ad lit., IX, 17; V, 23; III, 14, etc.), and the view-point of Robert Boyle at the end of this paper.

[11] Maier, with reference to the divine origin of magic, quotes: *Origines* 5, tract. sp. Math.; 23 Hom. sp. Numeri. Further Philo, Jud.; Περὶ τῶν ἀναφερομένων ἐν εἴδει νόμων. Opp. ed. Adr. Turnebus (Colon, Allobrog. 1613), p. 611:

" Vera magia h. e. perspectiva scientia per quam opera naturae clarius cernuntur." Compare with this conception of magic that outlined by Thorndike: " A way of looking at the world which is reflected in a human art . . . employing varied materials in varied rites often phantastic to work a great variety of marvellous results which offer man a release from his physical, social and intellectual limitations, not by the imaginative and sentimental methods of music, melodrama, fiction and romances or by religious experience or ascetism, but by operations supposed to be efficacious here in the world of external reality." *Loc. cit.*, II, S. 974.

[12] See Gaffarel, James (1601-1681, librarian to Cardinal Richelieu), *Unheard-of curiosities concerning the talismanical sculpture of the Persians, the horoscope of*

diligent student of nature, who is equipped with an extensive knowledge of her works and possibilities. Now if, at the right moment, he unites the active with the passive, he can obtain such premature effects as appear miracles to ordinary people, although he has achieved nothing more than an anticipation of time in the natural course of events. Thus there are always wonders in the world accessible for discoveries and inventions, so that continual progress is possible, while the needs of men increase proportionately. Nobody would have suffered if printing had not been invented.

This relation to magic which originated in the ideas of the Renaissance (Picus,[13] Paracelsus) has ruled the thoughts of religious scientists and physicians during the XVIIth century.[14] The example of Sir Thomas Browne, who believed in witchcraft, shows the possibility of a via media. He recognizes magic as a revelation of " honest effects of nature " and admits on the other hand that magic was originally conceived by the devil and by spirits which may or may not be evil. " Thus, I think, at first a great part of philosophy was witchcraft; which being afterwards derived to one another, proved but philosophy." That which we discover as " philosophia naturalis " is magic if it is taught by the devil or spirits.[15]

*the patriarch and the reading of the stars.* Transl. i. Engl. by E. Chilmead (London, 1650) : Amulets etc. should be made under certain constellations, " as that they shal have the power, *naturally* and without the aide of any demon or divel, to drive away noisome beasts, allay winds, thunder and tempests and to cure diverse kinds of diseases." — The treatise of Gaffarel contains a vindication of the Jewish and rabbinic writings which are much less dangerous than those of the heathen, allowed by the Fathers, and a refutation of the arguments against the Aristotelian doctrines.

[13] According to Inge, W. R., *Christian mysticism,* 7. ed. (London, 1933), p. 269, Pico regards magic as the " deepest mysteries and the knowledge of the whole of the nature with her powers."

[14] Further, to express it paradoxically, exaggerated scepticism could be a source of belief in magic and witchcraft. By his utmost scepticism as to the traditional Aristotelian methods as means of natural research Joseph Glanville was led to a vigorous defence of the belief in witchcraft, a fact which has been pointed out by Jos. Needham, *The Sceptic. Biologist, loc. cit.*, p. 196. According to Glanville there was not any valid argument against magic and witchcraft, because of the " vanity of dogmatizing and confident opinions."

[15] Sir Thomas Browne's *Religio medici,* ed. W. A. Greenhill (London, 1898), I, 31, p. 51 ff. For Browne's attitude to magic and witchcraft compare the excellent account of Sir Humphry Rolleston, Sir Thom. Browne, *Annals of Medic. History,* N. S. II, p. 7 ff., 1930. See also Jos. Needham, *Scept. Biologist, loc. cit.*, p. 195.

Even Francis Bacon recommends the trial of magic, " si forte subsit et lateat in aliquibus eorum aliqua operatio naturalis," as influences from body to body and spirit to spirit.[16] Although magic is overloaded with superstition and imposture, there remains a certain number of " consensus " which are proved by reliable experiments, e. g., the consensus — by virtue of their " occult " and specific powers [17] — between the magnet and the iron, between mercury and gold, between certain remedies and individual parts of the body, humours, diseases. Where great effects are produced by substances or virtues, inadequate according to their quantities, there occur " Instantiae magicae," i. e., examples of magic.[18] Such effects are produced by a specific poison, that is to say, a toxic substance, whose effects are invariably the same.

On the other hand we find in the official ecclesiastical viewpoint as represented especially by the Jesuits (*Del Rio*)[19] a kind of liberalism which refutes magic. This attitude is expressed in a book by Joh. Freitag [20] on the occult side of medicine. The treaty with the

[16] *Nov. Organum,* II, 31; *De augment. scient.*, IV, 3.

[17] *Nov. Organum,* II, 50.

[18] *Ibid.*, II, 51.

[19] About del Rio, see Pagel, W., *Joh. Bapt. van Helmont,* Einfuehrung in *die philosophische Medizin des Barock* (Berlin: Springer, 1930), pp. 93 and 99.

[20] Noctes medicae s. de abusu medicinae tractatus, quo universum medicastrorum examen empiricorum modernorum uberrima annona, uromantes s. lotiophysici . . . dentifrangibuli chirurgi genethliaci . . . myropolae pseudochymici, umbratici doctores Paracelsistarum sectae, magomedicastri, sagae et superstitiosam vulgo curam exercentes perstringuntur, de magia vetita et magorum suppliciis agitur, artis Paracelsicae fundamenta luculenter traduntur . . . et evertentur. Francof., 1616. Against empiricism and experiment: Cap. 5, " Experimentorum plaustra non facere artificem nec per solam experientiam addisci artem medicam." Galen's doctrine of humours and tempers explains more clearly biological facts such as the alteration of the character by the food, etc. The specificity of a remedy, its virtue, does not exclude humoralism. There may be sympathy or antipathy between the substance and one or the other of the humours. Thus the doctrine of sympathy and antipathy is applied to humoralism. Similarly, in the writings of Sennert and other contemporary authors, the new alchemy and the doctrines of Paracelsus are regarded as " ministra et famula " of the galenic, that is to say, rational medicine, e. g., in Christ. Horn, *De auro medico philosophorum,* i. e., de illo occulto salutari solari omnium mineralium vegetabilium et animalium corporum spiritu s. balsamo vivifico . . . dialogus scholasticus. Francof., 1615. With reference to Sennert's attempts to reconcile humoralism and the doctrines of Paracelsus, see Pagel, *loc. cit.*, p. 61. Compare the liberalism and scepticism of some medieval physicians regarding magic and sorcery as opposed to the official ecclesiastical dogma, which declared

devil is here accepted as the basis of all magic, and on the grounds that lunatics have never been known to make a compact with the devil, the author refutes the theories that witches are lunatics. A Christian must therefore prefer death to healing by magic procedures.

According to Freytag the only disease that gold will cure is covetousness. " Ars non adaequat naturam." The alchemist can not produce a droplet of blood artificially, but only a reddish liquor. He cannot make any " homunculus extra naturae ordinem a deo institutum atque coniunctione maris et foeminae fecundorum." The art of the alchemist is opposed to nature and therefore blasphemy.

Here we find the same contrast drawn between " Naturalia " and " Artificialia " to which Quercetanus [21] objects, when he, Quercetanus, maintains that the true chemical art must be founded, " quae naturam ipsam imitando metalla, transmutet."

Thus the art of chemistry is an " Opus naturale," if matter itself is a part of nature, because " decoquendo appetit, retinet, digerit, expellit, permiscit, corrumpit, generat et informat suo tempore lapidem cum quo natura informat metalla per ipsam permixtionem." And all that occurs " praecepto Dei omnipotentis." [22]

On the other hand, chemistry is also an art, not because art creates, implants and destroys forms, but because it serves nature in its efforts to make gold by such an indirect process as occurs when gold develops from base metals. The art of chemistry is able to imitate that natural process, but, unlike nature, is unable to produce gold directly.

common and natural processes and any disease under unusual circumstances as devilish trickery and work of demons: Diepgen, *Die Daemonen — und Zauberkrankheit bei den Theologen und Medizinern im Mittelalter.* Naturforscherverslg. (Nauheim, 1920). Janus., XXV, 1921, p. 112. — On the other hand, compare: Fehr, Joseph, *Der Aberglaube und die katholische Kirche des Mittelalters* (Stuttgart, 1857), illustrating the combat of the Catholic Church against heathen superstition.

[21] Jos. Quercetani, *Opera medica. ad J. Auberti de ortu et causis metallorum contra chymicos explicationem brevis responsio* (Lyon, 1591), p. 55.

[22] See also the *Diaeteticon polyhistoricon* of Quercetanus (Paris, 1606). The whole world, and man especially, demonstrates a deviation from " nature " (" Res a natura sua degenerarunt "), due to the sin of Adam. The degenerated, that is to say, unnatural things, are harmful for men, but God, by revelation of the Christian science of alchemy, has enabled man to become wise and to help mankind (p. 6 v.).

In conclusion: As a result of their scepticism with regard to the existing science as well as their religious convictions, and on the basis of their refutation of Galen's doctrine of qualities and humours, alchemists, such as Mich. Maier, the Rosicrucians, Suchten, Croll, Quercetanus, embarked on a course of independent empirical research. Their point of view is partly due to a positive appreciation of magic as a systematic imitation of nature by means of arbitrary variation of the conditions of natural processes.

On the other hand, the official deprecation of magic (Jesuits — *Del Rio* — Freitag, etc.) is united with a revival of humoralism and the rational explanation of natural processes by means of the ancient qualities. The procedures of alchemy and of "nature" are, according to these trends of thought, entirely different and incompatible. Hence the art of alchemy is blasphemy and imposture.

## IV

The conception of the world underlying the trends of thought described here is monistic. Things corporeal and things spiritual are connected in a graduated cosmos leading upward to God himself. The symbol of this transition from the finest corporeal to the spiritual, the intermediary between the two worlds, the beginning of all things, according to the tradition of the Pentateuch, is light. Light penetrates matter, giving it origin and form. "It animates all things, contains all things, supports all things, brings all things together, unites all things, it separates all things, it draws all things to itself; all that is, or is illumined, or is warmed, all that lives, or all that is created, or is fed, or is increased, or is perfected, or is moved. It purifies whatever it has transformed. It perfects all things, it renews all things, it preserves all things and protects them from annihilation. It is the number and measure of all things." Light is the image of the Deity, the world its coal. The terrestrial bodies gain in beauty and perfection according to their degree of participation in the light. Thus Franciscus Patritius in his metaphysics of light, his "Panaugia," sings of the world, which is entirely animated by the power and virtue of light.[1]

[1] Patritius, Fr., *Nova de universis philosophia* . . . in qua aristotelica methodo non per motum sed per lucem et lumina ad primam causam ascenditur . . . quibus

The rays are the messengers of light which accomplish all things. The rays of God are, according to the hermetic book, the realizations (ἐνέργειαι). The rays of the cosmos are the elementary properties (φύσεις), the rays of men the arts and sciences.[2]

Robert Grosseteste regards all activity in nature as dependent on raylike lines, angles and figures, and their reception by the surface of the substratum (reflexion or refraction).[3]

We may call the agent "Species" or "Similitudo," we can imagine its transmission from one body to another only by means of lines, angles and figures, which like rays are absorbed or reflected in a manner which varies according to the state of the surface and translucency of the object. The shorter the distance between the object and the agent, the shorter the rays and the more intensive the effect. Rough surfaces with unequal parts destroy the rays or diminish their force. All natural activity varies in intensity according to the differences in the lines, angles and figures. All unity comes from the perfection of light, all multiplicity from its division.[4]

Roger Bacon, in his "Perspectiva,"[5] devotes an entire chapter to the importance to the health and disease of men of the "Multiplicatio virtutum," as the result of lines, angles and figures. Both the hidden and the manifest occur according to the "mira potestas huius multiplicationis." In order to preserve health we must endeavour to avoid harmful influences from without, at least, we must try to avoid their direct action, which is caused by the radiation of rectilinear rays, even if we are unable to escape the

postremo sunt adiecta Zoroastris oracula CCCXX ex Platonicis collecta, Hermetis trismegisti libelli et fragmenta, Asclepii discipuli tres libelli, Mystica Aegyptiorum a Platone dictata, ab Aristotele excepta et praescripta philosophia (Venet., 1593). I Panaugia (De luce. de diaphano, de radiis, de lumine, de opaco).

[2] *Hermetis trismegisti clavis,* Lib. IV; Patritius, *loc. cit., Hermes trismegist.,* Lib. XII.

[3] Libellus Linconiensis de phisicis lineis angulis et figuris per quas omnes acciones naturales complentur (Norimbergae, 1503). Frontispiece: Radius reflexus and Radius fractus.

[4] "Omnia esse unum ab unius lucis perfectione. Ea quae sunt multa, esse multa ab ipsius lucis diversa multiplicatione." De luce s. de inchoatione formarum. Baur, L., "Die philosophischen Werke des Rob. Grosseteste," *Btrge. Gesch. Philos. Mittelalter,* 9 (Münster, 1912), p. 51 ff.

[5] Ed. Joh. Combach (Francof., 1614); *Spec. mathemat.,* p. 16; p. 49; Cap. 6, p. 61.

broken or reflected rays. Thus the rays of the sun bring death in summer and those of the moon at night. Saturn and Mars cause great harm, imparting the germ of corruption to things " ut experientia docet." The contagious diseases develop when a species contracted in unclean places increases (" multiplicatur "). The same emanation and increase of a harmful " species " occurs when a woman during menstruation, by her presence or glance, clouds a mirror, and when a man " malae complexionis " has an evil influence on his fellows.[6] The facts included in the " Perspectiva " agree with the wisdom of the Bible and therefore are of use to mankind.

Just as the light and the beams of the sun break through after driving away the clouds, according to Alfredus Anglicus,[7] the finest parts of the blood are animated and changed into " spiritus " within the heart and the arteries, when the life-giving warmth, by virtue of its expansion, opens the outlets of the blood and radiates through all the channels. Like the sun, the heart emits the beams of its virtue (" primae virtutis actum ") thus distributing vital force all over the body.[8]

There are many paintings depicting St. Francis receiving the " stigmata." These pictures show Christ appearing to the Saint with rays passing from His wounds to the corresponding parts of St. Francis' body. The painters have demonstrated the course of the rays in a naturalistic manner.[9] The idea of influence being conveyed in rays of light is common in XIIIth century paintings (Dorothea Singer).[9a]

[6] Compare the " spiritus " and " vapores " which according to an ancient tradition, reviewed by Arnald of Villanova, transmit influences from one person to another (Arnald, *De parte operativa*).

[7] " De motu cordis," ed. Cl. Baeumker, *Beitr. Gesch. Philos. Mittelalt.*, XXIII, 1/2 (Münster, 1923), XI, 3, p. 46.

[8] *Ibid.*, VIII, 3; XVI, 17, p. 94.

[9] See, e. g., Musée du Louvre, 1312 (or Firenze Gal. ant. e mod.) : Giotto, *St. François recevant les stigmates*. Cf. the collection of pictures made by Facchinetti, V., *Le stigmate de S. Francesco d'Assisi*, 1924; and *San Francesco d'Assisi nella storia, legenda, arte* (Milano, 1921). — In the pictures of Guercino, Baldachio, Macrino d'Alba, etc., the beams are missing, in the pictures of Tintoretto, Foppa, Cardi they are only outlined. Similar to the conception of Giotto are the pictures of Duerer, H. Fries, and one of the Scuola Umbro-Fiorentina (copied in the book of Facchinetti).

[9a] Personal communication.

The wisdom of the world is knowledge and cognition. All cognition has its origin in the mind, being primarily derived from the

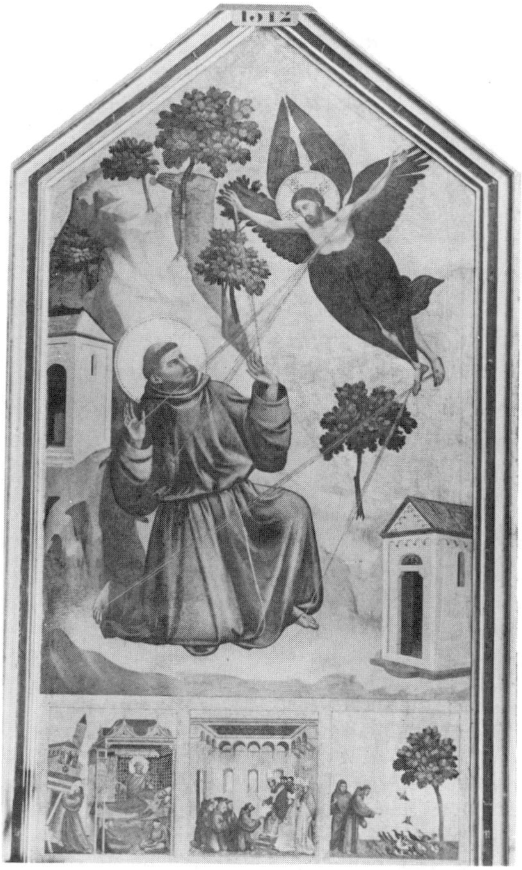

GIOTTO: SAINT FRANCIS RECEIVING THE STIGMATA. Paris. Musée du Louvre Nr. 1312. Naturalistic conception of light beams transferring celestial influences.

senses. The most important among these, on account of its subtlety and power, is sight. It was the first to experience light. By the aid and effect of light we are able to differentiate what is above from what is below or what is in the middle. Sight is succeeded by wonder, wonder by speculation, and speculation by philosophy. Philosophy, is therefore the legitimate descendant of light, of illumination, of wonder, and of contemplation. Light is simple, unity before multiplicity, the singular number before the division into two. Therefore it is in close connection with the Divinity, spiritually the image most resembling Him, physically His reflection in the mirrors of the stars. Thus light is the mediator between the Deity and material nature.[10]

The wonders of light are here regarded as metaphysical entities and are connected with each other in a general sense. If, however, man is the microcosm who, as one degree of its development, reflects the macrocosm, the study of optics promises to reveal laws which govern both the origin of things and the nature of man. The development of parts in a whole, wherein the integrity of the whole is preserved, appears to be strikingly illustrated by light and the laws of its transmission. Thus it was the metaphysical conception of the significance of light which may have stimulated the scientific study of the problems of physical optics. By means of the application of the principles of optics Marcus Marci of Landscron attempted to solve the problem of the origin of man.[11] His importance to the

[10] Patritius, *loc. cit.* A source of these doctrines typical of the XVIIth century is Comenius, according to whom light works up matter by loosening, warming and lightening it, whence all qualities are derived (*Physicae Synopsis,* Cap. II ed. Reber. Giessen, 1896, p. 88 and Addenda, *ibid.*, Cap. 5: "De primo omnium in mundo motore, luce s. igne," p. 420).

[11] Marci, the "Bohemian Plato," the "Hippocrates of Prague," was born 1595, studied 1610-24 at various Jesuit colleges and at the Prague University; 1627 he was appointed professor; 1647 physician to the Emperor Ferdinand III and "physicus senior" of Bohemia; 1654 "Pfalzgraf" with the title "Von Kronland"; 1662 Rector of the Prague University. He died in 1667. From his early youth he was accustomed to overtax himself and his weak bodily constitution. He wrote about sixteen books, e. g., the *Idearum operatricium idea* (1635), the subject of discussion; *De proportione motus figuram recte linearum et circuli quadratura ex motu* (1639), *Thaumantias, liber de arcu coelesti* (1648), *Philosophia vetus restituta* (1662), etc. See Biography in his *Liturgia mentis s. disceptatio medica, philosophica et optica de natura epilepsiae* (Ratisb., 1678), edited by his scholar, J. J. Wenc. Dobrcensky de Nigroponte. Further: Guhrauer, *Marcus Marci und seine philosophischen Schriften*; Fichte-Ulrici'sche, *Ztschr. f. Philos. u. philos. Kritik*, XXI, 241, 1852; Hasner, *Prager Ztschr. Heilkde.*, IV, 170, 1883; Hoppe, E. M., "Ein vergessener Physiker des XVII. Jahrhunderts," *Arch. Gesch. Math.*

progress of science is due to his work in physics, particularly in optics. In connection with the latter he successfully studied the division of light into colours and anticipated Newton's "experimentum crucis" by proving the homogeneous nature of the coloured rays (Hoppe).[12] Here a science is developing on the lines employed by the exact experimental scientists of a later era. This author is of special interest to historians of medicine and biology, because, in these spheres, he combined experimental investigation with an abundance of mystical and philosophical conceptions which could not fail to give impulse and colour to his scientific work. This combination of scientific method with mysticism gives him an intellectual and historical position similar to that of Helmont, to whose doctrines of archei and ideas he adheres, while his general application of the laws of light and radiation in all spheres, even of the animate world, places him among the light-mystics. Reference to his work is appropriate, as in it mystic philosophy is closely allied with a tendency towards exact science. At the same time, like so many of his scientific contemporaries (Harvey, etc.), he is emphatically a disciple of Aristotle. Nothing, however, shows the union of mystical and religious ideas with a mechanistic and scientific point of view so clearly as his "Idearum operatricium idea," a never completed pamphlet which contains his *speculative embryology, based on optical conceptions.*

The work first of all deals with the nature of the semen. Marci rejects, as too materialistic, the ancient hypothesis (Democritus)[13] that the semen is derived from all parts of the body. As a matter of fact, it is not a part *of* the body, but is attached *to* the body as something independent following its own inherent idea. If the semen were a mosaic of the products of the individual parts of the body —

*Natw. Techn.*, XXX, 1/2, 1927; Lehmann, E. M., "Gesundheitsbuechlein," *Anhang zur Otosophie* (Landskron, 1928).

[12] "Refractio superveniens radio colorato non mutat speciem coloris" (Thaumantias, 1648). See Hoppe, *loc. cit.*; cf. also his doctrines in mechanics, theory of motion, importance of elasticity, on the pendulum, etc. Further, Hauessler, *Mitt. Gesch. d. Mediz. u. Natwiss.*, XIV, 165, and against the over-rating of his achievements: Rosenfeld, L. M., "Untersuchungen ueber das Prisma und ihr Verhaeltnis zu Newtons Farbenlehre," *Isis*, 1931, XVII, p. 325.

[13] Agrippa of Nettesheym had taken the numerous divergent theories of the ancient authors on the origin and importance of the seed as the proof of the uncertainty of scientific medicine. *De incertit. et vanit. scient*, Cap. 82; *loc. cit.*, p. 428: *De medicina in genere.*

who should save the germ from becoming a confused chaos? The essential part of the semen is the independent epigenetically plastic "vis efficiens."

In the presumably vaporous material of the semen the soul-like force first of all designs the *whole picture* of the child to be, making a shadowy outline, not only of the exterior, but also of the internal parts. Therefore, before the existence of the individual members there is a peculiar model of the whole, composed of the most delicate substance. Between this stage of development and its completion in matter another intermediate species must exist. The work of this is to ensure the achievement of the idea, e. g., that a human being and not a man-like stone is formed.

The semen is fundamentally different from a machine, being related to living things, even though it is itself without the attributes of life, such as movement, feeling, alimentation. In the engine the result is exactly equivalent to the motor force put into it; in organic reproduction the result, that is to say, the soul of the new individual, is very often quite different from the soul of the parent.

Like the soul, the semen is immortal. This is evident from the existence of spontaneous generation, an event which occurs probably on account of the great surplus of semen formed. According to all experience, a small part of the semen suffices for reproduction. Obviously it is *monadically* constructed. Its entire virtue must be contained in its *smallest* parts, for as a shattered mirror breaks up the original single image into numerous small ones, so the semen, when broken into fragments, also has numerous centres, and this makes it evident that even a small portion of the semen can produce one or more embryos.

The soul-like vegetative principle in the semen forms the future character, transmitting resemblances and hereditary sins. The statement that all mankind sinned in Adam is explained by the fact of the enclosure ("Einschachtelung") of all living beings in Adam's seed. In addition to this "anima brutorum," which is contained in the seed from the beginning, there appears, at a later stage, the immediately divine "anima rationalis." It is the task of the vegetative soul to unite the corruptible matter with the immortal anima rationalis, the "vera hominis forma," wherein the individual returns to unity, the Many to the One and the realization to the idea.

How does the plastic force work in the semen? It is not entirely autonomous. Absolute epigenesis does not exist. On the contrary, its procedure is dependent upon the already traced outline of the whole. The plastic force works in " imo corporis recessu," in a geometrical centre of the future body corresponding to the heart of the true Aristotelian tradition. It operates " absque tumultu et instrumento," is worthy of the highest admiration, since the living being, in exquisite perfection, provided with numerous members and dissimilar parts, results from a single homogeneous entity. The time required for the work in the construction of the different parts is the same, for the " vis plastica " does not first draw an outline of the form and then complete the details in turn, but it activates regularly in all spheres. If the embryo be represented as consisting of concentric circles, the plastic force operates very slowly in the inner smaller circles in order that, even in the outermost circles, the whole process may be completed at the same time. Thus the force must be equally distributed, " esse totam in toto et totam in qualibet parte." [14] This theory of regularity is based on the assumption that the position of all parts has been previously determined; otherwise the same force could not form brain at A and liver at D. That it does not form brain also at D is due to the existence of the ideal outline of the organ contained within the general sketch of the whole organism.[15]

Marci illustrates the importance of the function of position in the development of the multiform organs from a uniform substratum by another comparison drawn from the study of optics. As the lens breaks up the rays of the single source of light into multiform images, so also here is the production of multiplicity from the single and uniform, the restriction of the infinite to the finite. The development of something distinct from the " confusa species " is also

[14] In spite of the regular progress of development in general an important organ such as the heart is completed before the whole. The " punctum saliens " of a bird's egg can be seen as early as the second or third day of incubation, " velut sanguinis concreti gutta." The tempo of the development varies according to the distinctness of the image projected from the centre.

[15] The whole conception foreshadows the modern so-called " Feldtheorie," as established by the work of Gurwitsch, Spemann, Mangold, Weiss, Joseph and Dorothea Needham, Waddington. See the review of Waddington in *Science Progress*, No. 114, Oct., 1934, p. 336.

comparable with the action of the lens, which " virtute refractionis," separates individual rays out of a bundle of rays.

The process of development commences when the anima of the parents, by imitation of its own species, draws the outline of the child. Then the anima operates as the plastic force according to the commands of the species which it has itself conceived. The process resembles that of perception which is nothing more than a kind of photography caused by the adaptation of the brain to the object by means of the impression of the senses. Thus the soul is her own ape.

The force of development operates from the mathematical centre of the fetal body. This point is fixed in definite relation to the centre of the parent body. As light gives off rays without itself decreasing, as the cornea outlines an image both as a whole and as a bundle of rays, the virtue in the centre loses nothing of its power and importance to the whole when it assists the parts in their development. It can be regarded as representing both " implicatio " and " explicatio."

The developing force in its activity resembles the process of imagination, but in its essence it should never be compared with processes, such as imagination, which are entirely connected with the brain. The brain does not penetrate to the interior of things, it can never see anything more than the surface. Even if we could split up everything into the smallest parts we should only see their surfaces, although these parts might be infinite in number.[16] For size, position, union of the whole with its parts, internal factors, are essentially decisive, such as the anima which " efficienter " forms the parts and the species which " exemplariter " designs them. External influences, however, can shape many things, as is seen in the case of deformed Chinese feet, artificially produced macrocephaly, trained plants.

Further, a conception derived from the study of Optics and applied to the whole process of development explains the occurrence of *deformities.* If the envelope surrounding the centre of the

[16] " Et tametsi interna viscera omnesque abditae partes detegantur, non tamen praeter superficies coloratas alia videremus, praeter-quam quod sectio partium numero infinitarum nunquam terminaretur." Even when the surface of the parts is very small, invisible channels in the internal parts have developed, by means of which the internal force distributes nourishment.

embryo is not uniformly opaque, the rays proceeding from the central point and transmitting the species may be abnormally refracted. If reflexion occurs, a limb belonging to the periphery may be pushed unduly near to the centre. Fundamental deformities, such as multiplicity of the whole fetal body, are said to be due to the multiplication of the centre of formation, i. e., the heart. On the other hand, abnormal refraction at the surface may possibly be the cause of an increased number of various limbs, the existence of more than the usual extremities, two heads projecting from the shoulders or additional heads springing from the abdomen. The latter abnormality is regarded as the result of a deflexion of the rays near the centre of the plan.

A particular form of refraction and deflexion of the rays proceeding from the centre and meeting with a medium which is too thin, causes giant growth. The reports of the enormous size of the ancients seem to Marci to be fables, since these reports are contradicted by the normal size of the mummies which have been discovered.

Thus the fundamental similarities in the majority of deformities become comprehensible, since in their formation they all follow the same laws of refraction. Irregularities of the surface, however, generally arise when the seed does not change at the right time into a homogeneous mass. For originally it consists of numerous transparent glass-like balls into which it has been changed through the effervescence which occurs during ejaculation. Later the enclosed spirits burst the walls, changing the seed into a homogeneous mass.

Deformities also occur as the result of external influence on the pregnant mother (birth-marks) or on account of the hereditary structure. Thus the thought of an apple by the pregnant mother can lead to the formation of an apple-like excrescence on the child. But naturally it is only the shape of an apple which is here imitated. The material composition of the excrescence is the same as that of the whole individual. A foreign species has forced the soul to work up the same material substratum into an abnormal formation. In normal development there is agreement between the working and commanding forces, the latter being the outline designed by the species. Once the process of development has begun it continues towards its goal without intermission.

The speculative embryology of Marcus Marci quoted here may be regarded as a typical product of the XVIIth century. It combines Aristotelian principles not only with mechanistic and physical explanations of the life processes but also with elements of mystic philosophy.

Light is the measure and model of development, the light-like unit, situated in the centre of the body, i. e., in the heart, governs the formation of the various organs. The messengers which carry its commands and transmit its activity to the surfaces where the parts are being formed, are like rays of light and subject to the same law of refraction. The transition from a confused species to the distinct formation, the termination of the infinite, may be compared with the separation of a single ray from a bundle of rays. Consequently deformities depend upon abnormal refraction of the rays due to irregularities of the surface. All this, however, is nothing more than an attempt to give to the general metaphysics of light a foundation of physical principles and to apply these laws to the fundamental processes of animate nature.

That Marci actually sees these processes under the universal aspect of a " Panaugia " is evident from his extensive dependence upon the physiological and pathological doctrines of Paracelsus and van Helmont, whose conception of the " Archeus " he accepts.[17] In van Helmont's opinion, light in its capacity of intermediary between world and individual, between infinite unity and multiplicity, is the symbol of the seedlike origin of all things in the world in general, and particularly in the moment of the origin of new life.

[17] Accordingly *Marci* in his paper on epilepsy (" Liturgia mentis ") suggests a particular " gaseous " species from outside like a poison, and not a primary disturbance of the humours, to be the cause of this disease. The poison operates by means of humours and vapors which are exuded and, like rays, transmit the effect. Such rays also cause fever. Poisoning signifies the reception of an idea transmitted by the poison. Either this idea causes death as the result of the extinction of the flame of life or the corruption of the seminal idea of the body, or the functions are damaged on account of the transplantation of the idea of the poison. The autonomy of the archeus is abolished by the penetration of the foreign idea. The same " magnetic " influence, that is to say, one connected with the imagination of a species, which causes an evil, also cures it. Human saliva which is able to cure snake bite when the wound is sucked, receives its curative virtue from the imagination of the healer, who does not derive this power from himself, even though such properties are hereditary. (Πᾶν ἐν πάντων. *Philosophia vetus vestituta* (Prague. 1662), Pars V: " De statu hominis praeter naturam ").

In the semen the archeus becomes " luminosus." Endowment with the " Lumen formale et vitale " by the Creator alone permits the existence of the living entity. All that is active pertains to light, both the action of poison and the command of the organism in its entirety over the subordinate organs.[18] Marci's estimation of the " hermetic " wisdom of Mose, which according to him greatly exceeded the knowledge of the Greeks who knew no more than four elements, corresponds to the view of Paracelsus and Helmont. Marci rejects the idea of the influence of demons, and, like Helmont, declares magic effects to be " effectus naturales " — notwithstanding the fact that magic can neither be taught nor learned and requires a peculiar kind of " saturnine personality."

In many respects Marci *dis*agrees with Helmont, in his aspiration for mechanistic pseudo-explanation and simplification. Thus his hypotheses bear certain resemblances in many ways to those of Descartes and de le Boe. This also applies to his schematic valuation of the flame-like character of the life principle,[19] as well as to his one-sided Aristotelian emphasis of the heart. On the whole, however, his dependence on van Helmont and the close connection of the metaphysical and mystical view with the science of optics are his most noteworthy characteristics.

[18] See my *I. B. van Helmont, loc. cit.*, pp. 22, 24, and my *Helmont, Leibniz, Stahl, loc. cit.*, pp. 26, 33 (on *Comenius*).

[19] He explains disease quite naïvely as being due to disturbance of the upward or downward movement of the *life flame*. Both types of disturbance can be classified according to the increase or decrease in these movements. The cause of disease is to be found in the material feeding the flame or in the flame itself. The fire and flame of life are distributed over the body, although there is a " focus perennis " in the heart. The persistence of that focus explains the reanimation of the apparently dead. In mountain sickness, e. g., a special " species " causes the sense of fear. Then the innate heat becomes too great on account of the accumulation of smoke and the flame of life is dimmed. A large, rapid, strong pulse shows the necessity for coolness and ventilation. Thus tremors, chattering teeth and bristling hair occur. The limbs become very cold, since too much of the spiritus returns to the heart. On account of the cold the nerves cause alternating contraction and relaxation in the innervated parts of the body. Compare the doctrine of Fr. Bacon, *Hist. de ventis, loc. cit.*, p. 167 — according to which like a flame the spirit of the body consumes its life and finally dries up the engine of the body entirely. See Croll, *Basil. chym., loc. cit.*, p. 105: As laying wood on the hearth preserves the fire, suitable arcana and remedies preserve the flame of life.

II

## V

The foregoing chapters have dealt with the individual trends of thought resulting from the conception of a uniform world on which the doctrines of Paracelsus were based, and have examined the negatively sceptical criticism expressed by Hirnhaim, who took as his model Agrippa of Nettesheym. It has been shown how, in the utterances of the alchemists and in the textbook of the Rosicrucians, religious scepticism with regard to existing rational and dogmatic science stimulated experimental work in medical biology. Chemistry, in particular, owes much to these tendencies, even if, for the time being, it must be satisfied with a close connection with religion, mysticism and magic. Finally, the example of Marcus Marci, in his embryology deduced from a speculative view of optics, has shown how conceptions relating to the metaphysics of light contributed to the mechanistic explanation of biological processes. In all these movements there has been one common element, the interdependence existing between the new scientific mode of thought and religion, each of which, at this time and particularly in the case of Paracelsus, was a source of inspiration to the other. The new conception of nature closely associated piety and experience, and both were regarded as immediately subordinate to the Divine Creator. It was in this sense that Comenius [1] recommended an approach to God and truth rather than to Aristotle and the opinions of the schoolmen in order to obtain a reliable philosophy: "Deo duce, ratione luce, sensu teste." It seems almost paradoxical that this religious contemplation played a part in the investigation of nature "iuxta propria principia" [1a] which is the

[1] *Phys. synops., loc. cit.*, p. 34 ff.

[1a] According to *Telesius*' main book ("De rerum natura iuxta propria principia"). Lynn Thorndike, *A History of Magic and Experimental Science during the First 13 Centuries of Our Era* (London, 1923), Vol. 2, 535, refers to Bernhard von Gordon: "Scire unumquodque secundum quod in propria natura se habet, hoc enim

basis of the aspiration for new realities. The emphasis of the spiritual as the active force and of all transitions from spirit to matter in a monistic conception of the world, finally led to the creation of the new notion of disease. Even disease must be regarded as a new reality, a real thing, caused by a " species " from outside (contagium) and not only the expression of the relation between things, as in the case of antiquity, when disease was explained as the result of an abnormal mixture of the humours. Here begins the " system " of diseases, the ontological and etiological notion, allowing their classification.

A conception of unity, the conception of a uniform world, which regarded all things as united as if by a magic chain, was applied even to the off-shoots and details of scientific and experimental research, where its stimulating influence is apparent. The picture of unity is more clearly defined in the writings of Paracelsus than in those of his followers, where it is partly concealed by the quantity of the recently acquired empirical material. Once again the XVIIth century shows us in the writings of Robert Fludd an attempt to describe the world as a mystical unity. His work is an irregular mixture of theological parables, directly applied to the explanation of natural processes, of cosmic metaphysics, on which are based chemical and physical hypotheses, and finally, of purely mechanistic descriptions of physiological and pathological processes modelled on the study of physics.

Although there are certain judicious statements betraying considerable medical experience, as well as a description of a cleverly contrived instrument, something between a thermometer and barometer, the preponderance of the imaginary explanations and an overdone conception of uniformity in the world make it evident that the

optimum et perfectum est genus sciendi," because God reveals his will in nature (*Lil. med.*, V, 12). Forty years ago Jul. Leop. Pagel, in the introduction of his " edit. princ." of the *Areolae of Johannes de St. Amand* (Berlin, Reimer, 1893, p. xi), pointed out Gordonius' attitude of independence, especially in his treatise on the " Theriac," and later on his opposition to an uncritical imitation of authorities (Pagel, J. L., *Die Concordanciae des Johannes de Sancto Amando,* Berlin, 1894, p. xi). Bernhard of Gordon, in his treatise on " Theriac," quotes the doctrine of Averroës, previously mentioned on the " Proprietas " (syn. with " Tota species," " Forma substantiae," " Virtus orbis." Ed. princ. by J. L. Pagel, *Pharmazeutische Post,* Wien, XXVII, 205, 1894, p. 259).

value of Fludd's work to the progress of science is to be estimated as slight and in no way to be compared with that of Helmont.

While the works of Fludd are unproductive of discoveries, they form a profitable study insofar as they reveal the stimulus given by the contemporary view of the world to research in medical biology. Indeed, it is probable that the religious basis of experimental research has nowhere found such lucid expression as here. The examination of Fludd's biology is also instructive on account of the remarkable similarity of his ideas to those of the biology of the so-called romantic period which reflects an important current of thought at the beginning of the XIXth century.

The study of Fludd appears to be an excellent starting point for the discussion of the question as to whether romantic medicine represents a body of opinions of independent growth, with its own methods, investigations and solution of problems, or whether it is merely the attempt of a fanciful generation to resolve the ancient problem of the unity of the world, spirit and matter by the employment of the method approved since the age of Neoplatonism or even more ancient times, that of unlimited speculation.[2]

The lifetime of Fludd[3] (1574 to 1637) almost coincides with that of Harvey, Bacon, Rubens, Kepler, and van Helmont. Like the last, he is called "per ignem philosophus" and like him, too, he belonged to a family of some importance, his father being Sir Thomas Fludd, Paymaster to the Forces in France and the Netherlands during the reign of Queen Elizabeth. Fludd studied in Oxford (St. John's), after which he travelled extensively on the continent, where he became acquainted with the works of Paracelsus. In this again he may be compared with van Helmont, whom disgust with his scholastic education and a thirst for new realities drove forth into the world, to follow Paracelsus. About 1604, Fludd returned to England, took his medical degree at Oxford in 1605,

[2] See Diepgen, P., "Alte und neue Romantik in der Medizin," *Klinische Wochenschrift*, 1932, p. 28, and "Virchow und die Romantik" (review of Pagel's "Virchow und die Grundlagen der Medizin des XX. Jahrhunderts"), *Dtsche. mediz. Wochschr.*, 1932, pp. 1256/58.

[3] See on Fludd: Craven, F. B., *Rob. Fludd, the English Rosicrucian*, 1902. Further, A. E. Waite, *Rosicrucians, loc. cit.*, S. 274. See further, Gassendi, *Epistolica dissertatio in qua praecipua principia philosophiae R. Fluddi deteguntur*, 1631. — Marin Mersenne, *Correspondance*, ed. P. Tannery, I, 1617-27 (Paris, 1932).

was admitted as Fellow of the Royal College of Physicians in 1609, and set up a practice in London. In 1616 appeared his first defence of the Rosicrucians, and a year later the theological and philosophical pamphlet on " Life and Death and Resurrection," under the pseudonym of Rudolf Ocreb. The end of the second decade of the XVIIth century witnessed the publication of his more important writings, polemics against Kepler, Mersennus and Gassendi. His collected works appeared in six volumes at Oppenheim in 1638. The church of Bearsted in Kent contains his monument.

Although in education and early life he has much in common with Helmont, unlike the latter, in his more mature work he appears to be interested not so much in laboratory experiments as in the practice of medicine. A study of his writings with the view of obtaining some idea of this practice, leads to the conclusion that it was essentially astrological, uromantical and theosophical. In accordance with his fundamental opinion, prognostication from the constellations of the stars plays a conspicuous part. Actually it is this astrology which leads to the incorporation of the old humoralistic doctrines in his system of medicine, which is but the construction of a biology and pathology out of the comparison of macrocosm and microcosm, a comparison which he industriously works out in great detail.

All this clearly distinguishes him from Helmont, whose life work was so important in the evolution of natural science. But Fludd, from his own tenets has elaborated *one* particular part of the work of Paracelsus, and that alone should ensure for him the interest of the historian. Moreover, he is a fertile source of information on the contemporary conception of the world, and the ideas current and possible in his time. Our description of his doctrines follows in essentials his *Medicina catholica.*[4]

The absolute unity of the world in God is the foundation of Fludd's system. God clearly appears as the chief chemist with nature as His laboratory. The truly wise man daily observes the work of His creative word, which, partaking of the nature of light, bestows origin and forms in the heart of the elements. It works " conveniente arte spagyrica." Thus our chemistry is simply an imitation of

[4] Francofurti, 1629.

divine creation in nature. Chemistry is both the search for God and the vision of God. It is " philosophia naturalis " and therefore theology. In the destruction of the specific individual form resulting in the general higher form it represents union with God.

Therefore true practical theology is nothing but mystical chemistry which furthers our attempts to uncover the divine light for our own benefit. The study of nature is the " mons rationalis " leading to paradise. Its aim is not the making of gold, but the cognition of things as realities, and of the truth. This rests with God alone as the true " perfectio." But since there is nothing in nature which He is not, a knowledge of nature leads to His truth. It is our right and duty to investigate nature, because His justice and truth exist on account of our justice and truth. " My truth will make known your eternal truth."

Access to nature is given by simple experience, which recognizes the healing power in the organs of the body (e. g., of pulverized skull bones) and demonstrates that by means of great concentration things may be perceived happening at the most distant places, two ideas of epoch-making importance, subjects of systematic dispute.[5]

This mystical view of the world which denies the importance of reason, accepts a pseudo-rational element in biology and medicine by the employment of astrological and mathematical deductions. If all being is dependent upon matter receiving form, the number three is of peculiar importance. It is the " principium formarum." Two lines make neither form nor figure. Therefore the triangle is the basic figure which cannot be resolved into other figures. Three is the number of the Godhead, consisting of God the Father, the " causa efficiens," the representative of matter containing the potentia of formation, God the Son, the " causa exemplaris," the representative of sapienta, the origin of forms by virtue of logos and idea, and finally the Holy Ghost, the " causa finalis " and " conservans," the representative of goodness. Hence the number three is nearest to the essence of God and therefore to perfection. It permits man to approach God's infinity, and, as the result of its most wonderful and secret truth, it conveys (" insinuat ") into

[5] Compare the account of the contemporaneous quarrel " de magnetica vulnerum curatione," Pagel, *van Helmont, loc. cit.*, p. 96 ff.

things the cause and principle of universality, which is absolute unity incompatible with diversity. On these theories is erected an arithmetic complete to the last detail of prognostication, which forms the principal part of the medical section of his work.

If the world is a unity and God infinite, Fludd is equally justified in having taken the stars and their courses as the measure of all "sublunary" things, and in having employed the principles of mechanics in order to provide a uniform explanation of natural processes including biology and pathology. Hence Fludd's neoplatonic mysticism finally resolves itself into a *simple mechanistic view.*

God influences things by means of his instruments, the angels, the essence of whose activity is the "Jesus spiritualis," the eternal wisdom which distributes forms and ideas, and is identical with the glory of the emanation of the eternal light. One of the most important of the angels, according to cabalistic tradition which Fludd accepts, is Michael, who commands the winds.

As mediators between God and nature ("virtus media") the angels perform all operations inaccessible to human reason which are the effects of the "proprietas occulta" in the things.

Matter is derived from the primary element, water. This hypothesis is based on the biblical story of the creation, and corresponds to the theory of van Helmont, etc.[6]

But matter never is the first cause. It obeys the word of God borne by the winds. These are the *causes* to which the student of nature must penetrate. The various winds are derived from the various characteristics of God, thus the east wind is "ex parte clementiae et miserationis," the north, "ex parte iudicii et severitatis," and in accordance with their origin is the result of their influence and their commands.

But the action of the winds on matter is not direct. As a rule they make use of special "Principes elementorum," immanent in elementary matter, i. e. demons, which, aided by the wind, change the air "in suam naturam." This is in accordance with the belief, common to all mysticism, that material changes are due to the trans-

[6] Compare Joel, *loc. cit.*, p. 56, who points out the agreement of all mystic cosmologies, especially those of the presocratic thinkers (Thales), with regard to the importance of water.

formation of matter by a dynamic principle into something resembling itself.

Fludd's demons are nothing more than the elements of the ancients which, without examination, he accepts with all the characteristics attributed to them since antiquity. The only difference is their spiritualization, which is achieved by the simple device of personification with the object of depriving matter of its preëminence: accordingly, Samuel is the spirit of fire, Azazel, of moist air, Mahazael, of earth, and Azael, of water.

Man was in absolute unity with the Divine until the fall of Adam. Adam was able to comprehend the essential nature of all things. The Fall was in the sphere of the number two. This was the beginning of all polarity and all extremes, such as light and darkness, activity and gravity.

Polarity conduces to the maintenance of stability in the sphere of comparable things, which, according to the well-known tradition from St. Augustine and the Areopagite until Kues, are equal in the infinity of God.

The doctrine of polarity is the source of our knowledge of the parallelism existing between *mac*rocosm and *mic*rocosm and decisive for all natural processes. Thus it is the basis of the whole of natural science.[7] Such universal analogies are

Heat-Movement-Light-Dilatation-Attenuation
Cold-Inertia-Darkness-Contraction-Inspissation

Sun-Father-Heart-Right Eye-Visus-Sanguis vitalis
Moon-Mother-Uterus-Left Eye-Mucus.[8]

As a result of the emphasis of the absolute unity of the world in God and this legitimate parallelism, in spite of his belief in the essential spirituality of things, Fludd arrives at a universally applicable mechanistic explanation. Therefore, his view of the world, which is a religious monism, a kind of philosophy of identity, gives

[7] See Giordano Bruno, *Della caus. princ. et uno*, transl. Seliger (Leipzig, 1910), p. 191. Whoever wishes to investigate the deepest secrets of nature, might observe the " Maxima et minima " by means of comparison with the opposite and contradicting entities. It is a profound magic to be able to produce the opposite after having discovered the point of conjunction.

[8] Compare Ptolemaios, *Tetrabibl.*, III, 11.

rise to a purely mechanistic theory, which itself is based on a uniform principle.

This principle is that of expansion and contraction. Since it is the key to the explanation of the world, Fludd calls it "Universale naturae in raro et denso mysterium."[9] The knowledge of this is derived from experiment, a "speculum experimentale," from which Fludd has deduced the general laws governing the behaviour of all natural objects, and has come to the conclusion that the activity of even the smallest atom is comparable with the activity of God.

The universal instrument demonstrating this mysterium is something between a thermometer and barometer to which we have already referred.[9a] It consists of a trough filled with water in which stands an inverted air-filled retort. The neck of the retort, which is immersed in the water, has graduated markings. When the globular end of the retort is warmed, the air within expands and displaces the water in a downward direction. The amount of this displacement can be read from the graduated marks on the neck. Conversely, the action of cold causes the water to rise.

The world of matter which we observe by the aid of this instrument, whether expanded or contracted, is always the same. Cold and heat are not differences, but merely degrees of a single quality. The

[9] Compare Fr. Bacon, *Hist. de ventis, loc. cit.*, p. 114: Historia densi et rari. Because the sum of matter always remains the same the expansion and contraction of the bodies is of greatest importance in order to avoid a vacuum. "Cum igitur sit res (si qua alia) *plane fundamentalis et catholica . . .*" Similarly according to Joseph Needham, *Chemical Embryology* (Cambridge, 1931), I, p. 130. Sir Kenelm Digby refutes all qualities and "faculties" in biology and like Galileo and Hobbes refers to a universal explanation of *two* virtues only, those of *rarity* and *density* which work by means of local motion. "Two treatises, in the one of which the Nature of the Bodies, in the other the Nature of Man's soul is looked into: in way of discovery of the Immortality of Reasonable souls." (London: Williams, 1663), p. 253. Compare Telesius, *De rerum natura juxta propria principia*, Prooem. I, 1 ff., and III, 34: "All natural effects are to be derived from heat and cold; their continual combat causes the different degrees of contraction and expansion by means of which matter appears."

[9a] The instrument described resembles Galileo's thermometer, the invention of which goes back to 1602. See J. J. Fahie, *The scientific works of Galileo.* Ch. Singer's *Stud. Hist. Meth. Science*, II, 1922, p. 219: "It was in truth a barometer as well as a thermometer, although Galileo did not recognize this." Compare the similar instrument constructed by van Helmont, and described in his treatise "Aer" 12.

air within the retort is not subjected to attraction in the sense of Aristotle; but there is active expansion and contraction of this active, because spiritual, element. Hence, even the great natural phenomena like wind, clouds and rain, are to be explained as the result of evaporation and condensation and not as the result of an attraction of the rarefied parts of water and air by heat, as Aristotle assumed. For the task of heat is not attraction but rather "pellere et propulsare." But if everything in the world occurs only on account of the evaporation and condensation of ever constant matter, there must be absolute conservation of matter. Therefore, there is no destruction.

The whole of Fludd's natural science and pathology is permeated by the ancient doctrines of the elements and humours which he actually accepts in their entirety and elaborates to the last detail. He even adheres to the belief of the ancients in the transformations of the same matter. Nevertheless, he emphatically states his fundamental *opposition to antiquity*. The ancients have missed the real causes, observing in their elements and humours only secondary causes. These correspond to the dead instruments used by the living winds as composers. According to Moses and Hermes, his most important sources of knowledge, everything consists of one thing only: water. Cold, heat, moisture, dryness are not qualities immanent in things; they are contained by the essence of the momentarily active angels, whose manifestation, as we have seen, is immediately dependent upon the divine influence.

With reference to individual points, Fludd is mainly concerned in refuting the ancient doctrines of crisis and pulse. The first is the result of inaccurate empiricism ("sine ulla ratione radicali"). Its chief error lies in the lack of consideration given to the true movements of the stars, the knowledge of which, derived from new charts of constellations, has made possible an entirely new system of prognostication.

Therefore Fludd is far removed from the decided rejection of the ancients, characteristic of Paracelsus and van Helmont, even though he, also, imagines himself as the creator of entirely new principles and the discoverer of the true cause of things.

Fludd's biology is based upon the hypothesis that life signifies participation in the world of ideas and forms, that is, in the universal soul. Life is therefore endowment with the specific function — species — and the faculty of reproducing this species. That the universal soul, in this sense, actually does exist, and that everything in reality is filled with God and ideas are proved by the fact of spontaneous generation, which refutes those who, like Fludd's opponent Mersennus, deny the existence of the universal soul.

Man, as a microcosm, contains within himself all parts of the macrocosm. Hence in him there are all stages of transition from matter to spirit. Since the world forms a ladder of the emanations of the Divine Being, life and soul in the human body are the rays of a higher sphere than the elementary sphere it contains, and these rays are the origin of the functions. Like the world, the body can be divided into an upper, middle and lower region. In the upper region predominates the superior, that is, the finest corporeal element, fire.

The middle region of the body, wherein heat and moisture prevail, corresponds to the element air, while the lower region producing chylus in the stomach, blood in the liver, and urine in the kidneys, corresponds to the element water. The more closely woven the tissues of the organs, the denser the spiritus which they produce. The spleen and the intestines excrete a pitch-like substance, the heart, the vital and almost invisible spiritus which is diffused by means of the arterial blood; the brain, the usually invisible rays resembling light.

The unity of the soul maintains harmony in this body, protecting it from diabolical duality, and therefore disintegration. Harmony expresses itself in the form of the metrical laws of music.

Just as the ancient elements play an important part in the whole of Fludd's philosophy, his biology is also based on the doctrine of complexion. From this the principal element of an individual body may be determined, and hence the constellation decisive for the individual. The close connection of the whole of Fludd's system with astrology demands such a study of temperaments and complexions. The predominance of black bile directs the attention to Mars, and the appropriate therapy in disease has to obviate the influence of this planet. Hence suitable medicinal herbs must be collected at the time when Mars in on the wane.

On the principle of his universal instrument, the thermo-barometer already described, Fludd explains temperament as the result of primary alteration in the temperature of the body. If this rises, the air in the body expands causing the movement of the

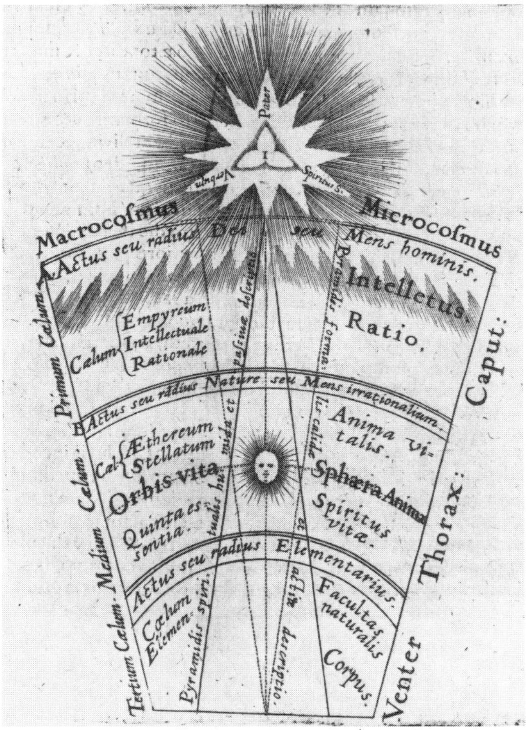


CORRESPONDENCE BETWEEN THE REGIONS OF THE BODY AND THE WORLD

From Fludd's *Medicina Catholica*

Compare the pictures in Charles Singer, "The scientific views and visions of Saint Hildegard," *Stud. Hist. Meth. Science,* I, 1917, p. 43.

humours. Then the relatively thin humor, black bile, predominates, giving rise to anger, heat, liveliness, nimbleness, fantasy, wakefulness. As an equator denotes, in the model, the balance of heat and cold, so, in the microcosm, it indicates the balance of bile and mucus. Therefore, there are only two temperaments, which are distinguishable according to the rise above or fall below the equator. Thus, also, according to the standard of the instrument, there are only two diseases of the body as well as of the soul. The deviations *above* the equator, denoting condensation of the air and the rise of the water,

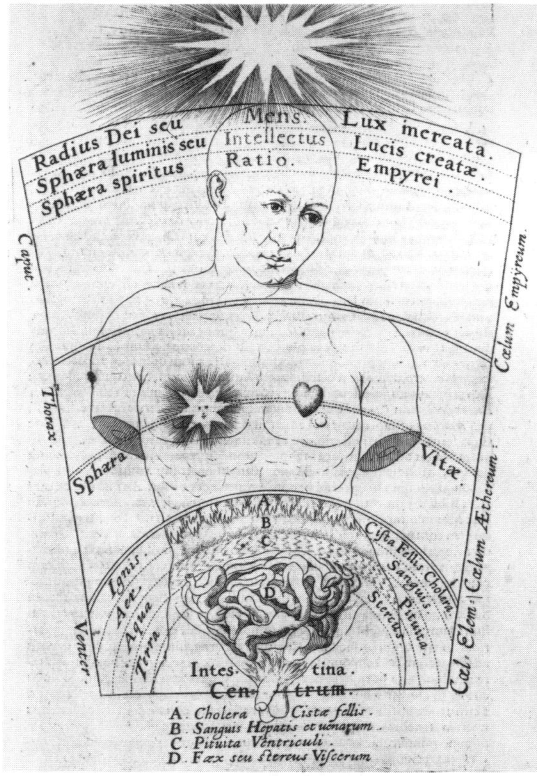


CORRESPONDENCE BETWEEN THE INDIVIDUAL ORGANS AND THEIR FUNCTIONS AND THE PARTS OF THE WORLD

From Fludd's *Medicina Catholica*

correspond to the predominance of mucus, which gives rise to epilepsy and all kinds of paralysis. The deviations *below* bring in their train bilious complaints and abnormal heat, of which inflammations, erysipelas, gangrene, pleurisy, are the signs. Fury and fear are the corresponding extremes in the spiritual sphere. Health consists " in temperamenti iustitia vel pondere." It embraces all vital functions in as far as they can be implied by "iustitia et perfectio." Disease signifies all manifestations of the vital functions when they are checked in their activity, removed from "Perfectio," or in any way debilitated or diminished.

The principle of polarity also explains the physiology of the pulse and the circulation of the blood. Expansion and contraction of the heart, as well as the parallel functions of inspiration and expiration, are manifestations of the polarity of the vital spirit causing function. And ultimately even these polarized fundamental functions are traceable to the contradiction between heat and cold. To the cold breath of the spiritus there is a corresponding contraction of the air, a rise of the water in the thermometer and systole of the heart, while conversely we find expansion and diastole. The normal pulse follows the laws of harmony in music, while the abnormal pulse, like all sickness, is dependent upon the influence of disease-bearing winds. If the east wind is the cause of the abnormal rise of temperature, the pluse is broader and palpable to four fingers. The pulse varies according to the phases of the disease and the corruption engendered by the heat of its cause in the part of the bodily substance which this attracts. The riper the pus, the calmer the pulse — a purely humoralistic and galenic theory which Fludd explains diffusely. The hard pulse is due to the north wind, which condenses fluids so that water hardens into snow and hail. Such a pulse we find in the tartaric diseases of Paracelsus, wherein the organs contain solid deposits representing the true anatomical change.

The result of this generally symbolical and analogical point of view is Fludd's definite acceptance of the new theory of the circulation of the blood. Like the world in its orbit, the blood circulates in its vessels, obeying the systole and diastole with a movement resembling the ebb and flood of the tide.

Such considerations confirm, according to Fludd, "exacte" (sic) the "sententia et opinio" of his friend, colleague and compatriot, Harvey, who was well versed not only in anatomy, but also in the deepest mysteries of philosophy. The theory which he demonstrates "consulte et prudenter . . . cum rationibus a philosophiae arca depromptis, tum multiformi demonstratione oculari " is that the movement of the blood is circular. How could it be otherwise, since it is absolutely certain that the spirit of life retains an impression both of the planetary system and of the zodiac? Thus, as the moon follows her unchanging path completing her journey in a month, she incites the spirit of the blood, and therefore the blood itself, by virtue of its " astra imperceptibilia," to follow in a cyclical movement. Every seaman is acquainted with the influence of the moon on wind and tide. Why should she not exercise a similar influence on the " microcosm " of man?

Like his biology Fludd's pathology is a strange mixture of humoralistic doctrines with ontological and aetiological ideas. As has already been shown, Paracelsus developed the ontological conception of disease by means of which he ousted the ancient humoralism. The new estimation of the external causes of disease and its localization in different organs caused a revolution in the ideas on the subject. Disease came to be regarded not merely as the one pathological condition [10] recognized by antiquity, varying on account of the differences of the properties of the individual organism involved, its mixture of humours, its temper and constitution, but as numerous pathological conditions all differing and classifiable according to their diverse causes and their respective seats. Fludd's medicine, which pretends to be a " medicina catholica," combines both points of view. Adhering to the ontological doctrine, he maintains that the cause of disease represents the essence of disease, and taking into consideration both the ancient belief in the influence of harmful exhalations (*Galen*) and the emphasis laid by *Paracelsus* on the importance of an aerial chaos of finest corporality, he decides that the causes of disease must be the *winds*.

In accord with these conceptions of Paracelsus, Fludd assumes the existence in the atmospheric chaos of " spiritus mali " and invisible seeds (" Seminaria invisibilia ") which penetrate into the body through the lungs and through the pores of the skin. Individually they partake of the characteristics of fire, earth, or moisture. In this idea we perceive the return of the ancient humoralism as an

[10] See my *J. B. van Helmont*, p. 112 ff.

essential constituent of Fludd's system, by which he is to be distinguished from Helmont. Moisture causes infections such as plague, measles, small pox and phthisis. Atmospheric substances with the properties of earth cause melancholy, stupor, as well as chronic infections, such as leprosy, scabies. Moist substances origi-

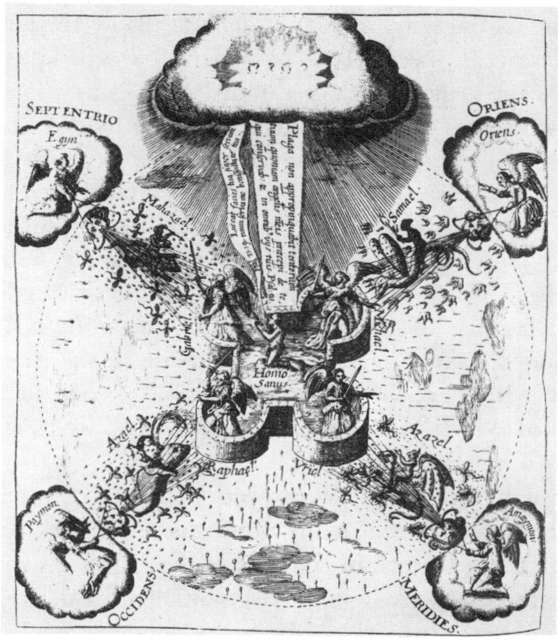


THE "HOMO SANUS" PROTECTED BY THE ANGELS FROM THE WINDS WHO, USING DEMONS AS MESSENGERS, SEND THE CAUSES OF DISEASES

From Fludd's *Medicina Catholica*

nate conditions like apoplexy and epilepsy. These causes of diseases are personified as the demons Samael (fire), Azael (moisture), Mahazel (earth) and Azazel (water), who make use of the winds in order to approach their object, the human body. Wind is, in this sense, the corporeal basis of all activity and new creation derived from the Logos. The winds are in the custody of the angels who may hold them fast or set them free. Thus the origin and development of disease are closely connected with the activity of the Deity. On the other hand, God does not create disease any more than the blacksmith, when modelling iron, creates the rust; disease is a mere by-product of creation, " consequitur creatum."

The pathological process originates in the condensation of air to a humour in the body. This humour influences either the blood or the flesh, just as the wind affects either the sea or the land.

Fludd illustrates the process by means of a simple mechanical device. A basin is horizontally divided by means of a diaphragm pierced in two places. Sand is poured through one of the holes with the result that the air, thus expelled from the lower part of the basin, escapes through the second hole. This air, having been dried by the passage of the sand, has properties resembling those of the north wind, for it is the north wind which conveys air with earth-like characteristics. When the north wind prevails, drought and cold predominate because of the addition of earth to the air. The same principle applied to man signifies that the air in the intestine comes into contact with particles of earth derived from the spleen, the tumefaction of which causes the earth-saturated air to rise, and this is the origin of melancholy.

By a similar mechanical construction Fludd demonstrates the development of catarrh and many other diseases. The different diseases are attributed to certain changes in the humours, caused by the prevailing winds. Leprosy and elephantiasis, which, judging by their external appearance, depend upon a condensation of humours, are ascribed to the congealing influence of the *north* wind. In accordance with this theory the *east* wind has a stimulating effect on bile and its corrosive properties. Thus acute inflammations such as dysentery, pleurisy, pneumonia, herpes and acute bilious complaints are some of the effects of the east wind.

Fludd has associated this doctrine of the causes of disease with the hypothesis of the decisive influence of the stars on men. Immediately subjected to the stars is a " Sal volatile " which is present in the air, and, according to the doctrine of Hippocrates and Galen, is attracted to the heart and brain, wherein it maintains the spark of life, this is the immediate seat of the human soul, as well as of the soul of the world, of which the former is only a part and emanation.

Thus it is a " Sal catholicum." All motion, whether in the macrocosm or in the microcosm, in air, sea, or earth, depends on the behaviour of this substance. The motility of the blood is due to its presence. In the human organism excessive expansion or commotion of the sal produces sweat and fever. Since the movements of the sal depend upon the will of God, fever must be regarded as a Divine message. The sal in the body undergoes innumerable changes. It is excreted as an ammoniacal earth salt in the urine, and, as such, is also obtainable from the bones, flesh, and blood. It decides the nature and properties of the urine. If it has a tendency to expand and to extend its own property of dilatation to other substances, the urine is darker in color. If it has a tendency to contract, the urine is paler.

This idea of the " sal volatile " as the origin of all motion apparently differs from Helmont's doctrine of the " Blas " [11] only in so far as it contains the suggestion of a material basis.

Fludd's *therapy* is the outcome of his firm belief in astrology which makes possible, on the one hand, a pedantic prophylaxis, and, on the other, a choice of remedies in accordance with the ascendant constellation. The general principle employed is that of " Contraria contrariis." The cause of disease brought by the wind " A " must be combated by remedies which have the properties belonging to the wind " B." Fludd, especially when confuting his rival Mersennus, points out that therapy is a part of magic.

Fludd's prognostication and semiology are an elaborate arithmetical mysticism, which is too complicated for further description.[12]

Fludd's system is, according to his own claim, a " Medicina catholica." In fact it embraces all conceptions of disease possible during his time: humoralistic and ontological theories, iatrochemical and iatromechanical designs, religious and metaphysical, as well as physical, chemical, and purely biological elements. By means of a dexterous employment of the analogies existing between macrocosm and microcosm, Fludd subordinates the heterogeneous elements of the philosophical notion of uniformity to the universale mysterium

[11] See my *J. B. van Helmont, loc. cit.*, p. 67.

[12] Compare the connection of arithmetical with geometrical and astrological mysticism in John Dee's *Hieroglyphica ad Maximilianum regem* (Francof., 1591).

which he sees in the faculty of the universal soul to expand and contract.

In Fludd's system, almost the whole of the ancient tradition of analogies in macrocosm and man is restored, which, according to the studies of Charles Singer,[12a] is expounded in the anthropology of Hildegard of Bingen and can be traced to the old Iranian cosmological physiology (Liebeschuetz). The " Kosmos-mensch " and the analogies of the regions of the human body with the parts of the whole world are the corner-stone of Fludd's system, as man is the centre of Hildegard's vision of the cosmos. The peculiar proportions of the man in the centre of the world, whose span is equal to his height, because the length and the width of the heavens are equal, are reconsidered by Fludd and illustrated by a special picture. Fludd's accentuation of the winds as the power governing the movement of the world and the stars, according to Liebeschuetz, is also derived from an Iranian or Hermetic source.[13]

The main features recognizable in Fludd's philosophy are:

(1) The adoption of the then " modern " ontological idea of disease. Disease is the " meteoron morbosum," that is, the morbid influence from without, which is closely connected with astral influences and the climatic effect of air and wind (" Meteoron ").[14]

(2) The inclusion of the whole humoralistic ideology as a dogmatic fundament of his system.

(3) The invention of various mechanical models to illustrate the mutual displacements occurring among the elements under the influence of a " sal volatile " which is inhaled and induces motion.

[12a] " The scientific views and visions of Saint Hildegard," *Studies in the History and Method of Science*, I, 1917, 1-55, espec. p. 43 (comparison of Hildegard's and Fludd's pictures).

[13] Liebeschuetz, H., " Das allegorische Weltbild der hl. Hildegard von Bingen," *Stud. d. Biblioth. Warburg*, XVI (Leipzig u. Berlin, Teubner, 1930), pp. 86 ff., 81 ff., 12 ff. L. refers to the paper of A. Goetz, " Persische Weisheit in griechischem Gewande," *Zeitschr. Indologie u. Iranistik*, II, 1923, 60, 167 ff.; Mich. Scotus, the Hermetic Asclepios and Ptolemaios. On the medieval tradition of the doctrine of the power of the winds (Isidorus, etc.) see Singer, *loc. cit.*

[14] " Quod iuxta intentionem nostram non sit inter meteoron insalubre et morbum discrimen." *Med. cathol., loc. cit.*, II, p. 76.

Thus Fludd pursues the method of analogy even in the details of his mechanistic explanation of the life process.

(4) The association of religious ideas with the mechanistic explanation of natural processes typical of the period of Baroque is demonstrated by such a figment of the imagination as " the winds,

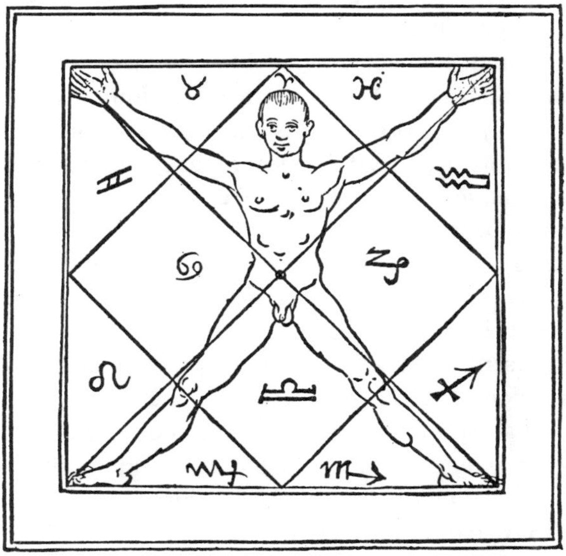

THE " KOSMOSMENSCH " IN THE CENTRE OF THE WORLD WITH HIS PECULIAR PROPORTIONS

(Span equal to height)

From Fludd's *Medicina Catholica*

Compare the graphic tradition of such " Melothesiai " in Ch. Singer's " The scientific views and visions of Saint Hildegard," *Stud. Hist. a. Meth. Science*, I, 1917, p. 43.

as the messengers of God, govern the air and influence its behaviour by transferring to it the commune mysterium of expansion and contraction."

(5) Finally, an essential feature of his doctrine is the purely cabalistic mysticism of numbers which culminates in his prognostication, his diagnosis from the difference of the strata of the urine in a glass, his doctrine of pulse and fever, and his therapy.

The study of Fludd's works immediately suggests a comparison with those of his contemporary Helmont. Both make use of analogies, but while this method of research with Fludd results in mere fantasy,[15] it has led Helmont to an extraordinarily well-founded vitalism which approaches reality. Both uphold the ontological conception of disease, the dogmatic entities of Fludd's system, the *winds,* being represented in Helmont's biology by the *gases,* which he discovered and connected with the doctrine of the contagium. While Fludd accepts the humoralism of antiquity without reservation, Helmont rejects both this doctrine and the ancient assumption that heat and moisture are the origin of life, demonstrating the vital functions as chemical processes. Therefore the comparison of these two authors appears to emphasize the achievements of Helmont showing that Fludd's doctrine deserves an historical interest only, because it reveals most clearly the religious ideas which inspired a mechanistic explanation of life and disease. Such an estimation is based upon present day standards and is unjustifiable from a historical point of view. Fludd and Helmont are products of the same epoch in the history of the human mind, and each has constructed a natural science which is subordinated to religion, the one more in the direction of the pantheism of the Renaissance, the other showing the tendencies of Christian mysticism.

Fludd and Helmont were children of the XVIIth century, the " reign of law " (Ch. Singer).[16] Therefore the idea of the harmony of the world, and the law of equality which governs it, finds its echo in their works. There are conceptions drawn from civil and legal affairs which both authors transfer to the sound and the sick organism. In the writings of Fludd, especially, such analogies are emphasized. " Justitia " is his expression for the " Perfectio " which is represented in the combination of the material (materia potentialis) with the ideal (lux formalis), a combination which is also a fundamental principle in Helmont's conception of the world. The " temperies vitae," that is to say, normal life, is destroyed, if the laws of divine justice, as represented by the harmonies in living

[15] Reasonable sentences such as: " In paralysi solent medici periti febrem martialem incitare " are rare.

[16] Singer, Ch., *A Short History of Medicine* (Oxford, 1928), p. 135.

beings, are violated. The "imperium" of health is disturbed and civil war (bellum intestinum) breaks out. During the time of peace, maintained by the physiological processes, concordia unifies the members of the body; if this harmony is absent, the autonomy of the body is unsettled by internal warfare and altercation "ita ut omnis iustitia ab illa oeconomia excludetur." Disturbance of this "Ligamentum pacis" in the body is an expression of a disturbance of the "nexus amoris antiquissimi" by which God, Logos and all creation are united.

The harmony of the body is the basis of its functions which originate in its anatomy, its "ratio constitutionis." It is the injustice of our sins which causes the disorder and strife, the injustice of our internal economy. Therefore disease is identical with uncleanness, sin, injustice. Like a judge in a court of justice, God decides on the critical days the life or death of the patient. "Ablato peccato," a paralytic recovered immediately.

Thus there is a "mysterium dierum criticorum." The number seven (= 3 plus 4) indicates the abolition of contradictions, being the expression of a combat between cleanness and uncleanness, light and darkness, beauty and ugliness, corpulence and emaciation, good and evil, life and death.

The crisis signifies the expulsion of the enemy from the invaded country. Similarly Avicenna has referred to the crisis as "separatio litigantium."

Like a regent, the beam of God in the seed governs the creation of the new organism.

The examples of such analogies taken from the civil and legal life could be increased. Their employment, which we also find in the writings of Marcus Marci, seems to be a typical feature of the biology of the period. According to Helmont the vegetative impulses derived from the centre of the organism have the same influence on the organs as the "nutus potestativus" of a guardian on his ward. They are not transmitted by material processes [17] and are like the command of an absolute dictator. Thus every effect due to any archeus is a "*potestas*." Disease is a "potestas peregrina" which is

[17] See van Helmont's treatise, *Ignota actio regiminis* and my *J. B. van Helmont, loc. cit.*, p. 68 ff.

foreign to the aims of the organism and therefore noxious. It subordinates the archeus of the organism to its own rule, forcing it to suffer war in its own country.[18] Similarly, according to Marci, the archeus of the body is subjected by the sting of the tarantula " alienis legibus."

Fludd's whole doctrine depends upon the fundamental conception of unity in the world. Thus the construction of analogies is his general method and his source of knowledge. It is the same sequence of ideas which characterizes the philosophy and biology of the romantic movement in the early 19th. century. This sees all things in the world, both corporeal and spiritual, as different aspects of the same unity. Spirit is but the highest degree of development in nature by means of which nature recognizes herself. Therefore, by its own method of speculation, spirit is enabled to apprehend natural processes in their true essence. The vision of parallelism and analogies in nature and in spiritual life is the paramount method of attaining to natural science. The idea of polarity and the deduction of all processes from one principle, that of the reconciliation of fundamental contradictions, such as light and heaviness, are the basis of this natural philosophy.[19] Contemporaneous experiences are combined with the construction of analogies to form a medicine or biology similar to that of the " Medicina catholica " of Fludd. As a matter of fact sentences taken from J. W. Ritter's Fragments,[20] which are definitely typical of the romantic movement, could be mistaken for excerpts from Fludd. E. G. " According to heat △ equal to force of expansion and cold ▽ equal to force of attraction, the limitation of both, matter, could be signified by ✡.[21] " Water is the chemical octave, the tones of which are the primary elements, and the chemical combinations of which are the accords.[22] " In order to produce substances, the contradictions must be restored, e. g. that

[18] Helmont, *Ortus imaginis morbosae,* 2, and my *J. B. van Helmont, loc. cit.*, p. 91.

[19] Compare my *Virchow und die Grundlagen der Medizin des XIX. Jahrhunderts* (Jena, Fischer, 1931), p. 10.

[20] *Fragmente aus dem Nachlass eines jungen Physikers. Ein Taschenbuch für Freunde der Natur* (Heidelberg, 1810). I am greatly indebted to Professor Martin Buber for having made me acquainted with Ritter and his work.

[21] Ritter, p. 33, No. 48.

[22] P. 39, No. 65.

of the sexes to the time in history when he, when she, really originated in the development of the world. It is a real cancellation of time, or, a putting back of the clock, and every organic creation is due to such a process. Nature is constantly referring to the time of creation. The higher the development, the further she has to go back." [23] "Every formation is due to polarity in space." [24] "Everything is a degree of a great scale: atmosphere — the world of plants — the world of animals — inanimate nature." [25] "Each drop of rain is a world, the dew contains many planets, the air is a sea full of celestial and terrestrial bodies." [26] "All force originates in polarity. Just as the sum of the living forces remains the same, the sum of living polarities does not change." [27] "Not history of physics but history *equal* to physics equal to history." [28] "The age of things seems to be expressed by their ability to be extended. Metals are very difficult to extend and they extend homogeneously. They are the oldest entities in the world. Then come salts, water, air, vapor. The last contains the force of youth, the first the rigidity of age." [29] "All individuals in nature are mediums of refraction for all beams of the universe. In man the beams of God are refracted, they are broken up, their colours being the harmonic interplay of his thoughts. It may be said that some thoughts originate in rays with a rectilinear course and that others are due to deflected rays. The heart is the rectilinear beam of God to man. The true man is the heart, because all the external world is refracted here. Life is a play of colors. Man should not take any color singly, when all are combined the complete picture of God is produced in him, as it appears in love, which is but the joy, love experiences in itself." [30] "Light is a contagium, it 'infects' space and space becomes light. Light is the highest organization with the lowest individualization." [31] "Tones originate in vibrations which return in equal units of time. Half the number of vibrations in the same time produce a tone an octave lower. Finally, there appear vibrations which last a day, a year, a life-time. We ourselves, and plants and animals, and, indeed, all life, may be comprised by such tones. Tone and life here

[23] No. 70.
[24] No. 76.
[25] No. 78.
[26] No. 83 B.
[27] No. 88.
[28] No. 170.
[29] No. 225.
[30] No. 256.
[31] No. 272.

become unity. In the future it will be of greatest interest to know the relation between the tone produced in the body by swallowing, the pulse, etc., or Volta's column and those large fundamental tones, or any one of them. The string of this fundamental tone will be the earth, whose density and velocity will determine the physical properties of the tone. This music might be heard as harmony only in the sun. The sun, like the whole planetary system, is a musical instrument." [32]

These examples from one typical exponent of the whole movement are sufficient to demonstrate the similarities in the fundamental view. It is the same method of finding analogies between all things and all forces in the world, which about 1820, as well as two hundred years before, in the writings of the followers of Paracelsus, forms the basis of natural science. How far the similarity goes, is demonstrated especially by the importance assigned to light and its beams, and their relation to man. It is the same fundamental conception which is elaborated by Marcus Marci in his speculative embryology. But the phenomena can be equally well observed as particular relations of tones and harmonies or as electric and magnetic phenomena. In this way Fludd endeavoured to work out from a knowledge of harmony the principles underlying the explanation of the similarities in macrocosmic and microcosmic phenomena. This parallelism between romantic natural philosophy and the mysticism of the XVIth and XVIIth centuries, as well as the ancient stoic and neo-platonic doctrines, is so obvious that it is recognized by the epoch of natural philosophy itself. Bouterwek observed the analogies and found the origin of this " materialization of reason and intellectualization of nature " in Aristotle's doctrine of the soul.[33] But Aristotle was a sober thinker, and it was not before his natural metaphysics was altered in Alexandria and by the Arabs (Abu Tschafar Ebn Tofail) that the vision of the absolute was connected with a state

[32] No. 360. Compare Novalis, who, in his " Fragments " applies the laws of harmony to the human body (*Schriften*, ed. Tieck and Schlegel, 4. edit., Berlin, 1826, II, p. 125). " Every disease is a musical problem, recovery a musical resolution; the shorter and more complete the resolution, the greater the skill of the physician."

[33] " Erinnerung an die Naturphilosophie einiger Arzte, Kabbalisten und Rosenkreuzer aus den vorigen Jahrhunderten," *Neues Museum der Philos. literat.*, 3, 3 (Leipzig, 1805).

of ecstasy, in which were realized the relation of the human soul to the stars, the identity of the Ego, as the recognizing subject, with the recognized object, and the power of recognition. Unity was seen in multiplicity, the individual was united with God. Bouterwek also referred to the correspondence between this doctrine and the doctrine of the soul of the world outlined by Averroës, the hylozoism and pantheism of Cesalpino, a follower of Aristotle, the metaphysics of light imagined by Patritius, the conception of Paracelsus and the sense of reality of this "kraeftigen Schweizers." Finally the philosophy of Leibniz is also said to have developed into pantheism and a doctrine of emanation because of the deduction of nature from absolute unity and the cancellation of the dualism of reason and nature. Fludd is mentioned as the forerunner of the idealists of the early XIXth century, because he differentiates between the forces of expansion and contraction and even goes so far as to call expansion the south and contraction the north of the universal.

The relations of romantic natural philosophy to Paracelsus and van Helmont are also shown by the renewed interest in these two authors.[34] J. M. Leupoldt,[35] one of the last exponents of natural philosophy, in his appreciation of Paracelsus and Helmont, expresses the opinion that it is unwise to deprecate doctrines only because they belong to the past. Their doctrine was, in their time, a just as necessary and natural expression of the inquiring human mind as any other, such as sophism, scholasticism and mathematical deduction, etc.

The romantic natural philosophy of the early XIXth century and the religious natural speculation in the XVIIth century have in common not only the general tendencies regarding the conception of the world and nature, but also the doctrine of normal and pathological life. Although the speculation on a special force of life as the distinguishing characteristic of living beings belongs to the romantic era, the same era is also marked by an equally strong distaste for such speculation. The origin of the reluctance to predicate a special

[34] See Lessing, Mich. Ben., *Paracelsus: Sein Leben und Denken* (Berlin: Reimer, 1839); Preu, Th., *Paracelsus* (Leipzig, 1838); Sudhoff, "Paracelsus-Bibliographie," *Acta Paracelsica*, I (München, 1930).

[35] *Die alte Lehre von den Lebensgeistern* (Berlin u. Leipzig, 1824).

force of life is to be found in a disinclination to interrupt the vision of nature as a *unit* by the introduction of a peculiar force in living entities. Thus Goethe sees the disappearance of the contradiction between the organic and the inorganic in a vision of a " Natura naturans " which is recreated in the mind. The creations of this nature are not fundamentally different from the act of spiritual knowledge. Nature in this sense " knows by magic." [36] Similarly, our knowledge of natural processes is identical with the production of the natural phenomena themselves. It is in this sense that Novalis declares: " All experience is magic and can only be explained by magic. Empiricism ends in a unique idea. . . . The active use of the organs is nothing but a magic mode of thinking which performs miracles, or an arbitrary use of the corporeal world; just as will is nothing but the vigorous magic power of thinking. The " physical magus " knows how to animate nature and to treat her arbitrarily as his body." [37]

As long as we lack valid proof that forces other than chemical forces act on the living body we are not justified in assuming new forces. (Ritter,[38]) It is the specific gravity of an organ which, according to Ritter, determines the quality and intensity of the vital functions. The higher the specific gravity of an organ, such as bones and nails, the slower the vital processes. If, supposes Ritter, referring to Kant, the decomposition of water is the vehicle of psychical activity, and the fundamental forces of life are included in water in a state of rest, it is possible that the Ego in its life activity acts upon the force of the decomposition of water.[39] Fr. von Baader also regards fluid as the basis of life. Fluid is the endowment of every living being as its innermost-heart of the heart, brain of the brain — animating the body, which otherwise is only a skeleton.[40] Accordingly Ritter considers the expression of the highest vitality as that with the lowest degree of cohesion, because this has to overcome the least individuality. The gases are nearest to

[36] See Hoffmeister, J., *Goethe und der Deutsche Idealismus. Einführung in Hegels Realphilosophie* (Leipzig: Meiner, 1932), pp. 35, 37, 9, 36.

[37] *Schriften*, ed. by Tieck and Schlegel, 4. Aufl (Berlin, 1826), II, p. 107.

[38] *Loc. cit.*, No. 393.

[39] *Loc. cit.*, No. 406.

[40] *Beitr. z. Elementarphysiologie* (Hamburg, 1797), p. 47 ff.

infinity, and volatile substances are the bases of life processes in animals and plants.[41] Accordingly, the psychical influences on the body are compared with the effects of poison, e. g. in Novalis' fragments.[42] " The soul is among the poisons the strongest. It is the most permeable and diffusible irritation; all psychical influences in local diseases and inflammations are therefore harmful." Similarly S. T. Coleridge [43] assumed latent life in all the organic world. This life is of low intensity, the inorganic world is asleep, dreaming, but not yet dead. Life means law of action, unity in multiplicity.

Romantic natural philosophy recognizes that matter and force are inseparable. If reason separates matter and force, the result is disintegration of the living organic being.[44] Force is a mere abstraction of reason without independent existence. On the other hand, the extreme materialistic view must be avoided which, e. g., supposes a fluid within the nerves, etc. (*Leupoldt.*)

Here we find relapses into archaic materialism which, in biology, had already been overcome by van Helmont. It was he who energetically rejected the theory of the origin of life in humid substances.[45]

Therefore romantic natural philosophy embraces two distinct doctrines: vitalism and materialism associated with pantheism.

The existence of *disease,* however, cannot be explained either by a *dynamic* or by a *materialistic* conception, for it is inherent in the solid, fluid and volatile parts, each of which can be the basis of pathological changes. But if life is derived from polarity, disease is a necessary consequence. In a state of perfect health life is impossible, because perfect health would be absolute unity, comparable with nothing, unlimited, and ideal activity alone.[46] Therefore one might die of excessive health, and life always requires a little illness. The same idea is similarly expressed by Novalis in his " Fragments ":

[41] *Loc. cit.,* No. 417.

[42] *Loc. cit.,* p. 125.

[43] *The Theory of Life* (1848). See Needham, " S. T. Coleridge as a Philosophical Biologist," *The Scept. Biol., loc. cit.,* p. 160.

[44] Leupoldt, *loc. cit.,* p. 130.

[45] His treatise " Humidum radicale," *passim.* See my *Helmont, Leibniz, Stahl, loc. cit.,* p. 21.

[46] Ritter, No. 407, *loc. cit.*

" The ideal of perfect health is of interest from a scientific point of view only. Disease is inseparably connected with individualization. The same is true for the human mind as for the doryphorus or the canon in art. It is by diseases that men are distinguished from animals and plants. . . . Perishableness and fragility are characters of nature combined with mind. They witness the activity and universality, the sublime personality of mind." [47] According to Fludd's doctrine, also, disease and health are opposite poles necessary for each other. Fludd symbolizes the conception of polarity by the image of God's face being turned towards or away from mankind.

Certain remarks of Ritter [48] recall Marcus Marci's comparison of life with a flame and his differentiation of diseases according to the disturbance in the movements of the flame or in the intensity of its heat: " Should not all diseases be divided into such as originate (a) in a deficiency of oxygen in relation to the amount of matter to be oxydized, (b) in the deficiency of matter to be oxydized and an excess of oxygen, (c) in excess of both, (d) in a deficiency of both." [49]

Finally, there are parallelisms between the ontological conception of diseases assumed by Paracelsus [50] and van Helmont, and partially supported by Fludd, and the theories maintained by romantic authors. Some of these are well known, especially the parasitological theory of diseases enunciated by the school of Jahn, Stark, and Schoenlein. According to the teaching of these physicians, disease is an entity which penetrates the body like a parasite and can be detected in the pathological changes. Like the patient himself disease lives as an individual autonomic being. Since disease is a living agent, it is subjected to the universal laws of the macrocosm and the microcosm. It is in this sense that we must regard the subordination of disease to the universal laws when our romantic natural philosopher Ritter gives expression to the opinion: " Epidemic diseases appear to break out especially in spring. Being animals, they revive at this time like all other organisms. Infection

[47] *Loc. cit.*, p. 123.

[48] 450.

[49] See chapter IV on Marci; compare Novalis' " Fragments," p. 119, *loc. cit.*, " Sollte Denken oxydieren, Empfinden desoxydieren? "

[50] Compare Mich. Bened., *Lessing*, *loc. cit.*, p. 118.

should be considered as a process of reproduction and the disease itself as the young. Some of these unions may remain unproductive and it is necessary to investigate how the sterility in any particular disease is connected with the general fertility." [51]

Such a statement might have been made by Paracelsus, for it was he who imagined disease as being born in the body,[52] as the result of an invading entity or a spiritual force which, through all transitions, is connected with the contagium, a thing of finest corporality.

Thus the parallelism between romantic biology and medicine and the natural philosophy of Paracelsus and his followers is both apparent and impressive. In order to make this clear quotations have been given above from the works of K. W. Ritter. The same conceptions are found in the writings of the majority of the biological philosophers in the period of romanticism. As far as the doctrines of life force and the conception of force and matter in general are concerned, reference may be made to my discussion on the parallelism between romantic natural philosophy and the ideology of Rudolph Virchow.[53] In this I endeavoured to show that according to the expositions of Hartmann, Reil, Burdach, Treviranus, Troxler, the romantic doctrine did not in the least accept the naïve theories of a special life force equivalent to other chemical or physical forces; the old conception of life force, which may be called ontological, is superseded by a critical estimation of living beings, the peculiar structure and mixture of which is the cause of the peculiar functions of life. It was especially the vision of the world and man as unity, fundamental to natural philosophy, which forbade the separation and isolation of living beings.

This all seems to justify the denial of a peculiar character to the romantic movement in the early XIXth century, and to exhibit it as merely a repetition of the tendency, typical of mankind and reappearing in all periods, to explain nature by means of speculation and analogies — no matter whether this occurs in Greek antiquity, during the Renaissance, in the XIXth century, or at the present day. In so far as the early XIXth century has produced a valid biological doctrine, it is said not to be " romantic," and in so far as it is said to be romantic, that is, devoted to speculation and

[51] *Loc. cit.*, 452. [52] Mich. Bened., *Lessing*, *loc. cit.*, p. 118. [53] *Loc. cit.*

phantasy, it is said not to have produced a valid biology.[54] According to this criterion, therefore, the speculative aspect of the period is separated from the scientific, so that it is necessary to consider each author (such as Reil, Purkinje, etc.) in different lights, and to differentiate in his scientific production entirely different phases.[55]

But even the study of romantic thought in the XVIIth century justifies an estimate of the romantic natural philosophy of the XIXth century as a movement with its own problems and solutions of problems. The very fact that it is sufficient to choose one author in order to explain the typical mode of thought of the period demonstrates that we are dealing with a peculiar movement differentiated from its predecessors and successors. No matter whether we examine enthusiastic natures such as Novalis, Baader, Kieser, Troxler, J W. Ritter, or more sober investigators such as Reil, Hartmann, Steffen, Purkinje, always the same ideology, even the same terminology recurs. It is, therefore, impossible to exclude certain individual authors from the movement on the grounds of the comparative exactitude of their expositions, which can be accepted even today. The similarities existing between all these authors and their conceptions result from the fact that the same subjects and the same theories continually reappear in the writings of both categories of biologists, the sober investigators, and the fanciful enthusiasts.

Some of the fundamental conceptions, continually reiterated in the romantic natural philosophy, are identical with those of Fludd and other followers of Paracelsus. But there is more similarity in the mode of thought derived from the use of analogies between macrocosm and microcosm, conceptions like polarity, the combination of speculation with empirical research, the careful observation

[54] Diepgen, "Virchow und die Romantik," *Dtsche. mediz. Wochschr.*, LVIII, 1932, pp. 1256-58. Compare my review on this paper in *Mitteilungen Gesch. Mediz. u. Naturwiss.*, 1933, Vol. XXXII, p. 42.

[55] S. Bettmann in a delightful address to the Heidelberg Medizinisch naturwissenschaftlichem Verein (February, 1933), gave a splendid account of *Purkinje* with special reference to the relations of his scientific work to the romantic ideas of his youth and old age. There are the same relations which I have had already noted between romantic philosophy and the scientific work of Virchow (*loc. cit.*), especially in the stress he laid on physiology. I regret very much that Bettmann's lecture has not been published.

of psychical influences on corporeal processes, the ultimate identification of body and soul, than in the real subject-matter and the results of research. The two hundred years between 1600 and 1800 witnessed a great number of discoveries and new ideas which were reflected in romantic natural philosophy. The influence of Haller and Stahl on contemporary trends of thought is sufficiently evident. Physiology, which is the center of romantic biology, is a science in no way foreshadowed by Fludd and the other Paracelsists, with the possible exception of Helmont. It is only necessary to compare the writings of Burdach or the romantic conceptions of Purkinje with those of Fludd, in order to demonstrate the fundamental difference between them.

The estimation of nature as a unity was the same in the early XIXth as in the XVIIth century. But how different are the conclusions drawn from this monadic conception! In the romantic period, spirit and nature are but different stages in the development of the uniform substance of the world, a development from lower to higher degrees. In that speculative basis originates a particular interest in all organic processes, an interest which gives impulse to the study of embryology. As a matter of fact, modern embryology is based upon the naturalistic speculation of the early XIXth century. Important results of empirical research, e. g., Oken's discovery of the identity of the vitelline sac in birds with the umbilical vesicle in mammals, and the communication of the vitaline sac with the abdominal cavity are to be found in the midst of speculations which remind us very much of Fludd. According to some hypotheses every animal consists of two animals, the one governed by the brain and the other by the genital system. These opposite animals have one neutral point in common, the umbilical cord.[56] On the other hand, the so-called "fundamental biogenetic law," according to which the history of the germ repeats the history of the tribe, is foreshadowed by Kielmeyer,[57] Ennemoser,[58] Sal. Levy Steinheim,[59]

[56] See Nordenskjöld, E., *Geschichte der Biologie*. Deutsche Uebersetzung (Jena: Fischer, 1926).

[57] Buttersack, "Karl Friedrich Kielmeyer. Ein vergessenes Genie," *Arch. Gesch. Med.*, XXIII, 3, 1930, p. 236.

[58] Bremm, Jac., *Der Tiroler Joseph Ennemoser* (1787-1854). Ein Lehrer des tierischen Magnetismus und vergessener Vorkämpfer des Entwickelungsgedankens in der Medizin (Jena: Fischer, 1930).

[59] Pagel, Julius, Salomo Levy Steinheim, *Janus*, VIII, 1903, pp. 233, 286.

in their speculative estimation of the conception of development. It is the natural philosopher, K. E. von Baer,[60] who corrects such notions, teaching that there is a biogenetic law only in so far as there is a greater similarity among the embryos of organisms than among their adult forms.

Whereas embryology is based on the general speculative vision of processes of development in the whole history of the world, comparative anatomy originates in the deliberate observation of the analogies and parallelisms in the cosmos. This science is derived from the conception of fundamental types, which are in connection with the so-called " Urphaenomene," such as Goethe imagines in the magnet, in light, and in the grain of seed, etc.

In that sense, Cuvier's doctrine of types, which rejects all transitions between the types and all speculation concerning them, as well as Geoffrey St. Hilaire's comparative anatomy, which is based on the assumption of one fundamental type, is an offspring of the romantic period. Finally, there are the genuinely romantic ideas of the progressive development from lower to higher stages which lead Lamarck to the establishment of modern theories on the origin of species.

In the doctrine of diseases it is the speculative notion of life which provides the groundwork for the knowledge that during disease the same vital processes are present as in normal life, and that disease is life under changed conditions. This law is absolutely fundamental for the whole of romantic biology, the centre of which is "*physiology*." It reappears in the writings of almost every representative of this era, e. g., as Jul. Pagel demonstrated in 1903 — in the writings of Sal. Levy Steinheim,[61] of Reil, Burdach, Hartmann,[62] and the representatives of the natural-historical school.[63]

Romantic medicine, therefore, has obtained its peculiar character through its entanglement with the peculiar aims and the state of knowledge in the early XIXth century. One may object to the term " Romanticism " as the designation of these trends of thought, because romantic speculation is ubiquitous and, in every age, has

[60] See Nordenskjöld, *loc. cit.*

[61] *Loc. cit.*

[62] See my " Virchow," *loc. cit.*, p. 15.

[63] Diepgen, *Deutsche Medizin vor 100 Jahren. Ein Beitrag zur Geschichte der Romantik* (Freiburg und Leipzig, 1923).

produced its own peculiar ideas in medicine and biology as well as in other branches of science. The extent to which the method of analogies is employed is shown by the example of Fludd and his " Mysterium " of polarity.

The romanticism of the XIXth century has also a strongly developed connection with religion. It may be sufficient to refer to the names of Joh. Nepomuk Ringseis and Heinroth and their religious pathology which regards sin as the cause of disease.

But the natural philosophy of the early XIXth century marks a particular period because of its close connection with the scientific biology and medicine of the second half of the XIXth and XXth centuries of which it is the philosophical basis. In the foundation of modern embryology, comparative anatomy and morphology in general, as well as in the cultivation of the physiological aspects, it propounds and resolves its own problems.

## VI

Mankind eagerly seeks after knowledge. Man devours knowledge like food whenever it is offered to him. But a very short time elapses before he vomits his indigestible fare. He seeks truth everywhere, but has never been able to give a sober and valid judgment on things.

Thus in the past the sceptic has always found himself in an isolated position; if he wished to proceed he had to begin from the very beginning, by doubting all statements about things and by investigating the things themselves, for this is the straight road to knowledge. But the more he pondered the more he must doubt; and this doubt finally led him to despair.

Nevertheless even then he adhered to his propositions. He applied to the scientists and obtained nothing but imaginary constructions, no knowledge of " Res naturales." By such fictitious tissues spirit can never be satisfied. Who can learn to understand that which does not exist, such as the atoms of Democritos, the ideas of Plato, the numbers of Pythagoras, the " Universalia " of Aristotle, his " Intellectus agens " and his " intelligentiae "?

Aristotle may have had his merits as an acute and ingenious observer within the narrow frontiers of human intellect. But did he really grasp the universal and nature in the fullness of her powers? Did he indeed never make any mistakes? Did he actually know everything and demonstrate everything without doubt and contradiction? Did he really never evade difficulties and problems? It is sufficient to remember that he was a man like ourselves.

But should we epigons, conscious of human and, therefore, our own weakness, disparage the efforts of these heroes of knowledge?

There is one way out of the dilemma. It must be admitted that we are able only to fight for truth, never to attain it, and even if we could attain it we should never be able to hold it.

Nothing can be achieved by logic. Vain is the knowledge gained from syllogisms. Knowledge is not an accumulation of facts in the mind, but if it were obtainable, it would be an internal conception of unity, that is to say, philosophy. Such philosophy would be withdrawn from the relativity of sensual, especially optical, perception. Such philosophy would be able to apprehend not only the outlines of things but also their true essence. Hitherto nobody has been able to attain to this knowledge. Everything beyond the senses is confused, veiled in doubt and darkness. But even in the senses there is no power of recognition (" Sensus non cognoscit ").

How could such power exist? Everything is in a state of continual flux. Innumerable are the changes occurring between dawn and sunset. With reason it has been said that no hour leaves man unaltered. The identity of a thing does not permit the addition or subtraction of even a single particle.

There are only two ways which can lead poor mankind to the knowledge of things unrecognizable " per se," that is, experiment and critical examination. Each is dependent on the other, neither can exist without the other. But even these parts do not lead to real knowledge, because experiment is fallacious and difficult, and even when incontestable, shows only the exterior of the process and never the " naturae rerum." This also applies to human judgment, because we are able to judge only what has been demonstrated by experiment. As far as the nature of the thing itself is concerned, there remains nothing but conjecture which so often has been proved erroneous.

Nevertheless, experiment has its value, for it leads to the collection of experiences which can never be achieved by deduction alone.

Thus, according to experience and experiment antidotes are mixed and their effects proved again and again in the individual case. That which seems logically rational is very often proved to be contrary to truth. By mere deliberation nobody would conclude that hemlock mixed with wine causes death more rapidly and more easily in men with warm and bilious temperament, than in those with cold complexion.

Experience therefore makes a wise and prudent man.

By means of such arguments the physician Francesco Sanchez demonstrates a scepticism [1] which appears to be entirely emancipated from religion, an attitude which results in an abolition of religious and metaphysical feeling in the mode of thought of the "Renaissancemensch." [2] It takes the form of a pessimistic resignation which finally arrives at the recommendation of experience as comparatively the most reliable source of knowledge. This scepticism does not give birth to the strongly imperative impulse to natural research which was actuated by the religious view of Paracelsus and his followers, because the latter enjoyed the illusion that they could apprehend the real essence of things through their conception of the world and their mystical union with God. Such human achievement, however, is emphatically denied by Sanchez. It is no more than a figure of speech when Sanchez occasionally introduces the will of God as the first cause of the long life of plants and refers to God's omnipotence as identical with the order in nature, its necessity and fatalism. Such things are withdrawn from our knowledge. We can only investigate the second, that is to say, the natural causes which are the outcome of the effects of the former. Among such natural causes Sanchez, in his doctrine of the duration of life, pays special attention to the ancient dogmas of humoralism and qualities. His work is nothing but a philosophical essay, unconnected with any achievement in biology.

Similarly emancipated from religion and mysticism is the point of view of the priest Mersennus.[3] By virtue of the establishment

[1] "Tractatus philosophici quod nihil scitur; de divinatione per somnum ad Aristotelem," in *Libros Aristot. Physiognomicon comment., de longitudine et brevitate vitae* (Roterod, 1649).

[2] See Dilthey, *loc. cit.*, p. 36.

[3] Mersenne, Marin, *La vérité des sciences contre les septiques ou Pyrrhoniens*

of a new idea of rational science he refutes both the sceptic and the religious alchemist. In a discussion on the truth of science he introduces himself as the Christian philosopher in argument with the Pyrrhonian sceptic and the alchemist. The Christian philosopher deprecates the expression of doubt in all science as well as the connection of science and knowledge with faith and mysticism.

The *alchemist* defends his own knowledge as being the most secure, because obtained by experience, which he calls: " La mère, la source et la cause universelle de toutes les sciences." It is the lack of experience which causes the errors and failures of the Aristotelian system. Whenever Aristotle did not investigate the things themselves he substituted imagination for knowledge. Thus he made nothing but negative statements on nature. Moreover, his intellectual honesty is open to criticism.

On the other hand the *Christian philosopher* emphasizes the fact that the doctrines of Aristotle even today represent that system which most nearly approaches the truth. There is no doubt that Aristotle makes some mistakes, such as his faith in the finiteness of the world, the origin of the veins in the heart instead of in the liver, and so forth. But, in general his views are well founded, and, within the confines of human knowledge, are the best imaginable. The principles of Aristotle are " intellectuel et raisonable." This is the ideal of the priest and mathematician Mersennus.

The alchemist who desires to go further than the rough empiricism dealing with external appearances only, must also take the Aristotelian conceptions into account. Even the finest elixir of the alchemist is finally nothing but a combination of a " forma " with " materia," and the physician has to assume these principles when he wants to explain his operations and the efficacy of his remedies. The sum of the experimental knowledge of Aristotle may have been less than that of the alchemists of today, but as far as the principles of science are concerned the greater experience of the latter does not enable him to proceed any further than the former whose experiences were of a nature so simple as to be easily attainable by every man without danger to his eyes, his time or his means.[4]

(Paris, 1625). For Mersenne see: Tannery, P., *La correspondance on Mar. Mers., publ. et annot.*, Corn. de Waard., I, 1617-1627 (Paris, Beauchesne, 1932).

[4] " Des examples familiaires qu'un chacun peut voir et experimenter sans perdre les yieux, le temps et l'argent par la fumée des charbons et des fourneaux."

If, however, alchemy is really such a sober experimental science as the alchemist maintains, why then those strange analogies of macrocosm with microcosm, why that mysterious comparison of chemical processes with those which have occurred during the creation of the world and the resurrection of Christ? Why quote the Scriptures in order to explain the chemistry of mercury, the acids, and gold? Why refer to mythical beings, figures such as Demogorgo and Pan, Saturn who devoured his own children, Jason and Medea, and at the same time pretend to remain a true Catholic? Solemn declarations of faith in God and mystical utterances are employed in the writings of many alchemists only in order to hide their lack of knowledge. Capable alchemists scorn such poor fools who, while pretending to be enlightened by God, sell their ignorance as science and truth. God save us from such people who desire to change heaven and earth in order to fill their own pockets at the expense of those who cannot detect their errors!

Why does the alchemist keep his doctrines secret? Perhaps he desires to conceal the large amounts of silver he spoils or perhaps he wishes to have the advantage of the rest of mankind. It would be much better if, instead of enjoying the magical effects of light obtained by occult methods and by pure accident, he and his kind would build up their wisdom into a reliable science, founding chemical academies whose presidents should ensure that chemistry becomes a science methodically applied for the benefit of the human race. Charlatans must be punished and excluded from that noble work, and the barbaric and dark expressions must be abandoned.

Here the *sceptic* interrupts the discussion remarking that the extraordinary knowledge of nature which the alchemists assume cannot be obtained by natural means,[5] because the alchemists have frequently betrayed the greatest ignorance in the world. Their doctrine concerning the seed of all things, the peculiar virtue inherent in things, the life of the metals and their purification and transformation into elixirs by means of fire are mere dreams. As a matter of fact, the world consists of a small number of simple

[5] Compare this sceptic point of view of alchemy with that of the official jesuit doctrine of del Rio, etc., and Freitag (mentioned previously), according to which the effects obtained by the alchemists are not entirely denied, but the aid of demons and the devil is supposed. See my *J. B. van Helmont, loc. cit.*, p. 96 ff.

elements, the different combinations of which are the cause of all diversity.

The *alchemist* replies that the secret mysteries of the alchemists have nothing to do with an intercourse with the devil, against whom they use the weapons of the Catholic Church, such as prayer, the Eucharist, and the Holy Cross. The secrets of the alchemists, obtained hourly by experience, can explain nature better than all the wisdom derived from the syllogisms of Aristotle, which are fed by the experiences of natural research. The alchemist is ready at any time to forsake a doctrine if convinced by experience of the contrary. There is nothing in the aims of the alchemists which is opposed to the dogmas of the Catholic Church, when they try to discern the part played by the soul of the world in everything, representing it as a volatile salt. Therefore it is not the composition but the effect of things which matters.

True alchemists recognize the excellence of the doctrine of Aristotle, especially his theory of motion, the denial of which would be equivalent to the denial of daylight at noon. Aristotle *himself*, in his paper called "Magisterium," made use of the analogy between macrocosm and microcosm, calling alchemy a "lower astronomy." He compared chemical substances with the fixed stars, and Thomas Aquinas assures us that he has obtained the indestructible essential of the four elements.

The *Christian philosopher*, however, denies the authenticity of the documents mentioned. The author of the Aristotelian book is a Christian believing in the Biblical account of the creation of the world, about which Aristotle knew nothing. Furthermore, there is no tradition to the effect that the Doctor Angelicus "se soit amusé à ces opinions du fourneau." The alchemists are accustomed to ascribe new ideas to ancient sages such as Adam, Abraham, Moses, Esra, and Hermes.

These extreme points of view, that of the sceptic who denies the possibility of knowing anything, and that of the alchemist who feigns an acquaintance not only with the exterior of things but also with their true essence, are repudiated by the Christian philosopher. Sense perception has its own department. Each sense has its own object in reality. Human thought, which arranges and makes use of the sensual impressions, is not deceived, since it originates in the divine light, the cause of the creation. This arouses in us meditation, exercise, experience, science. None of these can attain to anything without divine grace. Supernatural light increases the very narrow beam of our natural light to the knowledge of the divine being ("In lumine tuo videbimus lumen").

Therefore reason is the measure of truth; truth itself the judge of our thought. Thought corrects its own errors, when truth reveals the fallacy of the orignal conceptions. In a problem the truth is nothing but "la conformité de ce qui est proposé avec l'entendement."

The importance of reason is evident particularly from the part played by mathematics in all sciences and all points of view. To the alchemists, who so often refer to the mysticism of numbers, it is mathematics which teaches the harmonic proportion which God has implanted in His works. We perceive in ourselves the harmony of the four humours, when they compose the "temper of justice." As health is the result of the preservation of the harmonic proportions of the elements of the body, so this principle is observed by the wise governor of such a state as the French monarchy. Therefore it is important to know the harmonic proportions of our humours. Some physicians maintain that these are 1:2:4:8, which means that one part of black bile corresponds to two parts of yellow bile to four parts of phlegm to eight parts of blood.

Thus the discussion of Mersennus with the alchemist and the sceptic leads to the confirmation of reason as the absolutely necessary basis of all science, in contradistinction to the opinion of the alchemist, and to the recognition of the possibility of man's attainment to the truth as opposed to the arguments of the sceptic.

Man's reason is part of the reason of God, and, like everything in nature, is created by God. Science cannot possibly be built up of rough empiricism alone — notwithstanding the great importance of the experimental results of alchemy which are capable of forming the foundations of a science. For Mersenne Reason is discursive thinking by means of the categories of Aristotelian logic — not "reason" ("Ratio") in the sense of the general "Logos," which is innate in man as instinct, as is representative of the universal consensus in nature. This type of reason forms the basis, also of the

" religion of reason " in the stoic doctrine of *Herbert of Cherbury*, who is evidently influenced by Paracelsus and his " archeus." [6] Mersennus represents the viewpoint of the orthodox theology, which affirms reason and science, not that of Christian mysticism which denies both. It is characteristic that in medical biology he recommends mathematical deductions and returns to the ancient humoralism.

Like Mersennus, Francis Bacon separates religion from science.[7] He deprecates the construction of worlds and systems of philosophy from a small number of experiments in alchemy and physics. Free speculation and the construction of worlds, according to Bacon, is sin, and the outcome of a lack of reverence such as we find not only in ancient authors but also in Patritius, Telesius, Campanella, Paracelsus, and the alchemists. Instead of making careful investigation of the " seals " of the Creator, these philosophers have pondered on the " seals " of their own imagination. Instead of statements, hypotheses are made, experience is suppressed, man has triumphed over the works of God in his aspiration to be similar to God and to follow the commands of his own reason.[8] It is not the fire of the alchemists but the divine fire of human reason, which, in the realm of nature, has " to solve and to separate " skilfully in order to attain to positive results. Hence we must not rely upon miracles or natural magic which, like a soporific remedy, transports men into the realm of dreams and, by the fabrication of occult virtues and proprieties, detains them from the investigation of the true causes and all the good and real things which God has proposed for human research.[9] Similarly the discussion of the final causes has prevented the investigation of the physical causes. Therefore mankind has been satisfied with obscure and fictitious causes instead

[6] See Cherbury (1581-1648) and the stoic origin of his doctrines: Dilthey, " Weltanschauung und Analyse des Menschen seit Renaissance und Reformation," *Ges. Schriften*, II, 3 Aufl. (Leipzig, 1923), p. 248 ff., 260 ff.

[7] *Nov. Organ.*, I, 54.

[8] *Hist. natur. et experim. de ventis* (Amstelod: Elzevir, 1662). Prooem. — *De augment. scient.*, IX.

[9] *Hist. de ventis*, p. 118; — *Nov. Organ.*, I, 64; alluding to the construction of worlds from the Bible by Fludd is due to a " corruptio philosophiae ex superstitione " and " pro peste intellectus habenda " like the Pythagorean mysticism of numbers. *Ibid.*, I, 65.

of the real and natural causes.[10] Nevertheless, as already mentioned, Bacon did not entirely deny the achievements of alchemy, and admits a certain number of "instantiae magicae," which are proved by experiment.[11] He acknowledges the principal substances, sulphur and mercury, as symbols of the consensus of things.[12] To a certain extent the specific virtues are real, they may or may not be called "occult." Although the alchemists do not always attain to their aim they very often achieve other considerable results.[13]

On the other hand, Bacon refutes energetically the subjection of natural science to reason and logic which is obvious in the philosophy of Aristotle, who has committed the same crime as the alchemists and other empiricists by building up systems and worlds from his particular point of view.

Thus between mere empiricism and scepticism Bacon, like Mersennus, endeavours to found a scientific natural philosophy, but he seems to be disinclined to concede to reason and Aristotelian logic the high position it has obtained in the philosophy of Mersenne.

The recognition of the specificity of a substance, its peculiar innate virtue inaccessible to reason, was the fundamental principle of alchemy and was closely connected with the peculiar religious speculation which we have discussed. It was no less important a person than Robert Boyle who, standing on the borderline between alchemy and scientific chemistry, made this question the subject of a theoretical essay.[14] His conclusion that the specific virtue of a

[10] *De augment. scient.*, 3, 14.

[11] *Ibid.*, p. 49.

[12] *Nov. Organ.*, II, 50.

[13] *Ibid.*, I, 5; I, 73; I, 85. See Bacon's position with regard to Paracelsus and alchemy: Fowler, *loc. cit.*, p. 26 ff., and *passim*; further, the polemics of A. Ross against Bacon: "Arcana microcosmi or the hidden secrets of man's body discovered in an anatomical duel between Aristotle and Galen . . . with a refutation of Dr. Browne's vulgar errors, the Lord Bacon's natural history and Dr. Harvey's book *De generatione*" (Comenius, etc.: London, 1652), p. 251: "God will have us in some things rather *admire* his wisdom, than *know* his secrets . . . who can give the reason of that sympathy between the load stone and the iron? We see, there is a sympathy between some simples and some humours and between some parts of our body and some drugs." See the position of medicine in Bacon's system: H. Minkowski, *Archiv Geschichte Medizin*, XXVII, 299, 1934.

[14] *Of the reconcileableness of specific medicines to the corpuscular philosophy to which is annexed a discourse about the advantages of the use of simple medicines* (London, 1685). On Boyle's attitude to alchemy, see his *Chymista Scepticus*

substance is open to an atomistic explanation is one of the steps leading chemistry from the stage of prescientific empiricism to science.

Boyle insists that there is a specificity of substances which is not a matter of sorcery, but a quality which renders the substance in which it occurs more efficacious than an ordinary remedy in some particular case. This peculiar virtue is something which cannot be referred to the degree of any well-known property such as coldness, bitterness, and so forth; nevertheless its existence is evident from idiosyncracies, experience of the poison of spiders, the efficacy of emulsions of scorpions in the case of scorpion bites, etc., and similar instances quoted by Boyle from the works of Galen. The poisoned arrow of the Indians demonstrates that the quantity of a substance does not matter. Helmont's observation that water, after brief contact with mercury, is fatal to worms, even when there is no perceptible change in the weight of the water, is well founded.

Boyle is not disinclined to admit that there are things in nature inexplicable to our limited intelligence. But the atomistic theory of corpuscles is so simple and obvious that it is tempting to apply it in explanation of the specific efficacy of substances.

The body is a machine so finely adjusted that the efficacy of a substance is often due not so much to the substance itself as to the influence of one part of the body on another. This explains the diversity of the effects of specific substances and their validity in different diseases.

The effect of a specific substance consists (1) in a solution of the matter causing disease in such a manner that it can be excreted. The specific substance influences this matter on account of the suitability of its corporeal elements which must be so small that they can easily penetrate into the matter.

All conclusions derived by reason from an estimation of the known qualities of a substance are wrong, e. g., strong oil of vitriol is stronger in taste and dissolves more substances than aqua fortis. Therefore it might be concluded that like the latter, it dissolves silver. This, however, is not the case.

(Roterod., 1668). Ed. Faerber in Ostwald's *Klassiker der Naturwissenschaften*, vol. CCXXIX, 1930; Rob. Boyle in Bugge's *Buch der grossen Chemiker*, I (Berlin, 1929), p. 173; Needham, Joseph, *The sceptical biologist, loc. cit., passim.*

In any mixture the specific substance detects the substance to which its virtue is adapted. In a mixture of bone ash, Crocus Martis, sawdust, powdered sea salt and gold dust, water dissolves the sea salt only, while mercury will affect nothing but the gold.

The discovery of the circulation of the blood demonstrated that things which have once penetrated into the blood stream, are rapidly whirled into the most remote parts of the body.

These arguments apply also to the scepticism which denies the efficacy of amulets because they come into contact with the surface of the body only. All things emit very fine corpuscles which can penetrate into the skin through the pores; in this case they have greater effect than when they penetrate by the longer route of digestion. Instead of going through the door of the stomach the substances make their way through the keyholes of the skin directly into the blood stream.

(2) The specific substance can operate by neutralizing acidity which, according to Helmont, is the cause of many diseases. This result can be obtained either by substances endowed with positive hostility to acidity, such as alkaline salts, or, as a knife loses its sharpness, an acid corpuscle may lose its "prickling and cutting" power "by having its figure spoiled" by the action of an alkali. In this way chalk destroys the acidity of aqua fortis.

(3) The specific substance may precipitate the pathogenic matter, or

(4) it may strengthen the heart and hence the part of the body affected.

It is wrong to deride the doctrine of sympathy between an inanimate remedy and the living organ. The peculiar structure of the organs — and it is probable that the fluids are similarly constructed — and the varying sizes and quality of the corpuscles of some of the remedies point to the existence of an affinity between certain substances and certain parts of the organism. By fitting into the pores of an organ such substances can strengthen it, that is, increase its tonus, thereby enabling it to get rid of harmful matter.

In this manner even the most incredible effects can be explained rationally, e. g., the cure of scrofulous tumors by the touch of a dead hand, a cure which has been ascribed to Helmont,[15] but which is really of earlier origin, or a handful of powdered skull bones as an antidote to nose bleeding, or the healing virtue of amulets, etc.

The scientist Boyle therefore explains the effects of magic operations and of specific substances in a scientific manner. He agrees with alchemists and mystics that there are effects due to antipathy and sympathy. Furthermore, he is ready to admit the impotence of human reason, but in the corpuscular theory he finds an alluring possibility of explaining occult things.

Like the mystic empiricist he, the scientist, deprecates[16] the application of the categories of Aristotelian scholasticism, such as "ideas," qualities, "substantial forms," to the doctrine of chemical substances. There are not any independently existing qualities. They are distinctions created by reason only in order to conceal self-contradictions. Definitions have no importance for the knowledge of matter and its qualities.

The quality of a thing depends upon its peculiar figure and size. Thus quality is not a specific entity separable from matter. The solubility of gold in aqua regis, but not in aqua fortis is due only to the special texture of the gold and not to any inherent peculiarity, nor does the gold of today differ from that of the time of Plinius because he was ignorant of this fact. Therefore "forma" and "species" are but the "peculiar manner of existence of a natural body, its specifical or denominated state, its essential modification, its stamp."

Thus there is no difference between natural substances and those produced artificially in vitro. God, who put matter in motion and established the laws of motion, is the first, though not the immediate cause of forms.

Boyle therefore agrees with the atomistic school in his theory that the world consists of innumerable individual corpuscles, and with Descartes in his belief that God is the origin of motion.

[15] Boyle appreciates Helmont in general as an ingenious and reliable investigator, except with regard to his treatise on the magnetic cure of wounds, which Helmont's friends maintain to have been published by his enemies. *Sceptical Chymist*, Everyman's Library, p. 51.

[16] The origin of forms and qualities (according to the corpuscular philosophy); illustrated by considerations and experiments. 2nd ed. (Oxford, 1667).

But Boyle expresses disagreement with the atomists when they deny God as the creator of the world, and from Descartes when the latter accepts God as the origin of motion in matter but not as the creator of the individual things.

Accordingly, Boyle affirms the existence of specific aims in nature as revealed by the number, form, quality, situation and type of motion of the celestial bodies, and the coöperation of the parts of the animals and plants for the benefit of the whole organism.[17] To Boyle, Descartes' God seems to be too much subjected to the iron laws of matter, according to which the quantity of motion is never changed. He cannot understand why God should not pursue certain aims and thus demonstrate a change in His way of acting in natural things. Why should His unalterability be violated if occasionally He alters the quantity of motion which He has put into the world. Man is inclined to draw anthropocentric and geocentric conclusions. In spite of that, there is no reason to deny that he may be one of the causes why the beams of the celestial bodies are sent to earth. The eye of the fly and the structure of the muscle are the most striking examples of teleology in nature. To imagine a knowledge of all the purposes of God is arrogance, but to know some of them is no "presumption, rather it is a duty to take notice of them." Not teleology, but accident, is a product of human reason, because everything that happens is subjected to the fixed laws of the activity and passivity of matter. It is on account of our ignorance that we cannot recognize the true coherence.

Physiology, without the investigation of causes, would be useless, but a careful study of the causes cannot prejudice the observation of purposes. In regard to the latter it is necessary to avoid haste in drawing conclusions and in making too many affirmations. Much cannot be recognized in its purposes at this time. Asclepiades would have declared the valves of the veins useless. Harvey, according to a personal communication to Boyle, was led to his discovery by the reflection "that so provident a cause as nature had not so plac'd many valves without design." [18]

[17] *A disquisition about the final causes of natural things wherein it is inquired whether and (if at all) with what cautions a Naturalist should admit them* (London, 1688).

[18] This reminds us of the opposite views in philosophy of Harvey and Fr. Bacon,

The recognition of purposes is the form in which the religious conception derived from Paracelsus is adopted and cultivated by science — as Boyle's example shows. Joseph Needham was right to emphasize the importance of the " causa finalis " in the biological ideas of the XVIIth century.[19] The " causa finalis " is the most prominent of the Aristotelian conceptions, when the conflict begins between the new " experimental " science and the philosophy of the schoolmen.

This is the sense of the passage from Sir Thomas Browne's " Religio medici " to which Needham is referring. " Every essence created or not hath its final cause, and some positive end both of its essence and operation. This is the cause I grope after in the works of Nature; on this hangs the providence of God." [20] Browne regards Galen's treatise " De usu partium " as the great achievement because it investigates the purposes of God. " Has Aristotle been as curious in the inquiry of this cause as he was of the other, he had not left behind him an imperfect piece of Philosophy, but an absolute tract of Divinity." [21]

Reason is unable to follow in the tracks of the wise hand which brings the seeds of the most imperfect creatures, such as bees and spiders, to development and function.

" Thus there are two books, from whence I collect my Divinity; besides that written one of God, another of his servant Nature, that universal and publick manuscript that lies expans'd unto the eyes of all." [22] Here we find a genuine idea of Paracelsus. The heathen forgot God and adored nature as the principle of motion and rest, instead of recognizing therein the straight line of God's order and laws. Thus each natural process is no more and no less a miracle than any other. Creation, e. g., when it " produces effects before nature " is as miraculous as when it " produces effects against or above nature." It is due to our limited intelligence only that certain

who refuted the final causes entirely in the realm of physics. See Fowler, *loc. cit.*, p. 132 f. Sir Humphery Rolleston, " Harvey's predecessors and contemporaries," *Ann. Med. Hist.*, X, 4, 331, 1928.

[19] *Chemical Embryology* (Cambridge, 1931), vol. I.

[20] *Relig. med.*, I, sect. 14, ed. Greenhill, p. 25.

[21] *Ibidem.*

[22] I, 16, p. 27.

effects in the work of God are regarded as contradictions or against nature[23]

Mersennus like Boyle represents a religious point of view. But this is fundamentally different from that of the mystic alchemists; on the other hand, the viewpoint of Boyle is quite different from that of Mersennus. The latter, the Christian philosopher, emphasizes reason as the cornerstone of science when he endeavours to rehabilitate Aristotle and to restore his system as the basis of modern science. To Mersennus religion is the clerical dogma, the " fides " which is followed and supported by reason and intelligence. Boyle, the chemist, however, refutes the sovereignty of reason in empirical investigation and therefore remains in connection with the mystic alchemists. He tries to subject the empirical knowledge of the latter to a modern scientific explanation provided by the atomistic theory of corpuscles. This scientific method is the point where he approaches Mersennus who also does not deny the empirical results of alchemy and endeavours to use them for the construction of a new chemical science. Furthermore, Boyle represents a pious independent faith in God, but, like Mersennus, he does not advocate mystic pantheistic speculation which is also absent from the thoughts of Sanchez.

By the development of the experimental empiricism of the alchemists into science, mystic faith is either altered into " Reflektierten Glaube " or it returns to the ecclesiastical dogma. In alchemistic mysticism religion was the starting point for investigation. It was the source to which the desire for knowledge of nature can be traced. Knowledge of nature and religion represented an inseparable unit. Therefore natural science was rather revelation to the individual than science which generally forces and constrains (" Zwingendes Wissen "). Now science is emancipated. Science has its own sources and purposes. Its results are objective; they may confirm religion, that is to say, the cognition of the supernatural, the existence of God.[24] But its activity is no longer the

[23] I, 27, p. 47.

[24] Compare the characteristic of Boyle's religion in its relation to science given by Joseph Needham: " Boyle was constantly striving to mediate between his science and his religion, which he by no means held in separate boxes, and his efforts often seem in a quaint and theological manner to anticipate Kant's union of opposites in the transcendent." *The Sceptical Biologist* (London, 1929), p. 225.

result of a religious feeling of universality. The microscope demonstrates the delicacy and complexity of living structures, thus affirming the ancient cabalistic and religious doctrine of preformation. Leibniz and Henry More [25] are such philosophers who stress these confirmations of religious truths by the results of experimental science. But their position demonstrates how far the process of separation of science from religion has now gone.

Just as in antiquity, once again the process of separation of faith and knowledge, originally a unity, has taken place. Once again one source of natural science has been the mystic-religious speculation on nature.

I am greatly indebted to Sir Humphrey Rolleston, Bart., Mrs. Dorothea Singer and Dr. Joseph Needham for having kindly revised the manuscript of this paper and for having offered several suggestions.

*In this reprint the illustrations on pages 275, 276 and 279 have been reproduced from photographs kindly provided by the Wellcome Institute Library, London. The sources are:*

*P. 275: R. Fludd, Utriusque cosmi ..., tomus secundus de supernaturali ... microcosmi historia (Oppenheim: Bry, 1619), engraving on p. 82.*

*P. 276: Ibid., engraving on p. 105.*

*P. 279: R. Fludd, Medicina catholica, tomus I, tractatus 2, Integrum morborum mysterium (Frankfurt a.M.: Fitzer, 1631), engraving on p. 338.*

[25] On Henry More's relation to faith and science, see Powicke, F. F., *The Cambridge Platonists* (London and Toronto, 1926), p. 157 ff.

III

# The Religious and Philosophical Aspects of van Helmont's Science and Medicine

# INTRODUCTION *

Johannes Baptista van Helmont, a figure well known from all text books in the History of Medicine, Chemistry and Biology, is duly praised for his momentous discoveries.[1] He introduced the concept of " Gas," he was one of the first to use the balance in scientific, quantitative experiments. He devised one of the early thermometers. He taught the indestructibility of matter. He demonstrated acid to be responsible for digestion in the stomach and alkali for that in the duodenum. He is the founder of Biochemistry in that he studied and expressed vital phenomena in chemical terms. He proposed a reform of time measuring by use of the pendulum and devoted much work to the investigation of its laws. He is one of the founders of modern Pathology which he based on a study of the external agents and the anatomical changes in disease. His original anatomical, physiological and pathological research led him to a refutation of the " Folly of Catarrh," then the universal explanation of disease which was believed to be due to a flow of mucus from the brain straight through the base of the skull to all parts of the body, notably to the lungs and joints, causing pneumonia, consumption, rheumatism etc.[2]—As

* The author wishes to express his gratitude to Dr. V. C. Robinson, M. R. C. P., for kindly revising the manuscript and offering valuable suggestions.

[1] For the Chemical part of van Helmont's work I mention only: Metzger, H., *Les doctrines chimiques en France du début du XVIIe à la fin du XVIIIe siècle.* Paris, 1923, p. 165 ff. and Partington, J. R., Joan Baptist van Helmont, *Ann. of Science*, 1936, I, 359.—For the biological and medical part: Pagel, W., J. B. van Helmont, *Einführung in die philosophische Medizin des Barock.* Berlin, 1930; id., Van Helmont, Leibniz, Stahl, *Arch. Gesch. d. Mediz.* 1931, XXIV, 19; id., Van Helmont DE TEMPORE and the History of the biological concept of Time. With notes on the Greek concepts referred to in van Helmont, *De Tempore* by Helene Weiss. *Osiris.* In Press.

[2] The decisive part which van Helmont's work played in the abolition of the "Folly of Catarrh" has been fully described and documented by W. Pagel, *J. B. van Helmont.* Berlin, 1930 (with translation of van Helmont's treatises: " Catarrhi

a rule, it is mentioned that his treatises make dull reading as they are mixed with theosophical speculations, the account of dreams and visions. The usual method is to extricate from these the scientific detail which is valid today or should be regarded as stepping-stones of scientific discovery. The rest is " excused " with the spirit of the age. It was customary in his day to mingle matters scientific and philosophical. Then, the scientist, it is supposed, had to offer his new knowledge in a religious or philosophical cloak in order to be read or to be believed. In any case, van Helmont's Theology and Philosophy are not taken seriously. According to the usual accounts he must have lived in two worlds which are actually not reconcilable; there is the famous catchword of the " Two Souls in the same Body " and similar superficialities which serve to justify a summary dismissal of the " dark " chapters of his work.

While van Helmont's original discoveries and true scientific yearning are generally recognised among Historians of Medicine and Science, the position allocated to van Helmont in the History of Philosophy is still less adequate. Here hardly any knowledge or

Deliramenta," "Asthma et Tussis" and "Pleura Furens"). See also about Charleton's English translation of the Catarrh-treatise and van Helmont's merits in the refutation of the ancient Rheumatism-Theories: Riddell, Wm. Renwick, The Original Rheumatism. *Canad. J. Med. & Surg.* 1933, LXXIII, 128.

In spite of these, van Helmont's merits are still not sufficiently recognized. In a recent sketch of the History of Rheumatism, F. Klinge does not even mention van Helmont and gives full credit to Conr. Vict. Schneider who described the mucous membranes and confirmed the local origin of the Catarrh-Fluid therein, which was established before him by van Helmont. (Klinge, F., Der Rheumatismus. *Ergebn. Allg. Pathol. u. Pathol. Anat.* 1933, XXVII, 1).

Refutation of "Catarrh" in the old sense of a flow of fluid from the head to lower parts of the body is so self-evident to the present day observer that it is difficult to understand the long time interval which was needed until this concept was completely abandoned. The 1713-Edition of Castelli's *Lexicon Medicum Graeco-Latinum* says under "Catarrhus" (p. 146) that van Helmont in his "peculiar" treatise contended that the whole concept of "Catarrh" should be banned from the realm of Nature and medical consideration. "But this is not the place," the author continues, "to ventilate the jests of this importune reformer, although he has managed to find even to-day some followers." And this, after he has devoted one column to the various theories of "destillatio a cerebri intemperie frigida et humida et ab omnibus quae replent caput," or to a more qualified version, according to which each kind of flow from higher to lower parts in the body is understood as "Catarrh." This was printed about 70 years after the "Ortus Medicinae" and more than 50 years after C. V. Schneider's *De Catarrhis*.

understanding of his medical and scientific achievements is attempted—yet one disapproves of them. It is explained that van Helmont vigorously militated against the use of " Ratio," i. e. formal Logic and mathematical patterns. What can be expected from the scientific endeavour of a man with so strong an aversion against the elements of science and philosophy? [3]

[3] Nève de Mévergnies, P., *Jean Baptiste van Helmont, Philosophe par le Feu.* Bibliothèque de la Faculté de Philosophie et Lettres. Univers. de Liège. Fasc. LXIX, Paris. Droz. 1935.—

This book contains excellent bio- and bibliographical detail and promises to explain the deeper " philosophical " meaning of van Helmont's work which has not been recognized so far. The result is: van Helmont's " philosophy " is " Hermeticism," i. e. the belief in the transmutation of metals and a universal remedy such as " Aurum Potabile." The praise accorded to van Helmont as a worthy contemporary or predecessor of Descartes, Bacon, Boyle, Leibniz, Harvey, Glisson, Willis etc. is, therefore, not justified and the result of uncritical enthusiasm or local-patriotism.

Van Helmont's " hermetic " aspirations and belief are obvious to any student of his work. But it is hard to see how " Hermeticism " can be accepted as " Philosophy," i. e. metaphysics or epistemology. I agree with Nève de Mévergnies that it is necessary to trace the philosophical link which unites the parts of van Helmont's work to one whole and to study its significance in the History of Philosophy. To find this in " Hermeticism," however, is tantamount to deny any such significance. Why not follow up the metaphysical insight which van Helmont admittedly did possess (p. 149; 171), instead of dismissing it summarily in a footnote with the curious comment that " one swallow does not make summer "? A full account of van Helmont's real metaphysical and philosophical ideas and their comparison with those of " full time-Philosophers," notably of Leibniz, would have been the more correct and scientifically fair way.

Moreover, there is no proof that Alchemy was actually the basis of van Helmont's Cosmology, Metaphysics and Theology. The converse could be assumed with equal right and his " Hermeticism " derived from these. There is no need for " Hermeticism " as the explanation of what appears to the present day observer as " Bizarreries " and contradictions, in van Helmont's work. As soon as this is envisaged as an organic whole and not individual doctrines and discoveries are extricated from it, the " Bizarreries " disappear.

On the other hand there can be no honest interpretation and appreciation of van Helmont, unless his scientific, biological and medical contributions are thoroughly examined. His advanced Biology cannot possibly be dismissed with the remark that he did not understand the exigencies of matter and evolution, but simply transferred, to the realm of Life, his belief in the transmutation of metals which is all of a sudden brought about by the " Ferments." The example of " Spontaneous Generation " which Nève de Mévergnies gives in order to show that van Helmont was no " Biochemist " and indeed no Biologist at all, proves nothing. Aristotle, the first genuine Biologist, subscribed to the theory of Spontaneous Generation, a

Obviously no attempt at understanding van Helmont's work as a whole has been undertaken. We live in a period in which the clean separation of religion and science, of belief and knowledge, of vision and reason is felt to be the elementary premise of scientific activity, and so it does not occur to us that this was not always so and that the continuous affirmations of religious motives and purposes in van Helmont's scientific work might be more than figures of speech or symptoms of a morbid or archaic soul. In order to give a true

widespread belief in van Helmont's time which even Harvey's "Ex Ovo Omnia" did not refute.

Moreover, van Helmont himself has clearly separated spontaneous from normal generation. There is nothing in his concept of the latter which could justify a comparison with the transmutation of metals and the *sudden* action of ferments. On the contrary the process of normal generation is described as a very complicated series of events (Compare: van Helmont, Imago fermenti impraegnat massam semine 8 ff. for the separation of normal and spontaneous generation.—Process of generation: Archeus Faber 6 ff.).

Even if it could be proved that "Hermeticism" and the concept of transmutation are the basis of van Helmont's Biology, what would it matter? It would only show that the "dark" mysticism of the alchemical adepts, that "Magic," is the germ cell of advanced biological insight into the "specificity" of the living being and into the impossibility to demonstrate the "essence" of Life scientifically.

Even if van Helmont's knowledge and methods are to a large part Empiricism, this has more of a scientific "air" than the formal logic and humoralistic lore of the Schools. Nève de Mévergnies seems to regard the latter as "scientific." Van Helmont at any rate did not attack them because of their using "scientific" methods (in the modern sense) and because the "born" physician of his ideal would exclude or deprecate "Science." The opposite is the case. Van Helmont made systematic scientific and medical experiments, he combined their evaluation with the use of "Ratio" in the modern scientific sense and based all this on sound anatomical and physiological knowledge. In other words he was a true scientific worker. This is not the only attitude which he offers to the present day observer. But it is just as much *one* side of his personality as the attitude of the "Hermetic." The "scientific" Schools, however, he duly unmasked as unscientific, in that they followed methods inadequate for the study of Nature which to them was largely a battlefield of hairsplitting formal logic.

Nève de Mévergnies suspects van Helmont to have used religious and biblical language in the alchemical part of his work in order to avoid ecclesiastical persecution. This would mean that van Helmont was actually not as deeply religious as he appears to be. But why did he use the same religious language in almost each of his treatises, in those on Time, on the "Folly of Catarrh" etc. etc.?

It is easy to compile the "hermetic" passages from van Helmont's work and to demonstrate his adherence to the belief in Satan and witches. But to deny him, on account of this alone, the place which he duly deserves among the great early

historical picture of van Helmont as well as of the discovery of such fundamental scientific entities as " Gas " or " Ferment " or " Contagium," I think, it will be indispensable to investigate the inter-dependence and mutual motivation of van Helmont's religious-philosophical and scientific side.

I shall, therefore, follow a method directly opposed to the tendency to extricate scientific detail from the general philosophical or theological frame in which it is offered. It will emerge:

(a) that purely physico-chemical or physiological or medical entities to their discoverer meant notions of a wide cosmological and general-biological range which only a *religious* mind could adequately conceive, and

(b) that here is a classical example of the *active* role which religious motives, such as antagonism to " Ratio " played in the birth of modern Science during the seventeenth century.

scientists of the XVIIth century, is impossible unless the sum total of his truly scientific achievements is completely neglected. To van Helmont and most of his distinguished scientific contemporaries the " magic " virtues were just as much natural phenomena as " Gas " and " Ferments " and therefore objects of scientific research.

In any case, credulity and " Hermeticism " have in no way prevented van Helmont from making his momentous discoveries in Chemistry and Medicine and from indefatigable scientific work in the modern sense. I do not hesitate to believe that his religious conviction was a strong incentive for scientific work. Why should this diminish the significance of the latter? It is most bewildering to see some words of Bergson about the harmful influence of mysticism on science applied to van Helmont who was perhaps the only philosopher who closely approached and foreshadowed Bergson's concept of " Durée " in his " theo-biological " treatise *De Tempore*.

# I

## Van Helmont's Criticism of Methods and Substance of Heathen Natural Philosophy and of the " Schools "

A large proportion of van Helmont's work is polemical in character and chiefly directed against the Schoolmen who had based their learning on Aristotle's philosophy.

First of all it attacks their *methods*. At the Universities and Schools of van Helmont's time the study of Nature consisted of the academic discussion not of phenomena observed, but of their interpretation in terms of formal logic and of mathematical patterns which were uniformly applied to all fields of nature irrespective of the actual phenomena and their observation. It was sheer reasoning—Ratio—which pretended to make man omniscient by means of the art of discussion and combination. This kind of " Ratio," van Helmont says, will argue about questions such as: Why does light illuminate, why is water humid, why does it retreat from the immersed finger? The clearer a thing in itself, the more silly, remote and stupid the reason given for it. In this way of reasoning an immobile mover was introduced who should make motion and natural phenomena possible. A continuum of infinite indivisible points was supposed to be the underlying essence of Time; nebulous " Contraria " and " Similia," the universal action of heat, its combat with cold, the interaction of things humid and dry, sympathy and antipathy, the action of the stars served to explain processes in life and nature schematically. Phenomena had been subordinated to generally ruling principles such as that the " Generans " cannot be a part of the " Generatum " or that Nature is the initiation of motion in the moveable or that efficient causes must enter the object from outside—in short, science was a battlefield of formal logic and mathematical reasoning.[4] This is, in van Helmont's opinion, alien to Nature which deals with reality.

[4] On the significance of geometrical patterns in ancient thinking see Cornford, F. M., Greek Natural Philosophy and Modern Science in Needham, J. and Pagel, W., *Background to Modern Science*. Cambridge, 1938, p. 12: Geometry setting the pattern of all organised knowledge in antiquity, accounts for " the ancients defining the substance of things " whereas the moderns formulate sequences of events.

Truth is a real thing, reason an " Ens Rationis," a mere product of mental activity and therefore a Non-Ens. " Ratio et Veritas sunt disparata in radicibus." [5] Reason is by no means the highest function of the intellect, it is developed to a high degree of perfection in freaks of Nature, in the mentally deficient and in animals, notably foxes which outwit their enemies most skilfully.[6] Much more reliable than the logical conclusion is the knowledge of premises. In the end " ratio " is not more than the art of talking and arguing, given to man since the time of his fall, it is " defaecatissima " and a " worthless talker " (" garrula nequam "). It " dilutes, obscures, hampers, and smothers that noble activity of intellect by which knowledge is gained of the premises laid into us." [7] Van Helmont devoted a special treatise to the uselessness of the " Sermocinalia," entitled " Logica Inutilis." Most syllogisms are negations, science has to be positive, " cum sit positivi et de positivo." [8] Logic in no way adds to our knowledge, it does not provide any true " inventio," it but resumes something already known to the reasoning person, it is but arguing which serves to impress one's personal opinion on an audience by special adaptation and composition of words.[9] The same applies to mathematical patterns and considerations: It is not man who measures nature, but only nature itself.[10]

Formal Logic and Mathematics are particularly useless in the investigation of Life. We may disentangle individual phenomena or problems of Life and discuss them, but Life itself beats the human intellect. It is a sort of " light " descending from the " Father of Lights " and thereby outside the " Mundus intellegibilis," a term wrongly used by the Schoolmen for God who in no way " cadit sub intellectum nostrum." Like God himself, the " Powers of Life," its essence, direction and distribution are not accessible to our intellect. They are bestowed by God, distributed individually and situated in the non-intellectual, deeper layers of the soul. How little is motion and life itself affected by the blotting out of intellectual functions such as memory and speech! How easily is the weak intellect overcome by the morbid reactions of the Life-centre, such as syncope,

[5] Venatio Scient. 27.

[6] *Ibidem* 34.

[7] *Ibidem* 20 ff.

[8] Logica inutilis 11.

[9] Logica inutilis 23.

[10] Causae et initia natural. 41.

epilepsy, apoplexy, by life forces which emanate not from the brain, but from the actual seat of the soul, the mouth of the stomach! [11]

Van Helmont's refutation of formal logic and mathematical reasoning is the "negative" critical platform which he builds up for his original scientific methods and research and is largely actuated by *religious* motives. The domination of formal logic results from Hybris of the human mind which believes itself capable of mastering God's creation. It is the heathen Aristotelian doctrine, long ago refuted by St. Paul, but stubbornly followed by the Schoolmen.[12] Appropriate methods must be sought by which the creator and his intention in creating living beings—and that is reality—can be approached, as far as our "Docta Ignorantia" of matters divine and infinite will allow.

In van Helmont's age opposition to Aristotelian Philosophy and its application to the study of Nature was widespread. The "Novum Organum" sets out with the verdict: "Logica est inutilis ad inventionem scientiarum." Ramus, Taurellus, Telesio, and Campanella, Comenius, Stiernhielm [13] and others fight against Aristotle, against formal logic and for the "Propria Principia" in nature-studies, often achieving not more than a substitution of new syllogisms for the old ones. But the *religious motives* of the scepticism towards complacent human reason are nowhere as clearly expressed and illustrated as by van Helmont and his work.

His criticism does not stop at the *methods* employed by the Schoolmen. The *substance* of pagan philosophy so shamelessly adopted by the Christian Schools is still more the target of his fierce attacks.

The old Greek theory of the four elements, the four qualities and four humours was the chief pillar of seventeenth century natural philosophy. It was rejected by van Helmont—in the same way as he rejected the primitive attempts, by the "spagyric" school of the "Paracelsists," at substituting for the ancient four elements the three "principles": Sal, Sulphur and Mercury. Van Helmont endeavours

[11] Confirmatur morborum sedes in anima sensitiva 6.

[12] Venatio scient. 37; Logica inutilis 20.

[13] Compare Nordstroem, J., *Georg Stiernhielm Filosofiska Fragment med inledning och kommentar*. Stockholm, 1924. "Aristotelem, quem sectantur Ducem et Principem, hominem fuisse stultum et arrogantem; verbosum rixatorem, et contumeliosum derisorem." Vol. II, p. 93.

to show that all these elements and principles either do not exist or do not constitute matter, and that where they are, their function has been misunderstood. A few examples may be quoted: Bile which in ancient Physiology and Pathology assumes chiefly the role of a nocuous humour shortening life and initiating disease, is according to van Helmont's experimental and empirical knowledge a humour essential in digestion and life, a " Viscus nobile et vitale." [14] An " Innate Heat " and warmth in general are the essential life factors in ancient physiology, the agents which elicit and activate the development of seeds and govern the building up of the living structures and their function. Warmth is the factor responsible for digestion of food in the stomach.[15] Van Helmont's rejection of heat as the chief vital factor is the key note of his critical as well as his constructive work in science, biology and medicine. Heat is a *companion* of life, it is a " signum " of the modus operandi in warm blooded animals.[16] But it cannot be a requisite essential for life, since life is just as real in fishes and frogs as in the lion, in " cold " poppies just as in the " hot " pepper. It is not because our warmth cools off or because the mysterious " Humidum Radicale " in us is consumed that we die, but because we die, warmth disappears and humours dry up.[17] There is no heat innate in the heart or essential for the maintenance of the pulse. The heart of the frog expands and relaxes in the same way as that of any other animal, becoming pale in systole and darkening in diastole. The Schoolmen admit that the concept of " Heat and Fire in the Heart " is a metaphor—but Nature does not produce metaphors.[18]

In the jargon of the Schools warmth comes under the heading of " Accidentia," yet creative forces such as the production of " forms " and living entities as the developing chick have been ascribed to it.[19]

[14] Scholarum humoristarum passiva deceptio, Cap. II: Superfetatio supplementaria ad humorum fallaciam, 8 and 24.

[15] Aristotle, *De generatione animal.* II, 3 ed. Smith-Ross. Vol. V, Oxford, 1912, p. 736 b-737 a: " All have in their semen vital heat, which causes it to be productive; the heat of the sun and that of animals does generate them."

[16] Blas Humanum 15.

[17] *Vita,* ed. Amsterod. 1652, p. 585; ed. M. B. Valentini, Hafniae 1707, p. 691.

[18] Blas Humanum 16-19.

[19] Physica Aristotelis et Galeni ignara 7.

In van Helmont's opinion warmth may favour the production of "forms," it hastens the hatching of an egg, but it cannot generate anything but further heat. The axiom of the Schoolmen that any agent which predisposes to creation and development of a "Form" also produces that "Form," strikes van Helmont as not only wrong but also *atheistic*.[20] God alone creates the forms and substances. These differ from each other in principle as well as in their products; in other words they are *specific* in themselves and thereby completely different from heat which is a *general* medium and in no way specific.

The dominating role attributed by the Schoolmen to heat is but a symptom of their materialistic (and therefore atheistic) thinking. This recognises only *quantitative* and *locative* changes in the same everlasting and immutable matter as the causes of natural processes and phenomena. A "too much" (τὰ ὑπερβάλλοντα) or a "too little" (τὰ ἐλλείποντα), "Polarity," "Contraria" (τὰ ἐναντία), the combat between and the balance of cold and warm, dry and humid, attraction and repulsion of the uniform atoms and elements account for the course of nature, nay make changes possible. In van Helmont's opinion, the predominance of these heathen doctrines prevented the development of real science and truth and had a particularly devastating influence on Medicine. Therapy was directed against the fictitious humours, elements and qualities and thus led to indiscriminate bloodletting and purgation with the resulting decimation of mankind. If somebody pricks his finger with a thorn, neither bloodletting nor purgation will cure him, only the removal of the cause of the disease which comes from outside. Diseases differ from each other in the same way and as much as their external causes. But to antiquity there were no such things as diseases in the sense of individual varying in signs, changes and outlook with the nature of the causative agent and the particular organ involved. Not disease*s*, but disea*se* was the physician's concern, i. e. impaired function of the individual whose particular constitution was liable to upset his humoral balance.[21]

[20] Formarum Ortus 12.

[21] Sigerist, H. E., *Antike Heilkunde*. Munich. Heimeran. 1927, 1 ff. and On Hippocrates, *Bullet. Instit. Hist. Med.*, J. Hopkins Univ. Baltimore, II, 1934, p. 190 ff.

All this was bound up with a resurrection of the ancient belief in the stars and their profound influence on man's life, body and fate. Van Helmont recognises the whole system of diagnostic and prognostic tables which were based on this belief as pseudo-scientific and attacks it fiercely. To him the stars are time signals, they " necessitate " in that they indicate regular movement in the Universe. But, van Helmont asks with Plotinus, how can variety in nature, how can specificity be ever explained by uniform motion and its laws? Motion by which Aristotle defined Nature, must take place *in* something which exists and it is this something which has to be investigated.[22] The stars not possessing any " Ratio Causarum," can do nothing, nor can a Christian with impunity attribute to them duties other than to act as time signals.[23]

The materialistic theories of the ancients had been embellished by a senseless symbolism in which Sympathy and Antipathy and above all the Analogy between Macrocosm and Microcosm played a predominant role.

Paracelsus who like van Helmont was actuated by religious motives and decidedly opposed to Greek Humoralism and Materialism, had based his natural philosophy on the analogies between macrocosm and microcosm. His tradition was taken up, in the seventeenth century by Robert Fludd and finally by the Romantic movement of the early nineteenth century. Both Fludd and the romantic philosophers were deeply influenced by religious belief.[24]

[22] Physica Aristot. et Galeni ignara 2/3.

[23] Formarum Ortus 14; and: Astra necessitant, non inclinant nec significant de vita, corpore vel fortunis nati, passim; and: *De Tempore* 33. van Helmont admits, however, that the " Blas " in man not follows, but imitates the motion of the stars. Each viscus forms its own " Blas " " ad typum sui astri." Hence the Blas is called " Astrale." This explains periodical changes in the body, healthy and sick. Blas Humanum 5.

By " Blas " van Helmont understands an impulse originating in the stars which is responsible for air movements, winds, inundations, storms, etc. (" Blas Motivum "). It also distributes warmth and cold (" Blas alterativum ") and accounts for changes in weather. By " Blas in Man " all dynamic impulses are understood, especially distance action from one organ on the other, such as the effects of hormons—" Actio Regiminis." Van Helmont studied these actions carefully in diseases and described masterly neuroses of the vegetative system including hysteria and asthma. See Pagel, J. B. van Helmont, *loc. cit.* 1930, pp. 67 ff.

[24] On the Macrocosm-Microcosm symbolism in Paracelsus, Fludd and the

Van Helmont himself is fond of symbolical language. He recognises the role of the celestial bodies in initiating motion by means of the emanation of " Blas," he admits certain influences on man, e. g. those of the moon on emotions, on somnambulism;[25] he believes in the forces hidden in herbs, words and stones.[26] He nevertheless unceasingly deprecates the concept of the analogies between Macrocosm and Microcosm and indefatigably fights against the assumption of " Contraria " and " Similia " in nature.[27] Why? His antagonism against these theories is deeply bound up with that against ancient materialism and like this actuated by *religious* motives. If everything with us is governed by forces identical with those which act in the outer world, if the processes observed in living beings here are but replicae of what occurs anywhere in the great world and particularly in the celestial bodies, then no place remains for *specificity* in Nature. Specificity, however, is vouchsafed by divine creation which occurs but once bestowing on every being the features essential for its *individual* life. " Philosophies of Identity " which resort to one or two forces acting everywhere in nature in the same way must of necessity dispense with the specific forms, functions and purposes which van Helmont attributed to the living being and to life at large. To him life meant a modification of matter which the creator compels to act in certain ways which are different in each individual being. Van Helmont, therefore, reserved for things vital the " private " right and privilege of specificity as opposed to the general—" public "—institutions such as the forces of the stars, attraction and repulsion, sympathy and antipathy, heat and cold, wind and air of which all beings in nature partake.

The belief in the unique natural force accounting for all phenomena in nature is in no way necessarily atheistic or alien to religious think-

Romantic School and their biological theories see: Pagel, W., Religious Motives in the Medical Biology of the XVIIth century. *Bullet. Instit. Hist. Med.* 1935, III, 97-312.—Strunz, F., *Theophrastus Paracelsus; Idee und Problem seiner Weltanschauung.* 2nd Edit. Salzburg-Leipzig, 1937, p. 111 ff.

[25] Formarum Ortus 52 ff.

[26] *In Verbis, Herbis et Lapidibus est Magna Virtus.* Ed. 1652, p. 458. Ed. Valentini 1707, p. 544.

[27] *Natura Contrariorum Nescia.* Ed. 1652, p. 126; Ed. Valentini 1707, p. 155. On the other hand compare van Helmont's qualified recognition of " Sympathy " in *De Magnetica Vulnerum Curatione* 1 ff.

ing, and the explanations given by the romantic philosophers of the nineteenth century cannot even be called " mechanistic," since their symbolical and philosophical meaning is obvious. Fludd, however, embarked on a hardly concealed mechanistic view of Nature, inanimate and vital. He constructs crude mechanical patterns for every process and phenomenon including diseases and endeavours to reproduce all phenomena of life by means of a universal model, a mixture of a primitive barometer and thermometer.[28]

Van Helmont's vitalistic point of view leads him to reject these *monistic* concepts. He equally deprecates *dualistic* theories which create a gap between body and soul, thought and extension. He himself builds up vitalistic *Pluralism*. This sees the world composed of innumerable *" seeds "* which are neither spirit nor matter but have something of both. Products of immediate divine creation, they are characteristic by their *life*, i. e. their *specific* form, function and development. They are not unlike Leibniz' *Monades*.

[28] See Pagel, Religious Motives, *loc. cit.* 1935, p. 272: Fludd's universal instrument and crude mechanistic view; p. 286: Fludd and Romantic " Naturphilosophie."

## II

## Van Helmont's Original Work

### (1) *Methods:*

### *Illuminism, Docta Ignorantia, Empiricism, Pyrotechnia*

This brings us to van Helmont's original work, his *scientific* endeavour and achievement.

Van Helmont's method of thinking and inventing aims at not less than eternal truth which only divine illumination can give. He employs the highest faculties of which the human mind might be capable: The union with the object itself. "The intellect transforms itself, by migration, into the recognised object." [29] When, in this state of mind, divine illumination is acquired, all mental faculties melt into one "mere intellect," and the light of divine grace spreads over the soul. Then the intellect penetrates to the kernel of the objects, to the "Ipsa Rerum Essentia." There is no room for imagination which stops at the outer appearance of the objects.

The intellectual union with the object is the "Ecstasis" which makes "miracles" possible.[30] It is the "Binshikah" of the Rabbis, i. e. the state "In the Kiss" which they say is dangerous and identical with "peaceful death" such as that of Moses, but which in van Helmont's opinion is not dangerous and the most desirable state of mind. In this state we may be able to see persons who are far away, when a certain ecstatic power is excited in our blood by an irresistable desire concentrated on this particular person. Somewhat similar is the condition induced by certain poisons such as wolfsbane, although both originate in the seat of the vegetative soul, the mouth of the stomach, and not in the brain.[31] It is a sort of intuition which van Helmont has in mind. It operates without the eyes and without the recollection of things seen before, a vision in which will, love and desire take part.[32] Van Helmont describes some such visions which he had himself. After 23 years of vain desire to visualise his own soul, he succeeded at last in 1633. His soul appeared as a

[29] Venatio Scientiarum 48.
[30] De Magnetica Vulnerum Curatione 74 ff.
[31] Demens Idea 12 ff.
[32] Imago Mentis 34.

homogeneous light in a human shape, a " spiritual substance " with its own crystal-like " splendour." Van Helmont, then, knew that this apparition was identical with a small illuminated space which, in a visionary representation of his vocation to Chemistry, he had seen in the wall of his room 23 years before and which had shown him " something indescribable." [33]

The ultimate essence of Life, the " Lux formalis " might lend itself to ecstatic vision, otherwise it is beyond the reach of human investigation.[34] It is indescribable, since Life in itself is God.[35] It is the forming power of the " Seeds " hidden in the life principle (Archeus) of plants, animals and everything which multiplies by generation. It may thus be recognised by Ecstasis. It cannot be seen with our eyes. But God who taught Solomon and Adam the properties of creatures may open our internal eyes, the eyes of the soul which were given to St. Theresa, which man had lost with the Paradise.[36]

The intimate essence of life, inaccessible to scientific or rational discourse, may thus be contemplated.[37] Van Helmont's Docta Ignorantia, however, concerns only the Deity and what emanates from Him "" immediate et fontaliter." Not unlike Nicolaus Cusanus who introduced the notion of Docta Ignorantia in the same sense in which it was practised by van Helmont, the latter recommends and undertakes scientific research himself, on things accessible to human investigation, on concrete objects which are comparable and measurable.[38] Such research, however, must be empirical, based on observa-

[33] Imago Mentis 13.

[34] " Omnem arcet mortalium indagationem." Spiritus Vitae 19.

[35] " Cum vita in abstracto sit Deus ipse incomprehensibilis." Blas Humanum 23.

[36] Pharmacopolium ac Dispensatorium Modernum 14.

[37] " Vita ergo humana est lux formalis . . . neque enim vitae essentiam intimam aliter umquam describeret, qui vitas rerum formales etiam in ecstasi videret. Quia verba desunt et nomina, quibus haec dicantur, tanquam etymo a priori. Et licet Deus, alicui vitae essentiam in concreto ostendisset, suum tamen docendi honorem, nulli umquam tribuet creaturae." Blas Humanum 22/23.

[38] The advanced philosophical distinction which van Helmont makes between infinity and things finite and comparable, is noteworthy in the light of the attempts at minimising his merits in Philosophy (see before footnote 3). This distinction plays a special part in his treatise De Tempore where he refers to the " Finiti et infiniti nulla est proportio " (cap. 16). It may be asked whether van Helmont was influenced by the writings of Nicolaus Cusanus who stressed the distinction e. g. in his treatise De Visione Dei. The question is not unimportant, as one of van

tion and experiment, and not on syllogism and reasoning. The means by which scientific knowledge is acquired are: "Quaerere et pulsare,"[39] i. e. testing of nature by experiment. There is no knowledge of biological phenomena ("Archaei alteritates") other than "per nudam observationem."[40] Not book learning, tradition and conjecture based on inveterated formulae and tables will teach us the properties of herbs and remedies. On the other hand, sound observation and solid knowledge are gifts of divine grace which only the God-fearing will obtain. Religious life may thus actively support scientific research.

In nature studies man cannot go beyond observation, since we cannot formulate how transformations actually occur, for example that of the venous into arterial blood by means of the "ferment" intrinsic to the heart. No a priori statements on nature are possible to us.[41]

Van Helmont's method of choice in research is "Pyrotechnia," the application of combustion and he calls himself with pride: "Per ignem Philosophus." The ignorance of experimental chemical methods notably of "Pyrotechnia" marred the attempts of the ancients and of the Schoolmen.[42]

Fire is closely related to Light. They are different degrees of the same created entity. As Light acts on matter uniting with it and vivifying it, so fire combines with matter, converts and finally destroys it. In living matter the "Gas spirituale" of the blood ("Archeus") is the vector of the life-light and its vital impulses.

Helmont's famous experiments (see later footnote 65) was anticipated although not performed by Cusanus. I do not believe that van Helmont has simply copied this experiment, nor can I see how concepts common to all writers on "Mystic Philosophy" from Plotinus, Dionysius Areopagita and Boethius onwards can serve as a proof of dependence or plagiarism (see on the question: Prescott, van Helmont on fermentation. *Arch. Gesch. Mathem. Natwiss. Technik,* 1929, XII, 70 who is with Ch. Singer inclined to accuse van Helmont of plagiarism; Pagel, W., Helmont, Leibniz, Stahl, *loc. cit.* 1930, p. 42 and Partington, *loc. cit.* 1936, p. 376 who think that the dependence is not proved). It should be added that van Helmont's concept of Time differs from that of Cusanus.

[39] Logica inutilis 24.

[40] Pharmacopol. et Dispensat. modern. 14.

[41] "Eo quod naturae ipsae a priori non sunt demonstrabiles." Aura vitalis, p. 578.

[42] Complexion. atque mistion. elemental. figment. 40.

In the same way fire converts matter first into "Gas," i. e. smoke. Fire was created for the necessities of human life, it is the "blacksmith of the arts," it accelerates the maturation of seeds, the separation of things, in a time which otherwise would exceed that of human life. It opens up the arcana hidden in nature, it drives out the non essential admixtures, it separates the pure from the impure, the precious from the base, the nocuous from the useful, the crude from the mature. "Let us therefore exalt the Father of Lights, the Creator of Light." [43]

### (2) *Religious Motives.—Van Helmont and Paracelsus*

In van Helmont's time exponents of the religious approach to natural philosophy, notably R. Fludd, expressed in definite terms the idea that empirical research into Nature is tantamount to worship. God is seen as the chief Chemist with Nature as His Laboratory. He works "conveniente arte spagyrica." [44] This view is based on the conviction of absolute unity in the Cosmos, on a crude pantheistic creed to which van Helmont never subscribed. But he says that God formed man in his image. The Schoolmen when describing man wrongly have, therefore, failed in recognising God and themselves.[45]

There is, however, another strong religious incentive in van Helmont's scientific endeavour: *Religious Pragmatism*. It is the desire to help his fellow-creatures by detecting and opening up the divine resources in Nature, the hidden forces in herbs, metals and stones which God willingly reveals to the worthy. God has created Life, and for the sake of Life science should be promoted. In this light *Medicine* appears as the ultimate aim of Science, and Physics as the means for the conquest of disease. "Terminatur ergo Physica tota in usum vitae, inventionem causarum morbi et remediorum." For this ultimate and decisive object, so far, says van Helmont, "very little has been done, nothing known, a lot promised, still more neglected, expected for a long time and done in a wrong way." [46]

[43] Formarum Ortus 37 ff.—On the universal proficiency of the "Analysis by Fire" in early Chemistry compare: Faerber, Ed., Boyle, in Bugge's *Buch der grossen Chemiker* I, Berlin, 1929, p. 175, and Boyle's criticism p. 181.

[44] Pagel, W., Religious motives, 1935, *loc. cit.* p. 268 ff.

[45] Venatio scient. 36.

[46] *Promissa Authoris* I, 16 (ed. 1652, p. 9).

The invention of remedies requires knowledge of the forces in Nature, their mode of operation, application, preparation, distance action, varying with the special purposes and dependants of the individual organs. Only the Godfearing will eventually attain the art of prolonging life.[47]

*Religious* motives thus led van Helmont (a) to scepticism towards human reason and (b) to empiricism as the way to truth and reality. His religious attitude alone explains the so called contradictions in his methods, endeavours and achievements. We can now *understand* why the scientist who used the balance, who designed scientific instruments, who expressed his results so admirably in quantitative and chemical terms, who founded Biochemistry and Pathology on experimental knowledge,—why this man deprecated "Ratio," accepted magic effects and miracles as genuine natural phenomena and never completely concealed his ultimate doubts in the possibility of full human knowledge.

Van Helmont feels that his science is new and unheard of, a revolution against the recognised lore of the Schools of his time.[48] Moreover he is conscious of his advance on the doctrines of Paracelsus which admittedly stimulated his work and with which he agreed in their critical position against ancient natural philosophy and humorism. Van Helmont's harsh rejection of entities which, in his opinion,

[47] Praefatio to *De Tempore*, ed. 1652, p. 501.

[48] "Inaudita dum pando, anteriorum errores sicubi detexerim, id coactus egi, ne qui me sequentur, in salebras impingant et scopo veritatis orbentur." Ibidem;— For the sake of those who will come after him van Helmont has decided to start from anew and to detect the errors of his predecessors, notably of Aristotle who knew nothing of Nature as it really is, of Galen who is "totus excrementitius et ignarus" (Ius duumviratus 41), and of Paracelsus. Van Helmont is aware of the opposition which he and his methods will arouse from those who will blame him for intolerable boasting and severity in polemics, those who recognise nothing which has not been advanced by themselves and deride or fear all that is new. But progress must not be allowed to be suppressed for such reasons. When prepounding "Nova et Inaudita" van Helmont will not interpret the inventions of others nor quarrel with authorities, and he is conscious of himself as a new founder of medicine which, so far, has only been known by name. (Promissa Authoris II, 4/5). All this, however, is not his own merit. God who has made disease severer and more complicated than in the "good old times" when the medicine of our forebears sufficed, has implanted new knowledge of healing into the worthy. Hence van Helmont's vocation for Chemistry and Medicine.

are not really found in Nature, does not stop short of Paracelsus. Van Helmont's attitude towards him is, therefore, in no way "dishonest." There are many fundamental points in which van Helmont's work supersedes that of Paracelsus. The latter adhered to pantheistic symbolism, to the analogies between Macrocosm and Microcosm, to Sympathy and Antipathy. He introduced the three new *general* principles of Sal, Sulfur and Mercury, i. e. forces which act everywhere and in the same way. He was thus prevented from developing an advanced vitalistic view such as we find in van Helmont's work. Van Helmont's experiments are the recognised basis on which modern Chemistry developed, those of Paracelsus convey suggestions that he was in some way in advance of his time. Van Helmont actually discovered and differentiated gases, he demonstrated the decisive action of acid in the gastric juice, he established the principle of the indestructibility of matter—all this by legitimate scientific methods. Paracelsus outlined in symbolical language a "Chaos" which probably covered Gas-like substances. He emphasised the existence of special digestive properties in every organ of the body, but does not mention the action of acid in the stomach.[49]

[49] "Als ein exempel mit der speiss, die mag kein andere Hitz, Feur oder digestio in sein ultimam materiam bringen, als allein der Magen der Menschen, der hatt den Gewalt." (*Opus Paramirum* III, ed. Strunz, p. 186; Sudhoff, vol. IX, p. 134) ". . . es ist im Magen Mund ein andere digestion zu verstehen, wie im Mund" (*ibid., loc. cit.,* ed. Strunz, p. 188).

Van Helmont argues as follows (Calor efficienter non digerit sed tantum excitative 13 ff.) : If, as the Schoolmen believe, warmth is the digestive factor, intensive hunger and strong and molesting digestion should be accompanied by excessive heat. This is not the case. How can the same factor, viz. heat, be responsible for the most different digestions which take place in animals as unrelated to each other as man, dog, horse, fish, water animal and bird, each having its own kind of blood and excrement? These can only derive from different *specific* ferments ("proprietatibus formalibus"). If really heat was the factor of digestion, this should be better and more efficient in fever. The opposite is the case. There is no trace of digestion when food is brought into contact with a warm surface. Instead of being digested it putrefies. In van Helmont's opinion Paracelsus subscribed to the theory of heat as digestive factor and was ignorant of the specific ferment in the stomach. That is why he admired that certain very hard objects and even bone in the stomach of a dog are quickly absorbed or converted into chylus. "He who had the aspiration for the Monarchate in Healing, failed, having called this faculty admirable, knowing nothing about it and being ignorant of the ferments." (20) As early as a young boy van Helmont had learned that the "ferment" responsible for digestion in the stomach is acid. When feeding sparrows he often let them get hold of his tongue

On the other hand, Paracelsus recognised the importance of specificity in Nature, he sought for the "Seeds"[50] just as van Helmont, and arrived in Pathology at an early differentiation of diseases according to their external—specific—causes.[51]

with their beak and then noticed an intense acidity in the throat of the bird. This, he knew, was the reason of their greediness and good digestion. Later he saw that some acid sulfurous substance had reduced his glove partly to fluid which confirmed his conviction that acid is the principle of digestion in the stomach. Acid stimulates appetite. But it is a special and not any acid which digests in the stomach. ("Acidum esurinum, stomachicum, specificum et humanum: ita quidem per singulas brutorum species, specifice distinctum, quod ipsis sit appropriatum.") The specificity of the acid in each species of animals accounts for the fact that certain animals rather die than eat certain food, e. g. mice, field-mice and pigs detest beans. In conclusion: Warmth acts in a uniform way, the specific vital ferments act according to the exigencies of the species and living being in question. The vital faculty of transforming food "vere atque formaliter" van Helmont has called "*Ferment*" ("Eamque fermentorum nomine designavi" 30).

[50] "Also kompt der grunt in unser wissen und erkantnus, dieweil alle ding ein samen haben und im samen alle ding geschlossen seind. und die natur ist der fabricator in die figur, so gibt sie die form, die das wesen an im selbs ist, und die form zeiget das wesen an." Philosophia sagax der grossen und kleinen welt. Cap. 7 ed. Sudhoff, vol. XII, p. 176.

[51] Partington (*loc. cit.* 1936, p. 363) says that "the recent attempts to prove the great dependence of van Helmont on Paracelsus have gone too far and are often too vaguely expressed." Nève de Mévergnies, on the other hand, emphasises this dependence and refers particularly to the account of it given by the present author in his book on van Helmont (*loc. cit.* 1930). Here a multitude of conclusive quotations from Paracelsus and van Helmont has been adduced, and their relationship proved in no vague terms (e. g. Pagel, p. 15, 18, 34 ff., 39, 44, 48, 74, 77, 79, 84, 93, 112). The great progress achieved by van Helmont especially in Chemistry was pointed out at the same time (p. 10, 63, 110) and the passage quoted by Partington in favour of the dependence of van Helmont on Paracelsus (p. 41 of Pagel's book) was intended to and does prove the opposite, i. e. differences between the opinions of Paracelsus and van Helmont.

It is quite obvious for any impartial student that Paracelsus was remote from the attitude, methods and outlook of the modern scientist, i. e. the investigator of causality in the modern sense. Van Helmont definitely followed the ideal of the modern scientist, with no little success. Nevertheless, van Helmont realised the paramount importance of entities which are not accessible to causal analysis, especially in Biology, and subscribed, true to Paracelsus' tradition, to "Wholism," "Thinking in Analogies" and Symbolism. Hence van Helmont's recognition of "Specificity," qualitative differences of Beings, the particularity of Life, hence his "Pluralism" and refutation of flat "Iatrochemistry" or "Iatromechanism." The combination of research into the causes, as far as possible at his time, with wholistic biological Philosophy secures his unique and superior position in the History of Biology and in that of XVIIth century science and medicine.—Para-

### (3) "*Semina.*"—*Body and Soul.*—*Gas.*

The whole of van Helmont's work can be conceived as the search for the "Semina," i. e. the active principles in beings which are responsible for their *specific* form and function, i. e. the difference between them. These are not due to changes in the composition of matter, as believed by the Ancients. There must be positive entities which are created by God and in a certain way immanent in matter. The speculation as to how the non-corporeal is connected with and acts upon matter is the very centre of van Helmont's research which led him to his momentous discoveries in Science and Medicine. Again, its *religious* motives are obvious: It is the search for the *divine* spark in created beings with which he is concerned.

Van Helmont cannot agree with those who assume a gap between things corporeal and spiritual. Of course, there is inert matter, i. e. water, on the one hand and there are the seeds which bestow speci-

celsus has clearly anticipated the futility of the ancient elements and humoralism. His new "Tria Prima" (Sal, Sulfur and Mercury) are rejected in turn, together with the ancient elements, both by van Helmont and Boyle on empirical-scientific grounds. Paracelsus described in general outline results of daily experience, common sense and sound generalisation rather than products of deliberately planned scientific investigations which proceed from detail to detail and are found in van Helmont's work. Both Paracelsus and van Helmont subscribe to a system and Philosophy of their own, but the latter uses the equipment of the experimentalist to prove it. One example is Paracelsus' and van Helmont's position in Pathology. Both realise that there are disease-entities which differ according to their external causes, van Helmont's research is devoted to the detection of the causes which will teach him the remedy, i. e. how to remove the cause. In Paracelsus' Philosophy of Healing the specific character and cause of the disease are bound up with the remedy which indicates at the same time the cause—obviously the homoeopathic concept. I refer to R. A. B. Oosterhuis, *Paracelsus en Hahnemann, een Renaissance der geneeskunst.* Leiden, 1937. In spite of that, the emphasis laid on the specificity of disease in causes and character emerges clearly from Paracelsus' work, and forms another important link which connects van Helmont with it. I give a few quotations: "Wie vil genera mineralium so vil auch apostematum" (*Drei chirurg. Buecher,* 1. III, de morb. Gall., ed. Sudhoff, vol. X, p. 529).—"Ein natuerlicher, wahrhaftiger Arzt spricht: Das ist morbus terpentinus, das ist morbus sileris montani, das ist morbus helleborinus etc., und nicht das ist phlegma, das ist branchus, das ist rheuma . . . diese namen komen nicht aus dem grund der arznei . . . ." (*Paragranum* ed. S. VIII, p. 75). Recognising the specific character of disease, van Helmont rejects the homoeopathic idea as well as the galenic healing by "Contraria." There are other points in which van Helmont definitely differs from Paracelsus, e. g. in his refutation of "crises" (see footnote 131).

ficity, i. e. life, function, variety and transmutation on the other. We do not know how the creating God works, but there is reason to assume that the " Semina " are not unlike odours, which, we know, have a profound effect on living beings. Or they may be like light or flame by which matter is illuminated. The " illumination " of matter is brought about by an " odour " which confers upon it a " disposition for transmutation." The " Odour " is also called " Ferment " or " Image " of the thing which is to be formed or " Notion of what has to be done." [52] This entity acts on matter i. e. water, as van Helmont says, referring mainly to the authority of the Pentateuch and to some original observations and experiments which seemed to demonstrate that things, particularly plants and fishes, consist of water.[53] Water as such, however, is inert. It cannot generate anything out of itself. It is a " Gas lying on water " (" Gas obsidens aquam ") which receives the semen of a metal whereby the water is impregnated, condensed and gradually converted into a fluid mineral.[54] An " Odour " is not dispersed unless there is an " odorabile " present which is the " gas " of an object.[55] By the presence of the gas matter acquires a special condition by which it loses its coarse corporality and so to speak, meets the odour-like ferment half way, thereby becoming suitable for its reception.[56] Matter for this purpose is loosened and assumes a state not unlike that of putrefying substances. This is greatly furthered by heat. Matter becomes thus an "Aura " and is called "Archeus " as soon as it contains the image of the being. In some objects the "Aura " is very fine, in others, e. g. plants, it may be inspissated and appear as a juice or, in metals, as a dense homogeneous matter. It is in some way fluid (" Fluxibilis ") and has a certain " aspiration " towards the principle of life (the "Anima vivens ").[57] First, however, it forms the lower-vegetative-soul which is responsible for the—species-specific—shape of the body, but does not confer life.[58] The acquisition of the latter is greatly supported by the yearning of the Aura to partake of the divine light. The "Aura anhelat," it attracts the divine light (" splendour ") by

[52] Imago fermenti impraegnat massam semine 12.

[53] Complexion. atque mistion. elemental. figmentum 12; *ibidem* 30.

[54] Magnum Oportet 39.

[55] Magnum Oportet 36.

[56] Magnum Oportet 25.

[57] Imago fermenti i. m. s. 8 ff.

[58] Formar. Ortus 82.

breathing and thereby " comes to the light promised to its seed, then rests in the lower-vegetative-soul, unable to ascend higher." [59]

Not only when an object is formed for the first time, but also later, " ferments " act on the transformed matter, thereby trying to seduce the " archeus " from its own life plan and purpose. These foreign " ferments " act on the " sapor " and " odour " innate in things, i. e. on the spiritual nucleus of matter.[60]

Matter after having acquired the " ferment " or a " seminal property " of this ferment, and only such " disposed " matter is called " Gas." [61] Each body in nature contains such Gas. It is a spirit which under normal conditions is " concrete " or " coagulated like a solid body " and thereby kept dormant and detained. The whole body, however, may become volatile when it has combined with an appropriate ferment. This is seen for example in fermenting grapes, left lying about with their skin damaged. If the skin is intact, however, and the ferment thus prevented from access, they simply dry up without liberation of their Gas.[62]

A characteristic entity containing Gas is the " Semen," the germinal cell of every being in Nature. It is a substance, i. e. a piece of *matter* which contains the "Archeus," the " Gas spirituale " in which is hidden the " Ferment." [63]

Van Helmont himself establishes his discovery of " Gas " where he discusses matter, i. e. water. As far as their material part is concerned fishes are but water and can be artificially transformed into it. All plants and all flesh consist of water; stone, rock and clay are transformed into alkali salt, which, by addition of fat becomes water such as is seen in soap, lapis lazuli, etc. In this connection van Helmont reports [64] one of the first quantitative physiological experiments which became duly famous: the demonstration of the fact that a willow tree after some years of growth has consumed nothing of the earth. Van Helmont concluded that the substance of the tree must

[59] Formar. Ortus 66.
[60] Complex. atque mistion. elemental. figment. 40/41; Magnum Oportet 25.
[61] Complex. a. mistion. element. figm. 34.
[62] *Ibid.* 14.
[63] Imago ferm. i. m. s. 12.
[64] Compl. a. mist. elem. figm. 12; *ibidem* 30.

be derived from the water which was added to the earth at regular intervals.[65]

Conversion of bodies into water takes place after they have lost their specific seminal property, i. e. when they cease to be the well characterised entity which they represented before. If they are not immediately changed into water and forced to give up their fixed condition, for example by heating, Gas develops. In other words, Gas is a thing which has lost its concrete shape, but has not lost specificity. It has, therefore, actually lost nothing. It does exist and will never be consumed—as can be seen when charcoal is heated in a closed vessel; it may be heated until doomsday, yet will never substantially disappear. But it will be almost completely changed into a "wild spirit" (Spiritus sylvester"). It is "wild" because it cannot be held in an open vessel and it cannot be solidified unless it loses its "semen," i. e. specificity.[66] Finally it becomes water when by the action of cold at very high altitudes and after a long time interval it loses specificity and seminal properties. The extreme cold at the high altitudes of the sky also converts water into Gas (Gas aquae) by disintegrating its material composition, its solid (Sal), volatile (Sulfur) and fluid (Mercury) particles.

Gas is therefore, matter in a special form, it is "as far as matter is concerned from the element water." [67] But it is by no means matter alone. Matter in order to be Gas must retain specificity. Van Helmont clearly recognised—and here lies the main achievement of his chemical work—that Gas is, unlike air and watery vapour, no volatile medium common to *all* things, but something *specific*. It is the material vector of specificity which he believed he had discovered and demonstrated in every being in Nature. The Gas demonstrates empirically that particular alteration which matter undergoes when subjected to the action of a "Ferment." It shows that a deep substantial transmutation of matter follows and not only a different arrangement of the material particles without alteration of matter itself. The far reaching significance of "Gas" emerges from its role in living beings. We have seen that van Helmont attributed to it

[65] See before footnote 38 about the influence of Nicol. Cusanus.

[66] Compl. a. mistion. elem. figm. 14.

[67] *Ibid.* 28.

" seminalis proprietas " which it must lose in order to be converted into its original state: water. Since " Gas " contains the " concretum semen " it is capable of generation.[68] But above all the " Life-Spirit " in our arterial blood is Gas.[69] When it flees from the outer parts of the body they lose the appearance of living parts, such as seen in fainting, palpitation, syncope. The Archeus itself *is* Gas of the nature of a " balsamic salt," it can easily evaporate through pores, " munium agendorum atque familiae oblitus." Gas is therefore, not only the vector of specificity, but also that of " Life " in the widest sense.

It is thus that van Helmont feels the great progress which is due to his work—not so much because of the import of his discovery for Chemistry, but for the solution which he offered and empirically proved of the perennial problem of the action of the " spirit " upon matter. In van Helmont's concept the *immanence* of the dynamic principle in matter is emphasised—as opposed to its external and accidental action on it. Van Helmont achieved this immanence by spiritualisation and pneumatisation of matter. The great advance due to his work lies in the *empirical justification* of this tendency by the discovery of Gas. Gas was reality and truth, the elements and humours of the Ancients were fictitious. Gas was an empirical entity on which safely to base specificity in a vitalistic sense; whereas not more than a mechanistic pseudo-explanation was to be derived from the ancient concepts of imaginary changes in the arrangement of the material atoms. Gas showed how matter was enabled to unite with the divine spark of life, whereas the ancient theories did not require, nay rejected divine creation.

Van Helmont introduced a number of new entities which are represented in the diagram: By the action of the " forms " or " images " the divine light generates the dynamic principle in matter, the "Archeus." The "Archeus " forms out of matter the concrete objects in nature to which it confers specificity. The archeus is contained in the objects as "Aura," " Splendor," " Spiritus " or " Gas." All these represent organised matter. The Archeus in the " Semen " receives " Life " from God, with the help of the divine " fermentum " or " Odour." Developing material substance which

[68] Complex. a. mistion. element. figment. 34.
[69] *Ibid.* 40/41.

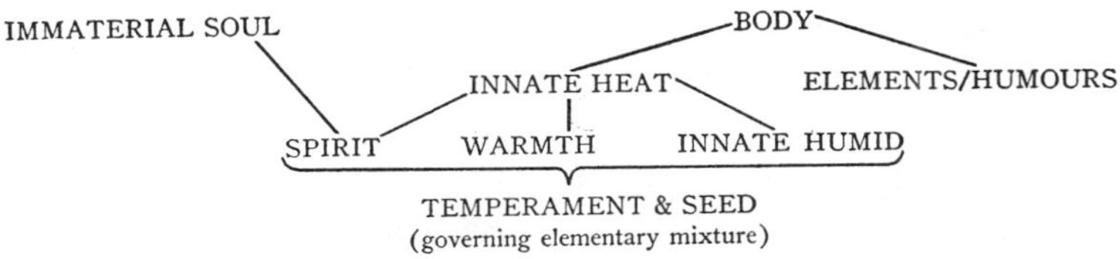


DIAGRAM ILLUSTRATING FERNEL'S CONCEPT OF MAN,
(for description see footnote 71)

as an example of the contemporaneous humoral and crude materialistic theory to which van Helmont objected and for which he substituted his new concept.

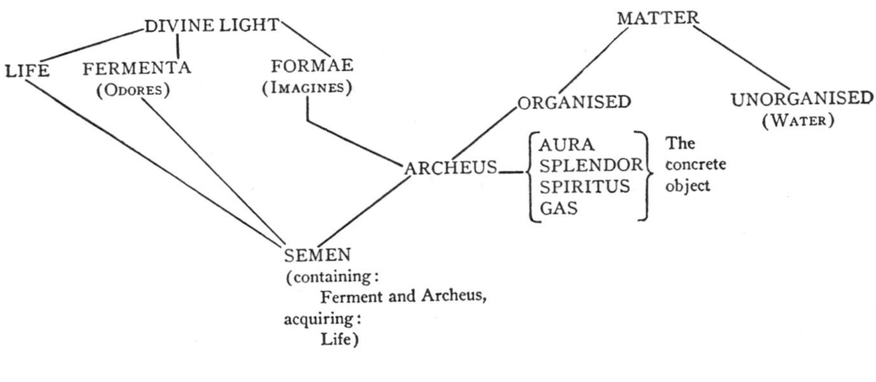


DIAGRAM ILLUSTRATING VAN HELMONT'S CONCEPT OF THE ORGANISATION OF MATTER

(a) contains the archeus with its aura, splendor or gas, i. e. " organised matter " and which is (b) endowed with the " Ferment " conveying Life is called " Semen."

### (4) *Matter and its Immanent Biological Impulses. Biological Specificity*

Why was it necessary for van Helmont to represent the interaction of things corporeal and spiritual in such a complicated way? In the writer's opinion, van Helmont's chief motive was to do justice to his biological insight into the exigencies of living matter and the immanence of the dynamic impulses, chiefly those of generation in it. To make matter a lifeless, passive non-ens which obeys the command of the omnipotent soul, could not appeal to him as Biologist and Chemist. On the other hand, his religious conviction would not permit of a monistic view in which matter alone was responsible for life, particularly as it could not account for specificity. If, however, an empirical foundation could be established for the " spiritualisation " of matter, then the action of non-material " Ferments " on it would not interfere with its proper function. Moreover, " spiritualised," i. e. organised matter could easily act as the vector and guarantor of specificity. Finally, van Helmont's solution is the view of a stratification of well defined biological entities in the individual. This forms a unit with different aspects (a) the " material " organisation in the form of Aura, Gas or Archeus and (b) the " spiritual " plan of form and function.

Gas has therefore a meaning reaching much farther than that of a chemical entity. It embodies a notion of general philosophical and cosmological import; it is a genuine offspring of van Helmont's religious system of Nature.[70] It cannot be isolated from its cosmo-

[70] The religious and theological background of the problem of the origin and action of " spirits " in the blood could be illustrated by many examples, notably the well known fact that it was this problem and its discussion in a theological work (" Christianismi Restituțio ") which provided the platform for the publication of Serveto's discovery of the lesser circulation.

The question of " what kinde of bodies shall those be after they be raised " was one of the practical catechism. In van Helmont's days H. Hammond, for example, described the " Spirituall Bodies " (I Cor. 15, 44) as follows:

" (1) In respect of the qualities *spiritualized* into a high *agility, rarity, clarity,* and such as will render them most commodious habitations for the soul, made par-

logical and religious background without endangering the full understanding of what van Helmont meant when he introduced and differentiated "Gas" as a new "Ens." Gas helps to build up the scientific representation of the mutual penetration of dynamic agents and matter. These are seen as a series with all transitions from finest corporeality—the odour of the "ferment"—to more and more coarse matter—Gas, and finally water. "Body" and "Soul" are different aspects of the same living whole, rather than entities inimical or subordinated to each other. Matter owes its shape and specificity of form to the same entity which is also responsible for its reception of life (i. e. function): to the Archeus or to the "Gas." This solved the problem of the "Qualitas Occulta" and Action of the "Tota Substantia" which hitherto was not accessible to scientific analysis, and had usually been explained by a "divine heat" in us (Fernel),[71] or by the action of the stars or by Sympathy

taker of that divine vision. (2) In respect of the principle of life and motion, which, in naturall bodies is some *naturall* principle, but in these is the *Spirit of God* which shall sustain them *without eating or drinking* etc."

It is thus that resurrection can be made *reasonable* to believe although we do not know how actually it will take place. (*A practicall Catechisme.* 5th edit. London, 1649, p. 302).

This shows the appeal which van Helmont's research on Gas must have had for wide circles of the clergy and indeed of the public, at a time when "Palingenesy" was a subject of discussion for the Royal Society. It is well known how the professors of "Palingenesy" such as Sir Kenelm Digby, Athanas. Kircher, Gaffarel, Schot and others believed that "Spirits" are a material product which is thrown off like a film or membrane from the surface of bodies. It is noteworthy that Lucretius to whom the concept of "Palingenesy" can be traced, assumed that the "soul" consists of "Perparva Semina" by means of which it is distributed all over the veins, viscera and nerves. It is thus comparable to the invisible and weightless "Succus et Odor Rerum" which consists of "Multa Minutaque Semina" (*De rerum natura* III, 214 ff.; ed. Creech, Oxonii, 1807, p. 160). The minute seeds, their distribution throughout the body as "Archei insiti," their "odor"-like quality and their condensation into a "succus," for example in plants—are concepts typical of van Helmont's "pneumatisation of matter" (see before and espec. Magnum Oportet 36, 39 ff.). On the whole, however, the differences between van Helmont's search for specificity in the "Semina," "Odores," "Spiritus" and the crude materialistic "generalising" concepts of Lucretius are obvious. On "Palingenesy" compare: Samuel Hibbert, *Sketches of the Philosophy of Apparitions.* 2nd edit. Edinburgh, 1825, p. 18 ff.; Smedley, E., Taylor, C., Thompson, H. and Rich, E., *The occult sciences.* London & Glasgow, 1855, p. 87 ff.

[71] *Universa Medicina.* Physiologia IV, 1 ff.: "Calorem quendam in nobis cunctisque viventibus inesse eumque divinum. . . . Animantium generi communi lege est

and Antipathy.[72] The union between Archeus (Gas) and Life (Ferment) is thus very close and made still closer by the introduction of the "Archei Insiti," i. e. the dynamic principles inherent in every organ, and indeed in the smallest particles of the tissues. Selecting from the stream of fluids the food suitable for the part in question and assimilating it into organ substance, the Archei Insiti act as metabolic centres. They convert the food which is offered to *all* organs into organ-*specific* material.

Thus, there is no room for Dualism. Stahl's system of "Animism" which is often regarded as the germ cell of genuine Vitalism, has separated matter and dynamic impulses ("Soul") by a wide cleft. Here the body is devoid of any right and action, it would continually decay but for the preserving power of the Soul. Life is preservation of matter from corruption. The Soul is not immanent

a natura tributum, ut insiti vi caloris vitam agant. . . . Spiritum quendam cunctis datum viventibus qui vitae calorem continet." Warmth must have a seat and vehicle in the body. The rapidity of its action and penetration excludes any fluid as seat and vehicle of the warmth. The very fine ether-like spirit seems to be the most suitable link between the "crassum corpus" and the "Animus." There are two groups of "spirits" in the body; The "spiritus stabiles et in unaquaque parte fixi," i. e. those which belong to the individual organs and tissues, and the three "errantes et vagi influentesque spiritus," offsprings of the three vital organs: liver, heart and brain (spiritus naturalis, vitalis and animalis).

The "Nature" of man, i. e. the first force and cause of our functioning and conservation, is the "innate heat" and consists of: (1) the prime humour, an oil-like fluid, (2) the spirit and (3) warmth. All these are contained in the "Seed." This "nature" of man is the "temperamentum" which is the result of the peculiar mixture of the elements and the perfusion of the divine warmth. (Physiologia, IV, 7.)

I have given Fernel's concept in detail in order to show the remarkable advance of van Helmont's scheme. It is obvious, however, that both have something in common, e. g. the differentiation of the spirit fixed to the organ and tissue—Archeus Insitus—and the general spirit—Archeus Influus—which in Fernel's opinion comes from liver, heart and brain, whereas van Helmont derives it from the stomach. There is also the tendency to introduce a link between coarse matter and immaterial soul, a link represented by matter of finest corporeality—the "spirit." But there is no emphasis laid on specificity, there is only the crude materialistic idea of mixture of elements with the "innate heat," accounting for the individual "temperamentum."

[72] A glance into the masterly collection of the theories of Elements and "Occult Virtues" given by Lynn Thorndike (*History of Magic and Experimental Science,* Vol. V/VI: XVIth century. New York, 1941, espec. Vol. V, p. 550 ff.) will reveal the differences and the progress achieved by van Helmont. It will also show where he stands on the shoulders of his predecessors. This particularly applies to Paracelsus (see Pagel, W., Religious Motives, 1935, *loc. cit.* p. 112 ff.).

in the body and its parts, it comes and directs it from outside. There is no cooperation on the part of the body. Motion, particularly obvious in circulation, is the universal instrument by means of which the Soul acts on the Body. Disease, disturbance of form and function, is an affair of the Soul alone, its main cause being: Emotions, abnormal circulation, Plethora etc. Material alteration of the body, anatomy, chemistry, morbid-anatomical and biochemical changes are of no interest; what matters alone is the mechanics of the movement of the blood and spirits, the influence exerted by the Anima. In building up his "Animism" Stahl might have been actuated by religious motives. He adhered to "Pietism," a special trend of Protestant thought in the early eighteenth century. Van Helmont, too used animistic notions and often identifies Archeus and Anima Sensitiva. The Anima is the Balsam which preserves the body not unlike the "Mummy" in Paracelsus' concepts.[73] The archeus directs and

[73] "Gas ergo vitale, quia lumen est atque balsamus, praeservans a corruptione ab primordiali geniturae adumbratione, incepit solari lumini adaequari." Complex. a. mistion. element. figment. 40/41. In this passage the function of the vegetative soul is directly attributed to the "Gas" in the blood, true to the old Hebrew tradition and to common contemporary opinion such as expressed for example by Harvey.

Similarly: "Est ergo spiritus vitalis, salinus ideoque balsamicus et custos a corruptione, idque non tantum ratione salis, quantum respecto luminis concepti in suo sale." Spiritus vitae 17. The venous blood produces when subjected to distillation a volatile "Spiritus salsus" which (unlike a similar substance from the urine) cures epilepsy even in the adult. This substance accounts for the conversion of venous blood into arterial "Spirit" in the heart, after the venous blood had been in contact with the air in the lung. It is this contact which allows the blood to become volatile without solid residuum ("Caput mortuum"). The air acts as "Aquarum Separator" by separating the watery vapour which is excreted, from the volatile spirit in the blood which is brought to the left heart and here converted into the "vital spirit." This vector of specific life forces and impulses is "Gas." Blas Humanum 45 ff.

One might interpret in the sense of Stahl's Animism, van Helmont's opposition to the sentence which he attributes to Aristotle: "Quemadmodum enim animae differunt, ita et natura ejus corporis differt." Van Helmont calls it "absolutely false and ignorant" to let any property of the soul take part in the body, although it might be linked up with the body (Phys. Arist. et Galeni ignara 4 ad Paragr. 3). Obviously van Helmont thinks of the vital importance which Aristotle attributed to heat (see before, note 15), but not to the actual unification of things corporeal and spiritual in the living being. Nevertheless van Helmont *has* expressed animistic concepts such as: "Clarum enim atque indubium est, quod homo nequeat se ipsum cognoscere, nisi prius animae cognitionem hauserit. Quippe sine anima est homo

commands bodily fluids and solid parts, it acts on them like a guardian on a child. This is particularly obvious in the functions which are today attributed to hormons. Van Helmont, however, emphasises hormonal and vegetative-nervous impulses in order to show that the genuinely vital functions cannot be explained by mechanical laws or the physiology of circulation. In van Helmont's system anatomical and particularly chemical changes in the living substance enjoy full attention. There is no special life-force which should be added to other forces in nature, there are only " seeds," and organised matter.

In many points, no doubt, van Helmont's doctrines of Life are related to the fundamental Aristotelian concepts of Eidos and Entelecheia. Like these van Helmont's Archeus is an active agent (ποιοῦν), inherent in the generating cause (αἰτία). It is often hard to see why van Helmont should attack these concepts. What van Helmont rejects is not infrequently the scholastic interpretation and mediaeval petrification of Aristotelian doctrines,[74] with the extensive use of formal logic and mathematical patterns which had largely replaced the knowledge of facts. No doubt, matter, elements, humours and humoral mixtures and above all warmth played the central role in the genuine Aristotle as well as the lore of the Schoolmen. Moreover, certain differences can be found between the Aristotelian Entelecheia and the Archeus. The former is not linked up with the free action of a living Creator. Entelecheia is more a philosophical and ontological entity than a real force in Nature seen in development and function. Van Helmont was bound to object, just as much on religious as on biological grounds. He went even so far as to connect the divine spark of Life with an " Odour," i. e. a substance of finest corporeality. Aristotle's concept would strictly exclude anything in the nature of a corporeal entity.

merum velut cadaver. " Tract. de Anima 3. Further passages from van Helmont see Pagel, Helmont, Leibniz, Stahl, 1931, *loc. cit.* p. 26, footnote and p. 45 footnote 2.

[74] See Weiss, Helene, Notes on the Greek concepts referred to in van Helmont *De Tempore. Osiris.* In Press. Here, the actual metaphysical and not only formal logical character of the Aristotelian concept of time is pointed out.

## (5) *Van Helmont and Monadology*

### (a) *The Principle of Life, Immanence, Quality.—Realism.*

Leibniz' " Monadologie " offers some aspects which show a striking parallelism with van Helmont 's system. It is surprising that this has not so far received attention. The reason seems to be that Leibniz rejected, expressis verbis, the "Archei " as far as they were supposed to act on the body as separate entity, altering the natural course of its mechanical and chemical processes.[75] Leibniz particularly objected to Stahl's "Animism." [76] This denied the existence or importance of any material processes or phenomena immanent to the body. As we have seen, van Helmont's concept differs widely from Stahl's Animism. Its object was to demonstrate and represent the " Energetic nature of Substance " (Glisson), the dynamical principles *immanent in matter* as opposed to those which might act on matter from outside such as Stahl's Anima. These immanent impulses exist of necessity in " organised matter." They are inherent in its smallest particles and therefore inseparable from it. Together with matter they form the individual being, and both represent two aspects of the same thing. Matter in this way is not subordinated to the soul but is the active vector of specificity. In van Helmont's concept a vindication of matter and its own sphere of action is achieved by its spiritualisation. This leads up to the scientific investigation of volatile substances, to substitution of the unreal elements and humours of the ancients by chemical entities such as Gas and to expression of vital reactions in chemical terms— in short to the search for real causes.

All this is congenial to Leibniz' Philosophy. Not abstract geo-

[75] G. G. Leibnitii Epistolae de rebus philosophicis ab anno 1699 ad me datae, in Frider. Hoffmanni, *Opera Omnia.* Genevae, 1754. Suppl. I, p. 55: Neque enim credo aliquid eum (Thomasius) in animo habere simile spiritui hylarchico Henrici Mori, qui et ipse doctrinam nunc communem impugnabat. Ego puto omnia phenomena naturae explicabilia esse mechanice, si quis caussas intelligat: etsi agnoscam, ipsa principia legum motus altiora esse, neque ex solis mathematicis considerationibus posse deduci: cum interveniat quiddam ἀπὸ τοῦ αγαθοῦ sive a caussa finali." (Sept. 23rd 1701.) See also Erdmann, Leibnit. Opera, 694 b; 702 a; 777 b.

[76] See the account of the controversy between Leibniz and Stahl in Pagel, W., *Arch. Gesch. d. Med.,* 1931, *loc. cit.* (Helmont, Leibniz, Stahl), p. 45 ff.

metrical synthesis of concept after concept and axiom after axiom is his method, but the organic development of observed facts out of a concrete principle, that of " Life." [77] Our mind, says Leibniz, undoubtedly contains in itself the germ of all truth. But experience is necessary to develop this germ. Otherwise mathematical deduction will never give us more than the " Possible " and not the " Real." [78] Mathematical patterns and rational thinking base their explanations on mere repetition of certain principles. Such repetition is an act of our mind. Reality, however, has to deal with the things as they are themselves, and no such repetition occurs here where everything is different in quality.[79] One may compare with this our quotations from van Helmont's writings on " Logica inutilis " and " Ratio." [80] Hence the " realistic " character of Leibniz' system. Its basis is the general idea of " Life," i. e. the specific differences of organic beings in form and function. There is no homogeneous reality in which the individuals are only modifications of an identical general medium or of a unique force and hence accessible to mechanical explanation. Each individual has its own force, developed and derived from its own " seed." The world consists of invisible Semina which, by the microscopical discoveries at Leibniz' time had become reality. As we have seen, the study of the " Semina " was van Helmont's chief concern. To find the general in the individual, i. e. in qualitative differences and in specificity was the idea of Leibniz' early work.[81] General phenomena and their quantitative graduation, such as modifications of motion and extension cannot determine an individual or a concrete object. Motion for example requires time in which it takes place. It could not explain anything if this is seen without time relation, e. g. in the smallest possible moment of time.[82] " Il faut," says Leibniz, "que les Monades aient quelques qualités, autrement se ne seraient pas même des êtres." [83] The same idea is expressed

[77] Compare A. Helfferich, *Spinoza und Leibniz oder das Wesen des Idealismus und des Realismus.* Hamburg und Gotha, 1846, p. 61.

[78] G. G. Leibnitii, *Opera Philos.* Edid. J. E. Erdmann, Berol. 1840, 171; 723 b. *La Monadologie* edid. E. Boutroux. Paris, p. 29/30.

[79] Erdmann 705 b.

[80] See before footnotes 5 ff.

[81] *Disputatio metaphys. de principio individui.* Lips. 1663.

[82] *Vernunftprincipien der Natur und Gnade,* her. Buchenau and Cassirer. Leipzig. Meiner., Vol. II, p. 436, footnote 482.

[83] Monadologie 8, ed. Boutroux, p. 144.

in van Helmont's polemic against the definition of natural objects as those which have the principle of motion and rest in themselves. Van Helmont says: by necessity an object must be before it moves, is moved or rests. The principle of Being precedes the initiation of movement or rest.[84]

Moreover, in van Helmont's opinion, this definition is directed against Creation. What, he asks, if God, after creation had added neither motion nor rest? Then, according to the above definition, creatures would have existed, but nature not:[85] Creation, however, is emphasised by Leibniz too. According to him, the monades show so intimate a connection of body and dynamic principle that they must have come into existence " tout d'un coup," i. e. by creation.[86] The firm belief in creation had prompted van Helmont's fight against the ancient materialistic theories: that corruption of one makes possible the generation of the other, that generation is simply a different arrangement of matter and due to accidental action of heat or to action of matter at all. Creation is the main point in which van Helmont disagrees with Aristotle's concept of Entelecheia.[87] To van Helmont creation means coming into being of seeds, in other words disposition of matter. Creation is also to van Helmont the unique act by which matter is endowed with form at once, the " tout d'un coup " of Leibniz.

### (b) *Vita media. Magnum Oportet. Perceptions.*

To the Monadologie there is no birth nor death, but only *dev*elopment of the seed and its *env*elopment and regression to smallest germs.[88] Van Helmont said: " Generation means nothing but

[84] " Necesse est ut aliquid prius sit antequam moveat, moveatur aut quiescat. Principium essendi praecedit initium movendi aut quiescendi." Phys. Arist. et Galeni ignara 2/3.

[85] Phys. Arist. et Galeni ignara 2.

[86] Monadologie 6, Boutroux, p. 143.

[87] Pagel, W., *J. B. van Helmont.* Berlin, 1930, p. 29.

[88] Monadologie 73, Boutroux, p. 61. In the same sense Leibniz' answer to Fred. Hoffmann who says in a letter to Leibniz: "Credidi semper nullum corpus, quatenus vi praeditum est movente et mobili, interire posse, et interitum corporis nihil aliud esse, quam tantum ejus mutationem in mixtione, constructione et motu, et sic animal ceu individuum sive certum corpus perire, ut corpus autem sive substantiam permanere, ipsas mentes vero in individuo subsistere." Hoffmann wants to know

the flow of the seed towards perfection, the maturation of properties, the emergence of hidden qualities, the consummation of schedule down to its end." [89] Accordingly the "Vita media" of things played a particular role in his system. As a rule natural objects do not perish but persist in a reduced form. The object does not return to a completely imperceptible stage, its "Vita prima," such as exists in the seeds,[90] but to a fluid form not unlike embryonic matter or the fluid precursor of metals and stones. When we take in animal or plant substance as food, their specificity persists in us with their "middle life," their "odour and sapour." [91] Meat or pigs fed on fish definitely tastes of the latter, yet it is genuine pork. The persistence of the middle life of things entering our body accounts for its gradual changes. This is the "great necessity in this valley of misery," the "Magnum Oportet" of van Helmont. It dates from the original sin when the human archeus lost the power of completely absorbing and transforming food and "properties of middle life." At this time "duality, alterities and vicissitude" crept into human life. Now, we suffer from the "tyrannis and multiplicity of tribulations and spines" inflicted by "alien ferments," i. e. from what is specific in objects outside ourselves. They act on the archeus, combine with it and thereby initiate new generations which often turn out harmful to our life and functions. The Archeus governs the metabolism of the body; as "Archeus influus" the general metabolism of the organism as a whole, as "Archei insiti" the local dissimilation and assimilation in the organs and tissues. These Archei are responsible for the gradual absorption of food material and its conversion into organ substance. An "alien ferment" might elicit in these Archei an "appetite, aversion or neutrality," i. e. seduce them from the obedience to schedule and enchant them with illusions. Consequently they cannot do their duty, the foreign material taken

whether this meets with Leibniz' approval. (Epist. Leibnit., *loc. cit.* p. 51. Halae, 1699). Leibniz replied (Hannover, 1700): "Arbitror ego, omnem substantiam, quae una vere est, seu monas et individuum esse et permanentem: massam autem corpoream non esse substantiam sed substantias, ut grex vel exercitus." See also Leibniz' letter to Hoffmann, Sept. 27th 1699, *loc. cit.* p. 50.

[89] Ignotus hospes morbus 38.

[90] Magnum Oportet 28; 40.

[91] Magnum Oportet 25.

in with the food or with the breath is not properly incorporated and residues will remain not unlike tartar in wine-vats. These are the anatomical changes which we see in the organs in diseases. The concept of the preservation of the " middle life " thus explains and emphasises the *gradual* course of changes in the individual being.

In Leibniz' philosophy the *gradual* changes of the monades are of equal importance. The multiplicity of things in nature, i. e. the other monades are represented in the individual monade by " small perceptions." [92] These are open neither to mechanical explanation nor to geometrical description. The varying clearness of perceptions accounts for the difference between the individual monades and their gradual changes.[93] The preceptions range from small unconscious and dim impressions to high mental faculties such as sensitivity, memory, imagination. A similar series of " impressions " which account for specific differences between objects and their specific action is found in van Helmont's concept of " Magic " in Nature. Not unlike the small perceptions the " impressions " are linked up in van Helmont's philosophy with the representation in the individual, of the variety in nature. All action and all properties of natural beings are caused by their imagination of their own forms. This is the " sensus rerum " which accounts for effects such as ascribed to " sympathy and antipathy." The imagination of forms is simple, " corporeal and ignoble " in objects such as constituents of matter (viz. Sal, Sulfur and Mercury). To this category of forms belong the so called " occult qualities " of substances such as sleeping draughts or laxatives. Like the " small perceptions " they do not lend themselves to empirical analysis and had been wrongly denied by the Cartesian philosophers. Higher faculties originate in the imagination of forms of composed bodies such as the magnetism of the magnet, the virtue of tinctures, meat, roots, leaves, fruit. These virtues are specific, e. g. for the leaves of the rose, but not for its blossom and cannot be derived from their simple material constituents. Still higher in order is the virtue by which an entity is produced and transmitted to the suitable object (" Sympathy "). This is the real magic effect by which every agent acts on *its proper object.* The

[92] " Perceptio nihil aliud est quam multorum in uno expressio " (Erdmann 438).
[93] *Vernunftprinzip. d. Natur u. Gnade, loc. cit.* 2; Monadologie 17, Boutroux 149.

correct result of the action is due to a "presentiment" of that towards which the agent deliberately "sprays out" its activity. This occurs "after *sensing* the object, exciting phantasy, dispersing an ideal entity and copulating it with the ray of the passive entity." [94] Thus acts the magic virtue of animals such as the basilisk, the mad dog, special fishes, a virtue often inherent in the blood of these animals. The highest virtue, however, is not bound up with corporeal forces and effects, but due to the excitation of the power of the internal soul by the Holy Spirit or by intense imagination or speculation. It is productive of "the most potent procreations, the most august impressions and strongest effects." [95] The same principle of grades and stages of perceptive representation is applied in the Monadologie: the coarser, the more material and "hylic" the monade, the less clear and conscious the representation of the other monades, the perception. The difference between monades lies (just as in van Helmont's concept of "Magic") in the degree of clearness with which they represent the outer world. There are as many degrees of representation and perception as monades.

### (c) *The Organs, the "Archei," the Soul.*

Together with the matter belonging to it, each monade forms a living being. The rank of the perceptions of which it is capable, depends upon the development of the organs. A similar high importance van Helmont has attributed to the organs. We have mentioned the part they play in van Helmont's physiology of metabolism and shall discuss their significance as the "seat" of diseases later. The high estimation of the organs led van Helmont to foreshadow the idea of specific sensual energy. This is the result of specific organ function. It is the same vital impulse ("Spirit") which is carried with the blood to *all* organs, but is adapted by the action of the latter to the particular local function without undergoing substantial changes. The "spirit" conveyed to the tongue accounts for the perception of taste, but it will cause no such thing in the finger. There will be as many essential modifications of the spirit as there are organ-functions.[96]

[94] De magnetica vulnerum curatione 152.
[95] *Ibid.* 157.
[96] Spiritus Vitae 29.

The monade in animals is the soul. This is subject to changes which occur pari passu with the metamorphoses of the body. But never will the soul leave this and enter other bodies, in other words there is no such thing as "metempsychosis." Body and soul form an indissoluble unity. This was emphasised both by Johann Baptista and his son Francis Mercur van Helmont, the friend of Leibniz.[97] The whole object of van Helmont's complicated representation of the Semen containing Forms and Archei was to demonstrate the close union of body and soul. This is in remarkable contrast with the later systems, notably those of Stahl and Hoffmann. The latter degraded the Archei to a purely physical "Ether" and nervous fluid. He did not pay much attention to the soul. The material substratum of the body is active in itself, it exhibits motion, secretion and excretion. The principle of Life ("Vitae ratio") should be searched for in the purely mechanical action of the body, not in its conjunction with the soul which is of general philosophical rather than of medical interest.[98] Stahl, on the other hand, understood motion as an immaterial substance and action of the soul, migrating into the body from outside. Bodies were parts of the purely passive matter which

[97] Pagel, W., *Arch. Gesch. d. Mediz.*, 1931, XXIV, 29.

[98] Hoffmann recognises the immanent dynamic impulses in the body and objects to the Cartesian concept of its passivity, a concept which shows the origin of Stahl's Animism: Descartes' philosophy. Leibniz had attacked Sturm who, with Descartes, ruled: "Corpora esse materiam, quae mere se habeat passive, omni vi movente destitutam, hanc vero immediate a Deo ipsi communicari, adeo, ut ipse infinita sua virtute materiam ubique actuet, moveat et per ipsam in universo operetur." Hoffmann supports Leibniz' point of view. According to him a mere passive ens cannot exist in reality and is not more than an abstract product of our mind. It is also impossible that a passive ens should be able to receive or retain any impulse coming to it from an outside source, viz. the Anima, or direct divine impulses. "Universalis Dei impulsus non ipse agit omnia, sed ipse excitat corpora, ut juxta vires suas a Deo ubivis extenso impenetrabili concessas agant: inducit rebus non motum ipsum, sed necessitatem immutabilitatis ad motum, cuius motus principium tamen ipsis rebus non est mere externum, sed internum." (Epist. Leibnitianae, *loc. cit.* p. 50.) The action of spirits and souls is free, independent and therefore irregular, that of the body "ex necessitate harmonice" and therefore uniform and regular.—Leibniz, in a letter to Hoffmann (Hannover, Sept. 27th, 1699) agrees that passive entia are never found alone nor can they exist by themselves.

As to Hoffmann's doctrine and its difference from that of Stahl see: Hoffmann, De differentia Doctrinae Stahlianae et Hoffmannianae, *Opera Omnia, loc. cit.* Suppl. I, p. 438 ff. and passim.

had constantly to be preserved from decay.[99] Both Stahl's and Hoffmann's views are dualistic, and remote from van Helmont's and Leibniz' natural philosophies.

The monade acts out of itself and from its own initiative, it has "Autarkeia" and "no windows" through which anything could enter into it from the outside.[100] Similarly van Helmont's Archeus acts by its own spontaneity, according to its innate schedule which runs down to its destined end. Nature is thus "ignorant of Contraria." Nothing can fundamentally alter the Archeus.[101] It might be disturbed, however, by illusions and "appetites" which "alien ferments" elicit in the individual. These will have no influence on the being unless directed by its own archeus. In the same way, natural changes in Leibniz' monades "viennent d'un principe interne, puisqu'une cause externe ne saurait influer dans son intérieur." [102]

True to cabbalistic and neo-platonic tradition van Helmont regards the "Form" of Life which divine creation bestows on the individual being as a light or spark. Leibniz speaks of: "Fulgurations continuelles de la divinité," which give birth to the monades.[103] It is divine perfection, the "essence" which is thus conferred, but limited by the receptivity, the empirical "existence" of the creature.[104] In a similar way van Helmont pointed to the original sin as the source of all the shortcomings of creatures.

[99] We have quoted before (footnote 73) passages from van Helmont which show an anticipation of some concepts of Stahl. The latter fights like van Helmont against humoral-pathology. Not the humours themselves, not "Dyscrasia," but anomalies in their motion and circulation are the cause of disease. This is a "Perturbata idea regiminis ipsius oeconomiae animalis," terms which are, no doubt, adopted from van Helmont and his "Idea Morbosa." (see *Theoria Medica Vera,* ed. L. Choulant, Lipsiae, 1831, Vol. II, p. 16). The structure and mixture of the bodily constituents are of no significance, since the body is subject to corruption at any time in the same measure. Moreover, according to old Hippocratic wisdom just the most vigorous bodies (athletes) and the best and "floridissimus" blood are most liable to corruption which may take place within a few hours because of the heat which is preserved in the lifeless body (*loc. cit.* p. 25). Fever is a healing process which does not occur "in malignis et contagiosis." In these "Urina sana, pulsus sanus, aeger moritur." (*ib.* p. 34). Fever is directly controlled by the "Animi Pathemata." In the same way inflammation is a healing process (p. 42).

[100] Monadologie 7, Boutroux 144.

[101] Van Helmont's treatise: Natura Contrariorum Nescia.

[102] Monadologie 11, Boutroux p. 146.

[103] Monadol. 47, B. p. 167.

[104] Monadol. 42, B. p. 162.

### (d) *Divergencies*

Some points may be mentioned in which van Helmont's concept differs from Leibniz' Philosophy. They are of minor significance. Leibniz adhered to the theory of "Preformation." Everything pre-exists in the germ in a minute compass. Development means growing of these minute elements into visible organs. Van Helmont, however, may be said to have advocated the "epigenetic" point of view. He compares the Archeus with a blacksmith who actually "perambulates through all recessus of the semen and starts to transform matter according to the entelecheia of his image. Here he locates the heart, there the brain, and everywhere appoints the resident governor for the realms determined by their exigencies, parts, destinations." [105] There is obviously no material preformation, but only a "preformation of tendency" in van Helmont's view.

The perceptions and impressions which van Helmont attributed to living beings are mainly those of their own specific forms and of "alien ferments" rather than a representation of all the other monades and indeed of the whole universe which Leibniz saw in the individual monade. It should be borne in mind, however, that van Helmont subscribed to Determinism. There is "Reason and an immutable root producing certain appointed effects." In the Universe and the Semina, Ferments and Archei are the instruments of this determination as they contain "Type, Form, Motion, Hour, Vicissitudes, Tendencies, Properties, Adaptations, Relations, Changes, Death" of everything in Nature.[106]

In Leibniz' concept the whole of the world space is filled up. Therefore, every motion in it must, of necessity, influence the whole and all of its parts. Thus, Determinism accounts for the representation of the Universe in the individual monade.[107]

Leibniz clearly separated his metaphysical principles from the explanation of individual natural phenomena which, according to him, have to be given on strict physico-chemical lines. Van Helmont, however, may not have accomplished or not even attempted such

[105] Archeus Faber 6/7.
[106] Causae et Initia Natural. 24 ff.
[107] Monadol. 61.

critical separation. In his " Philosophy " scientific and metaphysical elements are mixed up.

The views which van Helmont has in common with Leibniz are obviously those which are based on his religious conviction. This may throw a particular religious light on the origin of Leibniz' Philosophy.

### (6) *Central Regulation*

As we have seen, van Helmont's basic principle in *Physiology* was vitalism prompted by religious conviction. Religious motives are recognisable even in his work on individual physiological problems. Research on the stomach and its functions is of the utmost importance to van Helmont because he has found by casual observation and theoretical consideration that here must be the seat of the chief vegetative impulses and indeed of the soul, i. e. of the divine principle governing the body. Sad news takes the appetite away, fever impairs digestion in the stomach and elicits ructus indicating some putrefaction in the stomach.[108] Nightmares are caused by rich food, they make the person unable to move without impairing their sensual perception. This shows the essential role of the stomach in motion.[109] Syncope from carbon-monoxide poisoning causes, as van Helmont experienced once himself, a sensation around the mouth of the stomach.[110] All this demonstrates the action of the stomach on the brain. This action does not lend itself to a materialistic explanation by means of vapours and fumes which were supposed to emanate from the stomach. Even with an empty stomach certain remedies (e. g. Sulfur vitrioli) acting on this organ will relieve syncope. Thus, there is no place for vapours ascending from corrupting food left in the stomach. Neither do such ascending vapours exist, nor can vapours be condensed in the brain to fluid and flow down again thereby causing the multitude of the famous " Catarrh "-diseases.[111] Disturbances of the stomach like colic and stomach ache might be followed by paralysis of the limbs or by tetanus.[112] A huge hernia

[108] Jus Duumviratus 13.

[109] Jus Duumvir. 15.

[110] Jus Duumvir. 19.

[111] Catarrhi Deliramenta passim. See translation and commentary in Pagel, W., J. B. van Helmont, 1930, *loc. cit.*

[112] Jus Duumvir. 20.

beating all attempts at reposition in spite of continuous hot fomentation became soft and amenable to reposition at once when the stomach had been treated by a wine decoction with various seeds (Coriander, Anise, Caraway, Fennel).[113] Even the intellectual faculties are largely governed by the "Duumvirate," i. e. the combined action of spleen and stomach. A man who had taken Hyoscyamus in error remained "innocens et vesanus" although the drug had been removed from the stomach by means of a vomitive. There was therefore no question of fumes ascending from remnants of the drug in the stomach to the brain. Insanity in this case was in van Helmont's opinion entirely due to the action of the stomach injured by the poison.[114] Amentia makes a man insensitive to hunger and thirst.[115] Helleborus so beneficial in mental affections is a classical vomitive, a "remedium stomachicum." Stomachica also help in cough and asthma of the old people, thereby revealing the importance of the stomach for the lung.[116] The impulse to sleep is initiated in the stomach and then carried to the brain.[117] Affections of the uterus such as Hysteria, abnormal appetites in pregnancy, Epilepsia and others are primarily elicited in the "duumvirate" of stomach and spleen. In other words: the stomach contains like a bed the Anima and hence come all vital powers.[118] The "Duumvirate" watches over the "Symmetry of Life" by means of "tender modulation." [119] The stomach is thus the central organ profoundly connected with the action of the Divine in man. Hence the duty to examine its anatomy and physiology with particular scientific care and attention. Led by these principles, van Helmont not only discovered acid as the principle of digestion in the stomach, but also, what is less well known, the particular rhythmic movement of the pylorus. The pyloric movement follows its own laws. It is different from that of other orifices such as bladder and anus, in nature and rhythm. Not unlike the uterus the Pylorus is its own Monarch endowed with total power and governed by its own "Blas," i. e. an impulse to motion and alteration such as emanating from the stars.[120] It initiates vomit-

[113] Jus Duumviratus 20.
[114] Jus Duumvir. 22.
[115] Jus Duumvir. 24.
[116] Jus Duumvir. 62.
[117] Jus Duumvir. 54.
[118] Jus Duumvir. 58.
[119] Jus Duumvir. 52.
[120] Pylorus Rector 4.

ing when it closes and sends a wave of motion over the whole organ towards the oesophagus. Hence it is by no means devoted to a retaining function or connected with Galen 's " retentive dynamis." It knows what it has to do by its own discretion, e. g. to open and relax when acid digestion has reached the end point. It thereby regulates acid digestion, it " keeps the key " to the stomach. If it remains closed too long, the over-digested food is liable to cause corruption, " alienation " and disease. If it opens too early, insufficiently digested food will cause disturbances chiefly in the veins: Tremor, palpitation, fainting, acute fevers, tumours, arthritis may thus develop. As soon as new food enters the stomach the Pylorus closes again. If some of the old food is left in the stomach, its over-digestion will upset metabolism. Hence hyperacidity results from ravenous eating. If the pylorus fails to open and causes vomiting this is because it finds (" censet ") that it would be harmful for the whole body to let this particular food through. The pylorus is thus the " Rector digestionis." [121] It cooperates in concurrence with the bile, and diarrhoea, dysentery, haemorrhoids and various other intestinal trouble develop when this " consensus " of pylorus and bile is at fault. The pylorus is subject to emotions such as fury, for example when a limb has suffered severe injury, vomiting may follow as expression of the fury of the pylorus. This will be instantly relieved when the limb is put right. Poisoning may lead to general paralysis, due to the " indignation " felt by the pylorus. Pyloric spasm may cause exudation of greenish fluid into the stomach and eventually death. Postmortem examination shows in such cases the closed or strictured pylorus—in contrast with other muscular spasms which disappear after death.[122]

The minute and advanced observation of the stomach in normal and pathological life thus offers another example of the immediate scientific significance of van Helmont's yearning to find the seat of the vegetative and life centre, which meant to him the Divine in man.

### (7) *The Origin of Diseases*

The larger part of van Helmont's work was devoted to *Pathology and Medicine*. Religious pragmatism drives him to Medicine as the

[121] Pylor. Rect. 11.

[122] Pylor. Rector 29.

ultimate aim of science and he is conscious of his vocation as physician. What *is* Disease and what are its causes? This question fundamental to Pathology and Therapy had been left unanswered by contemporary Medicine which taught the "Artificiose altercari" but in practice was unable to cure headache or tooth-caries. If objects and phenomena in nature are entities by themselves, due to the development of a specific seed, diseases, van Helmont concludes, must be also such entities and due to a specific cause of their own, their specific seed. Pathology at van Helmont's time largely followed the ancient theory which regarded man himself, i. e. the mixture of his humours, his temperament as the chief cause of disease. This varies with the faulty humour, the humoral mixture, or the "quality" which, already in normal life predominated in the patient. To van Helmont, however, the disease-entity is something outside man, an "alien-ferment" which impresses its own schedule of Life on the Archeus of the Patient. It is thus an "Idea Morbosa" acting on our internal imagination, since all transmutations and indeed all action in nature are due to the imagination of a "Form," or as Leibniz would have expressed it, to the internal perceptions experienced by the "Monade." The "Alien Ferment" thus "contaminates" the Archeus, it acts as a "Contagium." Disease becomes identical with its external cause. Such causes are: the morbid impression conveyed with the bite of a mad dog, metallic and silica dust inhaled in mines, "Recepta" taken in with food or breath such as drink, Pharmaka, poisons, suggested ideas and above all the "Retenta," i. e. products of disturbance of one of the six "Digestions."[123] There must be as many diseases as causes. This ontological and aetiological concept of diseases paves the way (a) to their *classification* and (b) to *causal therapy*. Therapy of the Ancients was directed against the wrong humours and qualities, i. e. against man and his faulty constitution. It aimed at restoring the material balance of the body and thereby to cure diseases. In van Helmont's view therapy is directed

[123] Van Helmont differentiates six "digestions": (1) Acid digestion of food in the stomach; (2) its alkalinisation in the duodenum; (3) Digestion in the liver leading to production of venous blood (Cruor); (4) Conversion of Cruor into arterial blood in the heart; (5) Production of "Vital Spirit" in the brain; (6) Assimilation and conversion of suitable material into tissue substance in the organs and their "kitchens."

against the cause. After its removal the balance of the material constituents will recur automatically. The " contagious " cause had to be washed off from the archeus, to relieve it from the alien idea so that it might recover its genuine scope and schedule. Ancient therapy largely used dietetics, laxatives, venaesection and herbs—van Helmont's therapy is based on the powerful menstrua, the great " Confortativa et Restaurativa," the chemical remedies prescribed by Paracelsus, compounds of sulfur, antimony, mercury, metallic preparations. He by no means omitted purely empirical and " magic " prescriptions such as ram's testicle and blood against pleurisy and many other items of the " Dreckapotheke." " Magic " therapy in van Helmont's Medicine, however, is deeply bound up with the recommendation of immunological treatment which is far in advance of his own time and based on the knowledge of the beneficial effect of blood of convalescents.[124]

If disease is due to an alien ferment or idea coming from outside, it will combine with that part of the body to which it has a special sympathy or affinity. To open the way for the pathogenic agent into the body, it needs a propitious " imagination " on the part of the Archeus. There are as many archei, i. e. local governors ("Archei insiti ") as organs. Disease therefore is a *local,* an organ affair.

The ability to dissolve is one of the noblest effects which Nature achieves in mastering matter. The highest aspiration of the early chemist notably van Helmont was to invent a universal solvent, the Liquor Alkahest. The main function of the Archeus is to dissolve food material conveyed with the blood and to see that no crude residue is left. The Archeus thus acts as a " Custos," as the metabolic centre of the organ. Each organ has a " kitchen " [125]—the tooth at its root, the nail in its bed, the skin in its basal layers, the stomach in the spleen. Here the Archeus separates from the blood stream what is suitable for the particular organ and converts it into tissue

[124] De magnet. vulner. curat. 50: " Curatur autem tuto et celeriter, si sanguine cuiusdam, qui semel illo morbo laboraverit, foris vel tenuiter locus inungatur. Nempe qui semel a morbo illo convaluerit, sanguinem nedum balsamicum obtinuit, unde in posterius ab eodem morbo tutus sit."

Compare van Helmont's general and special Pathology and Therapy in Pagel, W., J. B. van Helmont, *loc. cit.* 1930, pp. 75, 77, 89 ff.

[125] Catarrhi Deliramenta 31.

substance. Disturbed in this function by the illusions emanating from an " alien ferment," the archeus will lack in its power to dissolve; it will fail in its watchman's duties. Residues will appear—the anatomical changes. Disease may be also provoked by the local Archeus eliciting abnormal acid in the cruor. For example, in the pleura the cruor turning acid causes spasms with subsequent tearing and ulceration of the pleural membrane. In addition the acid cruor coagulates and forms a deposit. This leads to local obstruction of pores and channels which should be free if normal function is to be maintained.

The local origin and development of diseases exclude the " Folly of Catarrh " and the action of " Vapours " which dominated Pathology for a long time after van Helmont's death.

Van Helmont thus became the actual founder of modern Pathology. It was he who taught the differentiation of diseases according to local changes (Morbid Anatomy) and external causes (Aetiology). His concept was in many points in advance of that of the famous " Father of Pathology " Morgagni who simply referred symptoms (not diseases) to anatomical organ changes. It is true that he thereby greatly furthered the art of clinical diagnosis.

I have endeavoured to show that the whole of van Helmont's Pathology down to his " Localism," Aetiology and new Therapy is based on his general philosophical and metaphysical view, on his concept of Semina and of disposed matter as the vector of specificity. Fundamental positions in Medicine thus grew out of his religious conviction, his belief in creation.

## (8) *Biological Time and Theology*

Van Helmont's religious conviction of Nature as the embodiment of created specific seeds led him to an ingenious anticipation of the modern concept of Biological Time. He propounds this in a treatise (*De Tempore*) which has never had the attention which it actually deserves as an attempt at linking up Time with the specific life forces of the individual. I hope to give a translation and commentary of this treatise elsewhere,[126] but wish to summarise it briefly

[126] Pagel, W., Van Helmont, *De Tempore* and the History of the Biological Concept of Time. With notes on the Greek concepts referred to in *De Temp.* by Helene Weiss, *Osiris*. In Press. Summary in *Isis*, 1942, XXXIII, 621.

here, because nowhere in van Helmont's work does the close interdependence of religious belief, philosophical outlook and scientific achievement appear as striking as here.

Like all treatises by van Helmont it sets out with the somewhat weary and extensive refutation of the doctrine of the Schools which is based on Aristotle's Physics.[127] Aristotle had linked up time with motion, Time counts motion, he had said. In van Helmont's opinion, however, time is no less an entity than anything else in nature. Days, hours and seasons are measuring units, invented by the human mind. They are not Time. This cannot be defined by mathematical construction of a continuum of infinite points, by the length or shortness, by priority or posteriority of something nor anything which can be measured. Real time which should be called " Duration " is created by God and inherent in the seed of each object in Nature. It determines the specific life rhythm and life duration of the individual by governing its motions. " For all variety of whatever alterations depends upon the slowness or celerity of motions. The duration of motion is therefore essentially, intimately and originally immanent in the seeds as their form and directing principle." [128] It is the variety of biological processes by which time may be gauged. As the seeds of the living beings are created by God from eternal times, time is eternal and devoid of succession.[129] It represents the creator in the creatures, but is not only the sum total of this something in all creatures; it has an existence independent of and above the creatures, it is something " absolute " and divine.

These religious-metaphysical considerations lead van Helmont to a critical examination of time measuring as actually practised in his days. He realises the fallacies of clocks which are subject to temperature influence and recommends the use of the pendulum. He discovers the significance of the length of the pendulum for its velocity and states that the duration of the swings is equal, although he believes that their range is diminished gradually.[130]

[127] *De Tempore* 1-16 and 20-24.

[128] " Duratio . . . seminibus quippe universis ab initio inest, nedum principium cuiusvis motus, sed et sua durationum determinata periodus, cuique motui propria; cum omnis varietas quarumcumque alterationum pendeat ex tarditate vel celeritate motuum. Igitur motuum duratio includitur seminibus essentialiter, intime originaliterque velut principium formale atque directivum eorundem." *De Tempore* 18.

[129] *Ibidem* 30.

[130] *Ibidem* 48-50.

The usual Aristotelian and scholastic concept of Time, the undue attention devoted to the movement of the stars in connection with the study and measuring of time, has secured the dominating position of the doctrine of " Critical Days " in Medicine, ever since early Pythagorean days. The constellation of the celestial bodies and particularly the influence of the moon had been made responsible for disease to take a favorable or unfavorable turn. Galen said that crises on a sixth day are dangerous and difficult to obtain, but easy and propitious on the seventh day, the sixth being similar to a cruel tyrant and the seventh to a wise and just king.[131] Here again van Helmont sees the Schoolmen resort to the analogies of Macrocosm and Microcosm and thereby to crude mechanistic and monistic explanations. These were bound to rouse van Helmont's opposition which was prompted by his better vitalistic and pluralistic insight and conviction.[132]

Ancient Therapy was expectative. It welcomed crises as an indication of the " Healing Power of Nature," its attempts to drive out harmful humours. In van Helmont's opinion crises should be avoided and cure accomplished before crisis sets in. There are no humours against which nature should " fight," there is no place for " Contraria " in Nature, there is only the pathogenic agent which should be removed by active intervention of the physician. Not constellation of stars, not critical days, i. e. regularities which are supposed to govern *all* diseases, but the *specific* rhythms and " life-times " of the different disease-entities should the Physician study.

Linking up time with the Divine spark of Life in the individual, with the time of life and the quality of the biological processes, van Helmont uses arguments reminiscent of those propounded in modern times by Bergson [133] and biologists and sociologists who deny that

[131] De diebus decretoriis I, 4; ed. Kuehn, Vol. IX, p. 785; I, 2, p. 774; II, 2, p. 846; II, 8, p. 875; I, 5, p. 792. Compare detail in A. M. Baumgarten-Crusius, *Periodologie oder Lehre von den periodischen Veraenderungen im Leben des gesunden und kranken Menschen.* Halle, 1836, pp. 54 ff. and also p. 264.

[132] *De Tempore* 52.

[133] *Time and Free Will. Essays on the immediate data of consciousness.* Transl. by F. L. Pogson. London, 1910, p. 107. Measuring time in the usual sense is counting " simultaneities." It is the internal process of organisation of conscious states which is real duration and produces succession. Bergson's time is

Time has the purely quantitative character of " astronomical time." Indeed, the speed of biological processes varies, for example with the size of the animal or with its age. As Joseph Needham puts it: " Mouse time must bear the same or a similar relation to elephant time as mouse spatial magnitudes to elephant spatial magnitudes.[134] The calendar of primitive people differs in agricultural, hunting and pastoral groups (Sorokin and Merton).[135] Biological processes form a clock by themselves which gives more and truer information about Time than the ordinary—conventional—time units. These indicate " empty," quantitatively equal periods which are unequal biologically and sociologically.

Nothing shows the whole character and scope of van Helmont's work as impressively as *De Tempore*. All that van Helmont designs, finds and teaches, he does for the sake of research on Life, for Biology, in the widest sense. For he regards Life as direct emanation from the creating God and therefore not only the noblest but also the only subject which opens the way to scientific and at the same time to eternal truth. Van Helmont's biological bent is due to his religious zeal, and his scientific achievement the fruit of his religious conviction.

thus much more bound up with the conscious self than van Helmont's Time which is the rhythm of the biological processes specific for the individual, its predestined life-time. Moreover van Helmont's Time has a theological significance as it is identical with eternity, unmeasurable and devoid of succession. Nevertheless there are striking parallels, e. g. van Helmont's argument that categories of space are introduced when we try to measure time (*De Tempore* 31).

[134] For " Biological Time " compare: Joseph Needham, Chemical Heterogony and the ground plan of animal growth. *Biol. Review,* 1934, IX, 79. Lambert, R. and Teissier, S., *Ann. Physic. & Physiol. Chemistry,* 1927, II, 212. As to " Sociological Time " see: Sorokin, P. A. and Merton, R. K., footnote 135.

[135] Social Time. *Amer. J. Sociol.*, 1937, XLII, 615.

# IV

## Paracelsus' ätherähnliche Substanzen und ihre pharmakologische Auswertung an Hühnern

### Sprachgebrauch *(henbane)* und Konrad von Megenbergs *Buch der Natur* als mögliche Quellen

### *1. Das ätherähnliche Präparat des Paracelsus*

Durch die Arbeiten des Vaters der *Chemiegeschichte*, Hermann Kopp, ist Paracelsus in der Entdeckungsgeschichte des Äthers heimisch geworden[1]. Nach Kopp scheint Paracelsus' *Spiritus vitrioli antepileptici* eine Mischung von Weingeist und Äther gewesen zu sein. Kopp führt die Stelle aus Paracelsus' Traktat *Von den natürlichen Dingen* an: «So ist das mein Proceß, daß der spiritus vini werde in dem Vitriol imbibiret, nachfolgend destillirt, wie ich angezeigt habe, von den feuchten und trocknen spiritibus.»[2]

Wie die Anhänger des Paracelsus diese Stelle auslegten, ergibt sich nach Kopp aus der wenig beachteten Vorschrift, die A. F. Pezoldt 1719 in den *Ephemeriden der Deutschen Naturforscher* für die Darstellung des «Spiritus vitrioli antepileptici Paracelsi et peculiaris sulphuris vitrioli anodyni» gab: «man solle calcinirten Vitriol mit Weingeist tränken und dann destillieren; zuerst gehe der Weingeist, dann die Schwefelsäure über; es verbreite sich dabei ein schwefliger Geruch; das Destillat soll man mit dem dritten Teil des rückständigen Colcothars nochmals destillieren: durch diese Operation

[1] H. Kopp, *Geschichte der Chemie*, vol. IV, Braunschweig 1847, p. 300. Siehe auch *ib.* p. 312.

[2] *Ettliche Tractatus.* I Von Natürlichen dingen, vom terpentin ... vom schwefel, vom vitriol, vom arsenik (? 1525), cap. 8, ed. Sudhoff, vol. II, p. 154.

wird ein durchdringender flüchtiger Spiritus gewonnen, der durch sein angenehmes Aroma konzentriertem oder Spanischem Wein nahekommt (hac encheiresi impetratur spiritus volatilis penetrans, odore grato vinum malvaticum vel hispanicum aemulans)».[3]

Für die weitere Literatur, die im Anschluß an diese Feststellungen von Kopp entstanden ist, verweisen wir auf die vom Verfasser gegebenen Darstellungen[4]. Wir möchten aber noch auf die neueste kritische und umfassende *Chemiegeschichte* von PARTINGTON hinweisen. In dieser ist der ursprünglich von Kopp zutage geörderte Sachverhalt übernommen worden[5].

Die einschlägige paracelsische Schrift, die wir zitiert haben, wird von SUDHOFF zu den frühen Werken von Paracelsus gerechnet und um etwa 1525 angesetzt[6]. In ihr hat Paracelsus seinem Präparat einen weiten Raum gewidmet – er spricht von der wunderbaren beruhigenden Wirkung, seiner Heilwirkung bei Epilepsie, einschließlich der prophylaktischen Verhinderung von Anfällen und – an anderer Stelle – von seiner Dämpfung der heftigen Paroxysmen bei der Hundswut[7]. Besonders bedeutungsvoll sind die theoretischen Folgerungen, die er aus diesen therapeutischen Effekten für die Entstehung der Epilepsie zieht. Entsprach es doch seinen iso- und homöopathischen Grundsätzen, anzunehmen, daß die Ursache einer Krankheit mit ihrem Heilmittel identisch sein kann. So sagt Paracelsus, daß die Ursache der Epilepsie ein *Odor stupefactivus* ist, der in die Zellen des Hirns aufsteigt. Dieser *Odor* unterscheidet sich von anderen Narkotika, wie *Hyoscyamus* (Jusquiamus), Opium, Mandragora, durch seine korrosiven und trunkenmachenden Eigenschaften. Dies aber ist der *Sulphur vitrioli*. Paracelsus fährt fort: «Welcher den selbigen isset nach den coniunctionibus

[3] KOPP, *l.c.* (in Anm. 1), p. 301–302.

[4] W. PAGEL, Review of K. SUDHOFF, Bibliographia Paracelsica (Neudruck), in *Bull. Hist. Med. XXXIII* (1959) 481. *id.* Das Medizinische Weltbild des Paracelsus. Seine Zusammenhänge mit Neuplatonismus und Gnosis (*Kosmosophie*, herausgegeben von K. GOLDAMMER, Band I), Wiesbaden 1962, p. 22–24. Siehe auch die dort zitierte Arbeit von TREVOR ROBINSON, On the Nature of Sweet Oil of Vitriol, *J. Hist. Med. XIV* (1959) 231–233 (die Substanz war wahrscheinlich eine Mischung von Diäthyläther und Diäthylsulfat).

[5] J. R. PARTINGTON, *History of Chemistry*, vol. II, London 1961, p. 150. Hier heißt es: "Paracelsus speaks of distilling spirit of wine with vitriol. This was probably ether, since he had just spoken of a 'sulphur embryonatum' in vitriol which is stupefactive, narcotic and with an agreeable taste. Chickens will eat it whereupon they sleep for a moderately long time and wake again without injury."

[6] SUDHOFF, *Paracelsus-Ausgabe*, vol. II, p. IX–XV (*l.c.* in Anm. 2).

[7] Wirkung bei den Paroxysmen der Hundswut: *Große Wundartzney*, lib. I, tract. 3, cap. 1., ed. SUDHOFF, vol. X, p. 170.

der gestirn, der falt in den fallenden paroxysmum. und die tiere, so etlicher art sind, als wislin, eichorn, auch die löwen, die fallen auch darein ...[8]» Im Leibe liegt Sulphur vitrioli – wenn dieser «exaltiert» wird durch Konjunktion mit seinem «Ascendenten», d.h. dem, was ihm in der äußeren Welt entspricht, dann ist die Krankheit fertig. Ihre Ursache ist nicht der Mensch, sondern der Sulphur in seinem Körper – die «Materie im unteren Himmel» – und ihre Aktivierung durch den von außen eindringenden gleichartigen «Anzünder» im «oberen Himmel».

Schon Kopp hat darauf hingewiesen, daß Paracelsus wohl nicht der erste war, der Schwefel mit Alkohol hat reagieren lassen, sondern daß dies schon von alchemischen Lullisten erwähnt worden ist[9]. Bei diesen aber finden sich keine Aussagen, die auf ätherähnliche Stoffe und vor allem deren organische Wirkungen hinweisen.

Paracelsus hat also vielleicht ein traditionelles Verfahren in seinen Dienst gestellt. Er hat aber dieses in origineller Weise ausgebaut zu einem Prozeß mit wiederholbarem Ergebnis, nämlich der Gewinnung einer für seine Zeit chemisch und pharmakologisch gut charakterisierten Substanz. Er hat nicht nur ihre chemischen Eigenschaften studiert, sondern auch ihre prophylaktische und kurative Wirkung bei Epilepsie und verwandten Zuständen erkannt.

Die chemiegeschichtliche Zuordnung des paracelsischen Sulphur vitrioli zu den ätherähnlichen Substanzen und Paracelsus' Stellung in der Entdeckungsgeschichte des Äthers ist somit durch die Autorität berufener Chemiehistoriker von Kopp zu Partington beglaubigt.

### *II. Paracelsus' Versuche mit dem Spiritus vitrioli an Hühnern*

In der Geschichte des paracelsischen Spiritus vitrioli verdient ein weiterer Punkt unsere Aufmerksamkeit: die Beobachtungen, die Paracelsus mit seinem Präparat an Hühnern vorgenommen hat. Diese Versuche haben Paracelsus die milde Wirkung seines Präparates im Gegensatz zu den landläufigen und giftigen Anodyna bestätigt: «das alle sulphura von den vitriolatis salibus stupefactiva seind, narcotica, anodyna, somnifera, und aber mit einer solchen proprietet, das an dem ort die somniferisch art, so

[8] *Elf Traktat* – 10: Vom fallend – Causa, ed. Sudhoff, vol. I, p. 143.

[9] Kopp, *Geschichte der Chemie, l.c.,* vol. IV, p. 299, mit Hinweis auf: Epistola de accurtatione Lapidis Benedicti missa anno 1412 Roberto Anglorum Regi, in Manget, *Bibliotheca Chemica et Curiosa,* Vol. I, 1702, p. 865.

ruwig und so milt hingêt, das on allen schaden sich abzeucht, nichts auf opiatische wirkung, als in iusquiamo, papavere, mandragora etc, sonder gar milt, tugentlich on all infectif ... zum andern hat er eine süße, das in die hüner all essen und aber entschlafen auf ein zeit, on schaden wider aufstont.»[10]

Ist Paracelsus in dieser sozusagen tierexperimentellen Ergänzung seines therapeutischen Verfahrens originell gewesen, und wenn nicht, läßt sich etwas über seine Quellen mutmaßen?

In dieser Frage verdanken wir einen neuen Hinweis den Studien von G. Eis[11]. Dieser verneint die Originalität des Paracelsus bezüglich der Heranziehung von Tierbeobachtungen. Es läßt sich, wie er sagt, «nachweisen, daß man schon viel früher Tiere (auch bereits Hühner) mit verschiedenen Substanzen (auch mit alkoholischen) betäubt hat». Dafür sei es nötig, die den Frühdrucken vorausgehenden Handschriften zu berücksichtigen. Eis verweist auf den Erfahrungsschatz der Fischer und Jäger, in dem die Verwendung von Tollködern von jeher eine große Rolle gespielt hat. In mittelalterlichen Handschriften werden von benutzten Pflanzengiften genannt: Bilsensamen, Schöllkraut, Eibennadeln, Tollkirschen, Eisenhut (die zum Vergiften von Wölfen geeignete Sorte hieß «Wolfswurz»), Fliegenpilze, Mistel, Herbstzeitlose, Meerzwiebel (Scilla noch heute als Rattengift benutzt). Die Beobachtungen waren zum Teil recht genau; z.B. wird in einem der zweiten Hälfte des 15. Jahrhunderts angehörigen Manuskript von einem Bilsenkrautköder für Fische bemerkt, daß die Lähmung zwei bis drei Tage dauert, während «alle möglichen Vögel», also auch – wie Eis schließt – Hühner, durch Weizenkörner, getränkt mit Rindergalle, Hanföl und Leinöl, nur auf eine halbe Stunde betäubt wurden. Von chemischen Giften werden in einem etwas älteren Codex gemahlenes Glas, Mausgift – wahrscheinlich arsenhaltiger Hüttenrauch – und sodann Arsenik und Bleiglätte zu Tierfang und Raubwildbekämpfung angeführt («Wolfskugeln-Rezepte»). Meister Egidius ließ pflanzliche, tierische und chemische Substanzen mischen, und wir finden auch Angaben bezüglich der Dosis, die auf Tierbeobachtungen beruhen müssen. Kugeln von der Größe einer Walnuß werden als für Wölfe, von Haselnußgröße als für Füchse tödlich angesehen. Eine Eintragung über die Betäubung zu fangender Rebhühner in einer weiteren Handschrift läßt sich für die Zeit vor 1500 ansetzen. Der Autor des Rezepts läßt Weizen-

[10] Von den natürlichen Dingen, cap. VII, vom Schwefel, ed. Sudhoff, vol. II, p. 133.

[11] G. Eis, Zur Beurteilung der Tierversuche des Paracelsus, *Forsch. u. Fortschr. XXXVIII* (1964) 16–20.

körner in Met sieden und sich damit vollsaugen – «das entspricht dem paracelsischen Imbibieren», sagt Eis. Außerdem wird das von jeher benutzte Bilsenkraut verwandt. Die Benutzung von Met in diesem Rezept zeige, daß, wie später von Paracelsus, Alkohol zur Anwendung kam, ebenso wie schwefelhaltige Verbindungen (nämlich rote Arsenik, $As_4S_4$, «arsenicum vel auripigmentum vel hüttrich», Realgar), z.B. durch Meister Egidius.

Unsere Kenntnis von den unmittelbaren Quellen individueller paracelsischer Lehren sind noch immer mangelhaft, und schon deshalb sind die Feststellungen von Eis von größtem Interesse. Es ist plausibel, daß Paracelsus mit Rezepten zur Tierbetäubung oder Tötung aus der volkstümlichen Überlieferung der Jäger und Fischer, aber auch ähnlichen in Gelehrtenkreisen überlieferten Erfahrungen vertraut war, und daß solche Kenntnisse bei seinen pharmakologischen Tierbeobachtungen Pate gestanden haben. Freilich handelt es sich bei den angeführten chemischen Substanzen im wesentlichen nicht um Narkotika, sondern um tödliche Gifte, im Gegensatz zu den Pflanzenmitteln. Die Verwendung von Met in einem Rezept und die mögliche Benutzung von schwefelhaltigem Arsenik in anderen Rezepten läßt sich kaum mit der bewußten Herstellung eines Destillationspräparates von Weingeist und Schwefel durch Paracelsus vergleichen. Schließlich handelt es sich um Rezepte zum Fange oder zur Tötung von Tieren. Hühner werden nicht spezifiziert, nur Rebhühner und «Vögel aller Art» («für tuben oder für was vögel du wilt»), worunter auch Hühner gemeint sein können.

### *III. Bilsenkraut – «Hühner-Tod» (henbane, hannebane, mort aux poules)*

Ich glaube, daß man ein präparacelsisches Paradigma anführen kann, das noch näher an die Verwendung von Hühnern bei der Ausprobierung eines Narkotikums durch Paracelsus heranführt. Ich habe darauf schon kurz einmal hingewiesen[12].

Es ist das altenglische Wort für Bilsenkraut *(Hyoscyamus,* Jusquiamus). Es heißt: *henbane,* zu deutsch: *Tod der Hühner.* Das früheste Vorkommen dieses Wortes ist durch ein Vokabular von ungefähr 1265 bezeugt[13]. Es

[12] W. Pagel, *Paracelsus.* An Introduction to Philosophical Medicine in the Era of the Renaissance, Karger, Basel/New York 1958, p. 277, Anm. 247.

[13] T. Wright, *Anglo-Saxon and Old English Vocabularies,* second edition by R. P. Wülcker, 1884, p. 559/9. Zitiert nach: *The Oxford English Dictionary* (13 vols), 1933, unter: Henbane. Der Verfasser ist für diese Angaben bezüglich Henbane Dr. F. N. L. Poynter, Bibliotheksdirektor der Wellcome Medical Historical Library, London, verpflichtet.

heißt dort: «Jusquiamus ... i hennebone.» Die nächste Erwähnung ist: Bartholomaeus Trevisa, *De proprietatibus rerum,* wo es heißt: "Aristotel ... seyeþ þat þe seed of hen bane is poyson."[14] Eine weitere Stelle aus dem 15. Jahrhundert lautet: "For the goute ... tak leves of the henbane."[15]

Das englische Wort *henbane* ist ins Französische übernommen worden. *Hanebane* wird als Äquivalent für *jusquiame* – Bilsenkraut – in Godefroy, *Lexique de l'ancien Français,* gegeben, als eine direkte Anleihe aus dem Englischen[16]. Die zusätzliche Angabe, daß es nicht vor dem Ende des 16. Jahrhunderts gebraucht worden zu sein scheint, ist m.E. fraglich, da man in der *Historia Stirpium* von Leonhard Fuchs schon 1542 findet: «Germanis Bilsamkraut, vel simpliciter Bilsen *(Gallis Jusquiame, ou Hanebane)*[16a].

Außerdem gibt es das Wort: *Mort aux poules,* wie es sich z.B. in Blancards *Lexicon medicum* unter *Hyoscyamus* findet[17]. Eine analoge Bildung fand ich in Toxites *Onomastica* von 1574. Dort heißt es unter Bilsenkraut: «Gall(ice): Hannebane, Endormie, Jusquiame, *mort aux oyes,* fibue de porc.»[18] Hier werden also nicht Hühner, sondern Gänse mit der schädigenden Wirkung des Bilsenkrautes epigrammatisch verbunden.

Nach alledem war die Giftwirkung des Bilsenkrautes auf Hühner dem mittelalterlichen Sprachgebrauch geläufig, und es liegt nahe, daß dieser Sprachgebrauch dem weitgereisten Paracelsus bekannt war, es ist nicht unwahrscheinlich, daß er für die Auswahl seines Versuchstieres bezüglich seines narkotischen Präparates bestimmend geworden ist.

[14] *Engl. Transl. XVII,* 87 (Tollemach MS), zitiert nach *The Oxford English Dictionary.*

[15] T. Wright and J. O. Halliwell, *Reliquiae antiquae.* Scraps from ancient manuscripts, vol. I (1841–1843), p. 55.

[16] Freundlichst dem Verfasser mitgeteilt von Dr. Gweneth Whitteridge, Edinburgh.

[16a] Zitiert nach *De historia stirpium commentarii insignes ... Leonharto Fuchsio medico ... autore,* B. Arnollet, Lugduni 1549, p. 790.

[17] *Stephani Blancardi Lexicon Medicum Tripartitum,* Editio novissima, Lipsiae 1777, p. 629. – Ich verdanke Dr. T. W. Stearn vom Natural History Museum, London, den Hinweis auf Rolland, *Flore Populaire,* vol. VIII (1910), wo «Mort aux Poules» als alter Sprachgebrauch für Belgien und den Haut-Marne-Bezirk angegeben wird, während in der Normandie das englische «Henbane» übernommen worden war. – Bei Blancard heißt es: «Gallice: Jusquiame, Hannebanne, de l'Endormi, la Mort aux poules.»

[18] *Onomastica II:* I. Philosophicum, Medicum, Synonymum; II. *Theophrasti Paracelsi,* Argentorati 1574, p. 255. – Nach Rolland, *Flore Populaire, l. c.* findet sich das gleiche in Adrian Junius, *Nomenclator omnium rerum nomina indicans,* 1577 (Mort aux oyes), und nach altem französischen Sprachgebrauch auch: Mort aux oisons – junge Gänse.

Es ging ja Paracelsus nicht darum, ein Tier mit seinem Präparate fangfähig zu machen oder auszurotten, sondern um den Vergleich seiner Wirkung mit bekannten Narkotika. Es war also eine echte pharmakologische Prüfung, und für diese mußten Hühner besonders geeignet erscheinen, da ihre Empfindlichkeit gegenüber Bilsenkraut durch den Sprachgebrauch sozusagen sprichwörtlich war.

### *IV. Konrad von Megenbergs «Buch der Natur» als eine mögliche Quelle*

Konrad von Megenberg (1309–1374) war der erste große Autor über Naturdinge in deutscher Sprache; sein großes *Buch der Natur,* um 1349 bis 1351, ist eine kritische Modifikation und zum Teil freie Übersetzung des *De natura rerum* von Thomas von Chantimpré ( ? 1204–1271/80). Konrad hat eine Reihe origineller Beobachtungen und auch theologische und astrologische Erklärungen beigesteuert[19]. Sein Buch war ungemein verbreitet, wie die große Zahl der Handschriften (17 in der Münchener Bibliothek allein) und Inkunabeldrucke bezeugt. Von letzteren gibt es sechs, die in Augsburg erschienen sind[20].

Konrad von Megenbergs *Buch der Natur* hat ohne Zweifel den *Liber principiorum,* das sogenannte *Spinnen- und Schlangenbuch,* das sich im paracelsischen Schriften-Corpus befindet, beeinflußt[21]. Es gilt zwar nicht als «echt», aber enthält anerkanntermaßen echt paracelsische Gedankengänge. In dem «echten» Buch *De imaginibus* hat Paracelsus zur Frage des natürlichen oder künstlichen Ursprunges der auf Felsen, Steine, Höhlen eingegrabenen Bilder Stellung genommen. Er hat sich für den ersteren entschieden und sich damit auf die Seite Konrads gestellt – denn dies ist einer der Punkte, in denen der letztere seinem Vorbild Thomas von Chantimpré kritisch gegenübersteht. Es ist nicht unwahrscheinlich, daß auch

19 Bezüglich der ausgedehnten Literatur über Konrad von Megenberg verweise ich auf: Ludwig Choulant, *Graphische Incunabeln für Naturgeschichte und Medizin,* Leipzig 1858, p. 99–122. – George Sarton, *Introduction to the History of Science Baltimore 1927–48,* vol. III (1947) p. 817.

20 Choulant und Sarton, *l.c.* siehe auch F. Pfeiffer, in seiner Ausgabe *Das Buch der Natur von Konrad von Megenberg.* Die erste Naturgeschichte in deutscher Sprache, Stuttgart 1861, p. V seq.

21 *Liber principiorum,* zuerst veröffentlicht 1570, in Sudhoffs Ausgabe, vol. XIV, p. 499 bis 512. Die Übereinstimmung mit Konrad bezieht sich auf die Heranziehung (in cap. 5, p. 503) von Techel, dem angeblichen Verfasser eines Steinbuchs. Siehe W. Pagel, Paracelsus and Techellus the Jew, *Bull. Hist. Med. XXXIV* (1960), 274–277.

dieses «echte» Buch des Corpus genau wie das «unechte» *Spinnen- und Schlangenbuch* von Konrads *Buch der Natur* beeinflußt ist[22].

War vielleicht Konrad von Megenberg auch eine Quelle bei der pharmakologischen Vergleichung, die Paracelsus mit seinem ätherähnlichen Präparat und bekannten Narkotika bei Hühnern vorgenommen hat?

Manches scheint auch dafür zu sprechen. Wir finden bei Konrad, daß Sperlinge – hitzige und zu Zorn geneigte Tiere – in manchen Ländern an Epilepsie erkranken («daz vallend leit»). In den meisten Fällen sei dies die Folge des Genusses von Bilsenkrautsamen («daz geschiht allermaist dâ von, daz si ezzent den sâmen iusquiami, daz haizt pilsensâm»)[23].

Damit hat Konrad eine rationale Erklärung für den im Mittelalter verbreiteten Glauben gegeben, daß Sperlinge zu Epilepsie neigen. In seiner Monographie über die Geschichte der Epilepsie hat TEMKIN diesen Punkt hervorgehoben und die Verbreitung dieses Glaubens schon vor Konrad belegt[23a].

Entsprechend heißt es weiter bei Konrad vom Bilsenkraut, daß sein Same gut zum Schlafen ist und daß Vögel, die das Korn essen, so fest zu schlafen anfangen, daß man sie mit der Hand fängt. Hier stoßen wir wieder auf den von Eis aus der handschriftlichen Tradition angeführten Tatbestand[24]. Beim Menschen, fährt Konrad fort, kann das Bilsenkraut tödlich wirken und Schlaftrunkenheit (Lethargie) und Vergeßlichkeit verursachen[25].

Wir gaben oben die Stelle aus den *Elf Traktat* des Paracelsus, in der er den die menschliche Epilepsie hervorrufenden Stoff mit der Wirkung von Bilsenkraut und ähnlichen narkotischen pflanzlichen Giften vergleicht. Zwar nennt Paracelsus in diesem Zusammenhange keine Vögel (auch keine Hühner), sondern «wislin, eichorn, auch die löwen». Außerdem legt er den

[22] *De imaginibus*, cap. 7, ed. SUDHOFF, vol. XIII, p. 373–375. Siehe W. PAGEL, *l.c.*, 1960 (in Anm. 21).

[23] *Buch der Natur*, lib. III, cap. 61: von der sperken, ed. PFEIFFER, p. 220.

[23a] O. TEMKIN, *The Falling Sickness*. A History of Epilepsy from the Greeks to the Beginnings of Modern Neurology, Baltimore 1945, p. 169, mit Hinweis auf Evang. Matthei X, 29 als möglichen Ursprung, ferner eine von VALESCUS von Tharanta an einem «epileptischen» Sperling ausgeführte Sektion *(Philonium I*, 18, Venetiis 1523, fol. 16 recto), ferner *The Ancren Riwle*, einen Traktat über die Regeln und Pflichten klösterlichen Lebens aus dem 13. Jahrhundert ed. und tr. J. MORTON, The Camden Soc., London 1853, p. 177.

[24] Siehe oben, Anm. 11.

[25] *Buch der Natur*, lib. V, cap. 44, ed. PFEIFFER, p. 404.

Unterschied dar, der zwischen der wahren Ursache der Epilepsie, nämlich dem Sulphur vitrioli, und den ähnlich, aber doch nicht genau so wirkenden pflanzlichen Narkotika, wie Bilsenkraut (iusquiamus), Opium, Mandragora, Schierling und dergleichen bestehen soll. Die Verknüpfung der Epilepsie mit dem Bilsenkraut sowohl bei Konrad wie bei Paracelsus bleibt aber eine beachtenswerte Tatsache. Vielleicht war es die Wiedergabe dieser Tradition durch Konrad, die Paracelsus bei seinen Darlegungen im kritischen Sinne beeinflußt hat.

Es gibt noch eine weitere Stelle bei Paracelsus, die in unserem Zusammenhang von Interesse ist. Paracelsus spricht hier von den Wahnsinnigen, die durch Speise oder Trank ihrer Vernunft beraubt worden sind («de vesanis ..., die do durch essen und trinken von irer vernunft komen und zerrütt werden»). Für diese gibt es zwei Kuren: eine «specialis» und die andere «sedativa». Die «arznei specialis» soll von dem gleichen sein, «davon das essen kompt». Angenommen, Katzenhirn sei imstande, Unsinnigkeit hervorzurufen, dann ist die spezifische Arznei gegen die letztere eine Substanz, die Katzenhirn vergiftet («töde»). Denn es gäbe einige Kräuter, die Katzen töten, weil sie gegen das Katzenhirn «sonderlich specificirt» sind. Es sind dann diese Kräuter, die die durch Katzenhirn hervorgerufene Unsinnigkeit spezifisch heilen. Für die sedative Kur werden Quintessenzen von Gold, Silber oder Chelidonium empfohlen, die mit Quintessenzen von Opium, Mandragora, Bilsenkraut (iusquiamus), Papaver, Lolch *(lolium)* vermischt sind. Dies sind die großen «Confortativa», die die Unsinnigkeit aus dem spiritus vitae entfernen, wozu einfache Purgativa unnütz sind. Das gilt auch von der Therapie der durch Zaubertränke verursachten Schäden, wie Liebeskrankheit, die «spezifisch» kuriert wird[26]. Vielleicht liegen auch diesen Vorschriften Beobachtungen an Tieren, besonders Katzen, zugrunde.

Von weiteren Parallelen zwischen den von Konrad von Megenberg überlieferten Traditionen und paracelsischen Lehren läßt sich noch manches z.B. in dem Kapitel von den «Wundermenschen», d.h. Schwachsinnigen, und Mißbildungen auffinden. Wir können darauf nur kurz eingehen. Konrad diskutiert die Ansicht, daß Wundergeburten wie die Onocentauri durch Vermischung des Menschen mit dem Vieh entstehen («daz diu wunder komen von den widernâtürlichen werken des menschen, die sich ver-

[26] *7. Buch in der Arznei.* Von den krankheiten, die der Vernunft berauben, Meth. II, cap. 5, ed. SUDHOFF, vol. II, p. 451.

mischent zuo dem vich»)[27]. Konrad führt seine eigene Meinung («nu sprich ich Megenbergaer») dahin ein, daß die Wundermenschen von zweierlei Art sind: «gesêlet und etleich niht». Die letzteren sind solche, die etwas von einer menschlichen Figur, aber keine Seele haben. Die «gesêlten» zerfallen in zwei Gruppen: solche, die körperlich, und solche, die seelisch abnorm sind. Für beide Formen ist die Sünde Adams verantwortlich zu machen. Zu den «gesêlten» Wundermenschen rechnet Konrad die kongenital Schwachsinnigen («tôren», «muriones») und die in Wildnis (Wäldern) zusammen mit Tieren Aufgewachsenen.

Weibliche Unkeuschheit bewirkt Teilung des menschlichen Samens, mit dem Ergebnis von Zwillingen, oder wenn sich der Same nicht vollkommen teilt, von Dicephali.

Ein weiterer wichtiger Punkt mit Rücksicht auf Paracelsus ist die Beziehung, die im Buch der Natur hergestellt ist zwischen der Entstehung der Wundermenschen und den Sternen oder genauer: der «stern-kraft in der muoter leib». Es ist diese Sternkraft, auf die die Beimischung tierischer Formen zu einer sonst menschlichen Gestalt zurückzuführen ist, z.B. die Geburt eines menschlichen Fetus mit Tierkopf[28].

Nicht-geseelte Wundermenschen können menschlichen Ursprunges sein («von den menschen geporn»). Ihre Entstehung beruht auf Sternenkräften, die durch Adams und unsere Sünden Gewalt über uns erlangt haben – ohne solche Sünde wären sie machtlos geblieben. Diejenigen, die nicht menschlichen Ursprungs sind, gehören zu den Affen und Meerkatzen – Wesen, die nicht «adamisch» sind.

Vieles bei Paracelsus verrät eine enge Verwandtschaft mit diesen von Konrad überlieferten Vorstellungen – obschon Paracelsus vielem davon seine eigene Wendung gegeben hat, meist in biologischem Sinne.

Paracelsus spricht auch vom Geseelten und Ungeseelten. Bekannt ist seine Theorie, daß die Nymphen und anderen «Elementargeister» «als Menschen ansehen zu sein, und doch nicht auß Adam» und daß sie der Seele entbehren[29]. Entsprechend gehören auch die Mißbildungen mit tierähnlichen Formen den ungeseelten Wesen zu. Ferner spricht auch Paracelsus wie Konrad von einer Spaltung, die sich im Samen vollzieht. Er

[27] *Buch der Natur*, lib. VIII, Von den Wundermenschen, ed. PFEIFFER, p. 486.

[28] *ib.*, p. 488.

[29] *Liber de nymphis, sylphis, pygmaeis et salamandris et de caeteris spiritibus*, tract. I, cap. 1, ed. SUDHOFF, vol. *XIV*, p. *118*, ed. ROBERT BLASER *(Altdeutsche Übungstexte*, vol. XVI), Bern 1960, p. 11.

sagt, daß der Mensch zweifach ist: ein Vieh und ein Mensch. Daher kann er viehische Gestalt erzeugen. Dies ist durch das Vorkommen von homunculus-artigen Monstra bezeugt. Diese kommen zustande durch Spaltung von Leib und Seele, so daß ein Geseeltes und ein Ungeseeltes – der Homunculus – entstehen. Im menschlichen Samen liegt das «Korn». Aus diesem wird «der Mensch, der die sêl hat». Ist das «Korn» nicht «ganz», sondern geht im übrigen Samen auf, als wäre es zerrieben und beigemischt, dann entsteht ein Monstrum. Der menschliche Same hat sich im Sperma «verloren», und dieses ist so zu tierischem Samen geworden. Die so erzeugte Mißbildung ist mithin tierisch und ungeseelt[30].

Die Beziehung zu den Sternen wird im Buch von den durch Sodomie Erzeugten berührt[31]. Es wird dort von einem von den Sternen herabkommenden Sperma – einem «Sterngeschoß» – gesprochen.

Im Buch *De lunaticis* heißt es, ähnlich wie bei Konrad, daß die Sterne keinen Einfluß auf uns haben, es sei denn, daß wir selbst ihnen einen Platz in uns einräumen[32]. Dies geschieht durch die Leidenschaften, also etwas Sündiges. Jeder leidenschaftliche Wille findet seinen Stern, der ihm zu Diensten ist. «... wil einer in der geschrift studiren, er fint sternen, die im leihen (auf zerrütten); wil einer kriegen, er fint auch also stern; wil einer hadern, kempfen, er fint auch stern; wil einer stelen, morden, rauben, wuchern, er fint stern, die im helfen und leihen im, dan die ding all seind viehisch.»[33] Hier wiederum liegt die Beziehung: Sünde–Stern–Tierisches zugrunde.

Narren, Monstra, Mißgewächs – wie Mörder, Kriege, Diebe, krumme Kinder, blind, taub, stumm und lahm Geborene –, alles das ist in die Welt gekommen, als der Mensch durch seine Sünde das Paradies verwirkt hatte und «zerbrechlich, tödlich», allem Elend und Jammer unterworfen wurde. Das machte sie der Einwirkung aller Sterne zugänglich[34].

Konrad spricht von der «Sternkraft in der Mutter Leib». Paracelsus sagt: «das gestirn in der eußern welt und das gestirn in der kleinen welt haben ir constellation oder confluenz mit einander, und ist ein lauf und ein wirkung nach art irer coniunction, das gestirn, die kraft, die entpfengnus

[30] *Liber de homunculis*, Philos. Magna XVII, ed. SUDHOFF, vol. XIV, p. 325 seq.
[31] *Liber de natis animalibus ex Sodomia*, ed. SUDHOFF, vol. XIV, p. 384 seq.
[32] *De lunaticis*, tract. III, cap. 1, ed. SUDHOFF, vol. XIV, p. 60.
[33] *ib.*, p. 63.
[34] *De generatione stultorum*, lib. I, tract. 1., ed. SUDHOFF, vol. XIV, p. 76–77.

zu machen, so die massa in irem gewalt ist[35]. Anderweit heißt es: «... von der matrix, dieselbig hat ir astra und hat derselbigen corpora. darumb dieweil nun der mensch aus der welt ist und muß die welt sein, das ist die microcosmisch welt, so nimpt er sie aus der mutter ...»[36] Und später: «nun seind der matrix astra zu solchen krankheiten dermaßen geschaffen ...»[37].

Die meisten dieser Vorstellungen lassen sich auf Quellen zurückführen, die viel älter sind als Konrad und Paracelsus. Sie gehören zur Sphäre des Neuplatonismus und der Gnosis. Das gilt besonders von der Rolle der Sterne bei der Übertragung des Tierischen – tierischer Leidenschaft und Gemütsverwirrung, aber auch tierischer Form. In dieser Vorstellungswelt nehmen die Sterne die Rolle bösartiger Dämonen, Unterschöpfer und Führer (Archonten, Demiurgen) an. Die Übertragung des Bösartig-Tierischen geschieht durch ein – minderwertiges – Pneuma, das sich der Seele auf ihrem Herabstieg vom Himmel anhängt, ein «Prosartema» oder «prosphyes pneuma», einen Gegenspieler («antimimon») der Seele. Dies geht schließlich im Begriff des Astralleibes («siderischen Körpers») auf, der bei Paracelsus eine so große Rolle spielt[38].

Für das Schöpfen von Anregungen zu diesen und ähnlichen Vorstellungen war mithin Paracelsus nicht auf das *Buch der Natur* angewiesen. Aber dieses hat sie in deutscher Sprache übermittelt. Es war zu Paracelsus' Zeit überaus populär und weitverbreitet. Es läßt sich mit Sicherheit als Quelle für eine Schrift und mit Wahrscheinlichkeit für eine andere des Paracelsischen Corpus aufweisen. Es ist daher nicht unwahrscheinlich, daß es auch für die Kapitel von den Wundermenschen, Homunculi, Monstra und die Rolle der Sterne bei ihrer Erzeugung als Quelle gedient hat. Auch Paracelsus spricht viel vom *Buch der Natur*, das der Arzt im Gegensatz zu den Büchern der Gelehrten zu studieren hat[39].

[35] *Philosophia sagax*, lib. I, cap. 2, ed. SUDHOFF, vol. XII, p. 49.

[36] Von hinfallenden siechtagen der Mutter (Hysterie), *De caduco matricis*, paragr. II, ed. SUDHOFF, vol. VIII, p. 327.

[37] *ib.*, p. 329.

[38] S. PAGEL, *Das medizinische Weltbild des Paracelsus, l.c.*, Wiesbaden 1962, p. 40 seq., 54 seq., 117 seq.

[39] «Denn das will ich bezeugen mit der natur: Der sie durchforschen will, der muß mit den Füßen ihre Bücher treten. Die Schrift wird erforscht durch ihre Buchstaben, die Natur aber durch land zu land: als oft ein land, als oft ein blatt. Also ist Codex naturae, also muß man ire blätter umwenden.» *Defensiones und Verantwortungen IV*, ed. SUDHOFF, vol. XI, p. 145–146. Paracelsus spricht auch schon vom *Buch des Körpers*, und zwar

*Zusammenfassend* können wir also annehmen, daß Paracelsus manches von seinem Wissen über das Bilsenkraut und seine betäubende Wirkung auf Vögel aus Konrad von Megenbergs *Buch der Natur* geschöpft und daß dies als Anregung für den Vergleich seines Präparates mit pflanzlichen Narkotika bei Hühnern gedient hat. Außer den Erfahrungen der Jäger und Fischer und ihrem Ausbau seitens präparacelsischer Gelehrter, wie sie von Eis angeführt worden sind, lassen sich das *Buch der Natur* und der englische und französische mittelalterliche Sprachgebrauch für Bilsenkraut («Henbane», «Mort aux Poules») als mehr direkte Quellen für Paracelsus vermuten.

Paracelsus hat nicht im luftleeren Raum gearbeitet. Er verdankt Grundlegendes der von ihm so geschmähten Antike – sowohl den klassischen Medizinern und Philosophen wie auch dem Hellenismus, vor allem in Gestalt des Neuplatonismus und der Gnosis. Er hatte auch mittelalterliche Quellen für die antike Tradition und neue, im Mittelalter und oft kurz vor ihm, gemachte Naturbeobachtungen. Aber allem hat er eine originelle Wendung gegeben und es in seine makro-mikrokosmischen Theorien eingefügt. Im vorliegenden Falle würde diese originelle Wendung in der Benutzung empirischer volkstümlicher Überlieferungen zu einem echten pharmakologischen Versuch gelegen haben.

vor VESAL, der als Schöpfer dieses Ausdruckes gilt (L. EDELSTEIN, And. Vesalius the Humanist, *Bull. Hist. Med. XIV* [1943] p. 547–561, 556, mit Bezug auf VESALIUS, *Fabrica,* lib. VI, cap. 16, ed. 1543, p. 600: «quae Galeni placitis penitus renituntur, et vere paradoxa ex hominis haud mendaci libro deprompta sunt ...). *Buch des Körpers* bei PARACELSUS, *Labyrinthus medicorum errantium – Vom Irrgang der Ärzte,* cap. 4, ed. SUDHOFF, vol. XI, 1537/38, p. 184. Siehe auch: W. PAGEL und P. RATTANSI, Vesalius and Paracelsus, *Medical History, VIII* (1964), p. 316. Über KONRAD VON MEGENBERG als Vorläufer im Gebrauch des Wortes *Buch der Natur* und andere Vorläufer (BONAVENTURA u. a.): E. R. CURTIUS, *Europäische Literatur und Lateinisches Mittelalter,* Bern 1948, p. 321–327 (auch für: *Buch der Kreaturen, Buch der Welt* und ähnliches).

# V

## PARACELSUS AND TECHELLUS THE JEW

In his qualified censure of Paracelsus, Daniel Sennert takes him to task for his leanings towards magic—as indicated for example by the words of praise which Paracelsus and his followers found for Techellus.[1]

Techellus is indeed mentioned in the Paracelsean Corpus as "a great teacher in Israel and true naturalist." He is given great credit as the only extant pure source of the very ancient knowledge of the magic effects of stones with carved images. Most of this "Highest Art, Magica and Cabalia" fell into oblivion, owing to "inexperienced and wanton sophists" who would not heed the fact that God revealed more in the Light of Nature to His people, the Israelites, than to anybody else after the time of Christ. Techellus was despised because he was a Jew, and for this reason only a small part of his works has been preserved.[2]

This praise accorded to a Jewish naturalist forms a remarkable contrast to the many passages in which Paracelsus denies to the Jews any originality and merit in Medicine.[3]

On the other hand, the same Paracelsus said that Christians surpassed the Jews in lying—a vice to which Greeks (including Aristotle) had an

[1] Daniel Sennert, *De chymicorum cum Aristotelicis et Galenicis consensu ac dissensu* (1619). Paris, 1633, IV, p. 50.

[2] *Liber principiorum Theophrasti Paracelsi,* cap. 5, ed. Sudhoff, vol. XIV, p. 503. In: *De pestilitate,* ed. Sudhoff, vol. XIV, p. 597, the "Techellische Philosophia" is credited with the indication of a seventh point at which plague manifests itself in the human body—in addition to the six points already known. In the Huser Folio edition, Strasburg, 1616, vol. I, p. 326, the word "*techellisch*" is replaced by "*tellurisch.*"

[3] According to Paracelsus, there is no ancient Hebrew tradition in medicine. God taught it to all peoples and in all tongues: *Von den Imposturen* (*Von der französischen Krankheit drei Bücher Para*), 1529, lib. I, cap. 14, lib. II, cap. 15, ed. Sudhoff, vol. VII, pp. 98, 127. Even the Kabbalah, so often extolled by Paracelsus as the source of knowledge of the Invisible, was according to him not an original Jewish achievement, but Persian in origin and only adulterated by the Jews: *Philosophia sagax,* lib. I, cap. 6, Probatio in scientiam necromanticam, ed. Sudhoff, vol. XII, p. 156. Against Rabbi Moses and his book "Nebolohu": *Von den Imposturen,* lib. I, cap. 14, *loc. cit.,* p. 98; *Drei Bücher der Wundarznei Bertheonei.* Vorrede, ed. Sudhoff, vol. VI, pp. 45-46.

inborn inclination.[4] In fact, all that Paracelsus has to say against the Jews accords with his attitude towards contemporaries and ancient medicine in general and does not necessarily contradict the praise granted to Jewish mysticism and Kabbalah—currents as unorthodox as his own philosophy.

Techellus only occurs, however, in two treatises that are strongly suspected of being spurious.[5] The very restriction of Techellus references may support the suspicion—more so than the contradiction between the praise accorded to this Jewish naturalist and the deprecation of Jewish medicine in general, for the Paracelsean treatises abound with contradictory statements.

At all events, Techellus has a place in the Paracelsean Corpus connecting him with a literary question of some importance, namely the spuriousness of at least one treatise. This justifies the question: *Who was Techellus?*

The answer is provided by Conrad of Megenberg's *Buch der Natur* from the middle of the fourteenth century. For a detailed account of this work and its author the reader is referred to Ludwig Choulant's *Graphische Incunabeln für Naturgeschichte und Medicin.*[6] The eleventh book of Megenberg is dedicated to stones and metals and contains a chapter on stones with carved images. This is followed by the *Techelsbüchlein* on the same subject—it is called " *büchlein eines grossen meisters in der jüdischheit der hiesz Techel.*" This is almost verbally the reference found in the *Liber Principiorum Theophrasti Paracelsi.* Moreover, like the author of the latter, Megenberg defends Techellus against his own " master "—the author of the original work in Latin which Megenberg purports to translate: Thomas of Cantimpré. In fact this is one of the pieces of evidence which, according to Choulant, show that Megenberg did not

[4] Draft for the dedication of a book on syphilis to King Ferdinand, possibly for the IVth part of the *Wundarznei,* ed. Sudhoff, vol. X, p. 485. *Grosse Wundarznei,* lib. II, tract. 2, " Beschlussred," ed. Sudhoff, vol. X, p. 347.

[5] The *Liber principiorum,* first appearing in 1570 and treating of Snakes and Spiders, was, according to Sudhoff, a product of the stir created by the publication of the *Archidoxis* (the " Archidoxensturm ") which made any Paracelsean item—however spurious—a highly coveted possession (Paracelsus Edition, vol. XIV, pp. XXVIII-XXIX). As long ago as 1889 Sudhoff admitted, however, that some general terms in this treatise are very much reminiscent of Paracelsus' manner (E. Schubert und K. Sudhoff: *Paracelsus Forschungen,* II, Frankfurt a.M., 1889, p. 137, note). *See also*: K. Sudhoff: *Bibliographia Paracelsica,* Berlin, 1894 (repr. Graz, 1958), p. 181 sub No. 113, p. 208 sub No. 124.

[6] Leipzig, 1858, pp. 99-122. For more recent literature on Conrad von Megenberg, (c. 1309-1374), George Sarton, *Introduction to the History of Science,* Baltimore: Williams and Wilkins, 1927-1948, vol. III, 1947, p. 817, may be consulted.

content himself with merely translating this work. Arguing against Techellus, Thomas had regarded all carved stones as the products of art. Megenberg, siding with Techellus, maintains that they can be natural.[7]

The author of the *Liber Principiorum Paracelsi* therefore appears to have used as his source the work of Megenberg in which also much material was to be found about his main subject: Snakes and Spiders.

Thomas said that he appended to his work his translation into Latin of a treatise by a Jewish naturalist (" physiologus "), Thetel or Techel, on stones and their magic effects.[8] He does not say, however, from which language the translation was made. Techel is probably identical with Zethel, Zachel or Zael, the author of astrological treatises,[9] and may ultimately stand for Sahl ibn Bishr, a Jewish astrologer of the ninth century.[10] Perhaps, however, " Techellus " never was a concrete person, but merely a name to indicate a doctrine.[11]

There is little to add about the significance of a treatise on the magic effects of carved stones and images for Paracelsus himself or any of his followers. The " Gamaheu," the carved stone, is the universal instrument in which the magician preserves supernatural (sidereal) forces and virtues and through which he transfers them to other objects.[12] In the book *On Images* Paracelsus enlarges on the miraculous pictures found engraved

[7] " nun spricht der meyster disz buchs im Latein das ich zu teutsch pring er wene das dem büchlein (sc. Techel's) auch nit gar sey zu glauben—aber der meister redet als ob die stein ire pild nur von kunst haben und nit von natur. Das ist nit war." Choulant, *op. cit.,* p. 104.

[8] M. Steinschneider, *Die hebraeischen Uebersetzungen des Mittelalters.* Berlin: Kommisionsverlag des Bibliographischen Bureaus, 1893, p. 237, espec. note 922. Lynn Thorndike, *History of Magic and Experimental Science.* New York: Macmillan, 1923-1958, vol. II, 1923, pp. 389-390 and Appendix II on some manuscripts of the treatise of Thetel on Seals. The text of: *Cethel aut veterum Judaeorum physiologorum de lapidibus sententiae* (Thomae Cantipratani *Prooemium de sculpturis lapidum*) is found in: Pitra, J. B., *Specilegium Solesmense,* tom. III, Paris, 1855, pp. 335-337. On the manuscript tradition of the various versions of the name Cethel, *see ibid.,* p. 335, footnote. The versions: " Cheel " and " Theel " appear to be of particular interest with reference to " Techel "—" Techellus." *See also*: Conrad von Megenberg, *Das Buch der Natur.* Bearbeitet von Hugo Schulz. Greifswald, 1897, p. VIII: " Wer der Jüdische Gelehrte Tethel gewesen is, habe ich, trotz vielfachen Suchens und Nachfragens nicht herausbekommen können."

[9] Thorndike, *loc. cit.,* p. 390.

[10] G. Sarton, *op. cit.,* vol. I, 1927, p. 569 and vol. II (2), 1931, p. 593.

[11] For suggestions in this respect see the present author in *Paracelsus. An Introduction to Philosophical Medicine in the Era of the Renaissance.* Basle and New York: Karger, 1958, p. 214, note 43. This must be supplemented by the material contained in the present article.

[12] Paracelsus, *Philosophia sagax,* lib. I, cap. 6, *In probationem artis magicae,* ed. Sudhoff, vol. XII, p. 133.

in rocks, caves, and secret passages, also on those in small stones, pebbles, and " gamahei." Such images seem to be works of art, but in reality have grown naturally through the ordinance of God and convey their own " great prophetic message," which will be understood by " magi and chiromantici." [13]

Here, then, we have a *genuine* treatise in which Paracelsus takes pains to advocate Techellus' point of view. Could it be used as a piece of internal evidence in favour of the authenticity of the *Liber Principiorum*? Not only the latter, but also *De Imaginibus* may have been based on Megenberg and his defence of Techellus. At all events, the doctrinal contents of the former treatise lose little in Paracelsean authenticity by the invocation of Techellus, and the question of the genuineness of the treatise does not seem to lend itself to an easy solution.

POSTSCRIPT: Of authors mentioning Thetel since the XVIth century only two may be cited:— 1) Rudolph Goclenius (1572-1621) has in his *Mirabilium Naturae Liber Concordias et Repugnantias Rerum in Plantis, Animalibus, Animaliumque Morbis et Partibus manifestans* (Francof. 1625, p. 258) *Imagines seu sigilla Thetelis.* It begins: " Thetel vetustissimus Doctor tractans de sculpturis lapidum, ait, has sculpturas in convenientibus lapidibus repertas, maximam habere virtutem. Hominis imago sculpta in Iaspide. . . ." This is followed (p. 260-287) by *Sculpturae Salomonis.* 2) Ernst Theodor Amadeus Hoffmann (1776-1822), the deep and witty romantic writer, describes how the " uncouth " and interfering " Genius Thetel " removed the body of the " Blumenkönigin Gamaheh " through the firmament to Samarkand—a journey on which " Meister Floh " clinging to Gamaheh's Brussels lace fell into the focus of Leuwenhöck's " magic instrument " and hence straight on the nose of the observing magician who immediately placed him on a Russwurm Universal Microscope. (Hoffmann, E. T. A., *Meister Floh. Ein Märchen in sieben Abentheuern zweier Freunde.* Frankfurt a. Mayn: Fried. Wilmans, 1822, pp. 57-59; 90-91 and passim).

[13] Paracelsus *De imaginibus,* cap. 7, ed. Sudhoff, vol. XIII, pp. 373-375.

# VI

## PARACELSUS AND THE NEOPLATONIC AND GNOSTIC TRADITION

### Introduction

Even a casual glance at the voluminous works of Theophrastus Paracelsus (1493–1541) cannot fail to show that his contributions lay in many fields: in medicine and chemistry, in mineralogy and meteorology, in epistemology and the knowledge of man as part of the cosmos, in theology and *magia naturalis* including alchemy, astrology and divination. It is not difficult to extract from his work a number of observations and results that can be regarded as stepping-stones in the development of science and medicine. What is not so easy is the demonstration of the link which joins these progressive views and findings with the non-scientific ideas and sentiments with which the *Corpus* of the Paracelsian writings abounds. The proto-scientific as well as the non-scientific parts are products of the same mind and of the same cultural climate —the era of the Renaissance. One of its outstanding features was the revival of Hellenistic philosophy—the doctrines of the mythical Hermes Trismegistos and of neo-Platonism. Associated with this revival there was the attempt at reconciling it with Christian doctrine, whereby belief seemed to acquire support through philosophical and symbolical knowledge—a new type of *Gnosis*. Paracelsus was bound to reflect these general trends of his era. Indeed

"Hermetic" and neo-Platonic speculation as well as Christian belief and symbolism can be recognized in his philosophy without much difficulty, and it has often been said that Paracelsus was influenced by these trends of thought. The detailed examination of this point, however, does not seem to have had sufficient attention, nor has its possible role as a link between the scientific and non-scientific part of the work of Paracelsus been appreciated so far. On the other hand there is a danger of overrating these influences and of overlooking the original way in which Paracelsus made use of traditional lore, and the distinct differences that exist between his ideas and those of Hellenistic philosophy and symbolism. Such differences have been rightly pointed out—we shall discuss them below. The extensive application of speculative and symbolic elements and their association with the faithful observation of nature alone mark Paracelsus out as an original and indeed as a unique figure. Yet a study of his parallels and contacts with the Hermetic tradition is still called for and likely to help in the understanding of Paracelsus—disposing eventually of the unsatisfactory cliché of the "two souls" of Doctor Faustus that has been applied to him far too often.

In the present paper no more can be given than a first sketchy collection of doctrines that appear to be characteristic of Hermeticism, neo-Platonism and Gnosticism and to have found access to the Paracelsian *Corpus*. They will be discussed in the light of their significance for Paracelsus' own natural philosophy and medicine.

## Basic Ideas Characteristic of Gnosticism and neo-Platonism

### Matter and Spirit

Gnosticism may be said to present basically a dualist view of the world. In it the dark waters of the material world are set in sharp contrast against spirit, soul and divinity. The former owes its existence to the fall of a lesser deity and embodies original evil as opposed to good. This dualistic idea is symbolized and illustrated in the Gnostic diagrams of the Cosmos. Here we see our world surrounded by detachments of evil forces, the *archons* or *demiurges* who formed it in the abyss of the waters, the *chaos* that was uncreated and aboriginal. It is through the circle formed by the *archons* that the divine element in us, the soul, has to grope its way back to its divine source after death. Knowledge of certain watchwords will enable it to do so—a knowledge that is furnished by the *Gnostic Magus*, by *pneumatic* man who vanquishes the forces of evil and leads the soul to the heights in which divinity dwells[1].

[1] W. Bousset, *Hauptprobleme der Gnosis*, Göttingen, 1907, pp. 361 seq. H. Leisegang, *Dante und das christliche Weltbild* (Schriften d. Deutschen Dante-Ges. Heft 6), Weimar, 1941, p. 17; pp. 21–26. G. Verbeke, *L'Évolution de la Doctrine du Pneuma du Stoicisme à St Augustin*, Paris et Louvain, 1945, pp. 287 seq.: Les Gnostiques.

Though probably inspired by oriental, notably Persian concepts, Gnostic dualism is essentially informed by Platonic *idealism.* It was Plato who appeared to a Father of the Church as the "Patriarch of the Gnostics", and Gnosticism stood for "Christian Platonism"[2]. The distinction that had been fundamental in Platonic theory, as notably propounded in the *Timaeus*[3], was between that which *is* and never *develops* on the one hand, and that which *develops* and *is not* on the other, between archetype and image, between *Eidos* and *Eidolon,* between the eternal world of the Ideas and the world of fugitive shadows and appearances that is ours.

Similarly neo-Platonism adhered to this basic dualistic view. Yet it emphasized at the same time the principle of continuity in the cosmos. To uphold it meant to bridge the dualistic gulf somehow. This was achieved by a closed system of emanations leading from the highest divinity down to coarse matter, to stone, metal and dirt. Intermediate beings had to be introduced. One such intermediary—a *"tertium quid"*—is the *astral body.* It is a *Pneuma,* i.e. of finest ethereal corporality, enveloping the soul proper which is not a "Pneuma", as it is immaterial[4]. Maintaining soul to be purely spiritual and

[2] See L. Noack, *Philosophie-Geschichtliches Lexikon. Historisch-biographisches Handbuch zur Geschichte der Philosophie,* Leipzig, 1879, p. 314 sub: *Gnostiker* and with reference to Tertullian.

[3] *Timaeus* 27C–29D. Prelude. The Nature and Scope of Physics. Quoted from F. M. Cornford, *Plato's Cosmology. The Timaeus of Plato translated with a running commentary,* London, 1937, pp. 21 et seq.

[4] No more than a casual reference can be inserted as to the parallels with Eastern speculation, notably that of the *Taoists* who can claim our special interest because of their significance for Chinese alchemy. As Joseph Needham writes, they "recognized a considerable number of spiritual essences, even godlings, in the human body-soul complex, almost as many indeed as the limbs and viscera of the human organism itself, but there was no place other than earth for them to inhabit as a coherent entity, and after death they simply dispersed, some rising to join the pneuma (*chhi*) of the heavens, some sinking to mingle with that of the earth, and others disappearing altogether". *Elixir Poisoning in Mediaeval China. Janus* 1959, XLVIII, p. 245. See also *idem* in: *Science and Civilization in China,* Cambridge, 1954 et seq, Vol. II, pp. 153, 333 and 490. "At death the three *hun* souls rose up to mingle with the universal pneuma in the empyrean, while the seven *pho* souls sank down to mingle with the material of the earth. The *hun* souls were connected with the *chhi,* or pneuma, the *pho* souls were connected with the seminal essence, the *ching,* and the *hsüeh,* or blood . . . —a polypsychical ideology . . . in the development of Chinese philosophical organicism. . . . Of course, whether there could be the slightest connexion between these old Chinese ideas and the neo-Platonic traditions in the West, he would be a very bold man who would attempt to say". (J. Needham in a personal communication to the present author of 3 November, 1958.) See also: H. Steininger, *Hauch- und Körperseele und der Dämon bei Kuan-Yin-Tze,* Leipzig, 1953.

immaterial, neo-Platonism made its stand against Stoic Monism and Materialism—in this the soul had been visualized as a *Pneuma*, a breath of finest corporality[5].

The soul receives its envelope or vehicle (*ochema*) or "chariot" when passing downwards through the stars and returns it to the latter when after death it retraces its steps to achieve reunion with divinity. It belongs to the stars, it is truly an *astral body*[6]. Its position as a being intermediate between spirit and body was best expressed by Marsilio Ficino (1433–99) who said that it was not body and almost soul, and not soul and almost body[7]. This neo-Platonic thesis in its Ficinian formulation can be regarded as a doctrine fundamental to Renaissance philosophy. It was verbally repeated by Agrippa of Nettesheym (1487–1535)[8] and introduced into the works of many others.

The astral body was one of the means by which neo-Platonism preserved its basic dualistic attitude without sacrificing the idea of cosmic continuity, coherence and unity[9]. "Steps" with innumerable transitions lead from God, the One, down to matter which forms the last and lowest step. As such, matter is still spiritual, although disguised by a thick material cover. Nature as a whole is seen as a "sleeping spirit". In its realm, Being and Action perform the task that is given to Contemplation in the realm of the spirit[10]. The individual object in nature exists not by virtue of its coarse material body, but by its spiritual kernel, the spark that is invisible to the eye. It is the latter that gives the object its specific form and schedule of function; indeed it is the vector of specificity. This commanding role of the spirit makes possible the

[5] F. Rüsche, *Das Seelenpneuma. Seine Entwickelung von der Hauchseele zur Geistseele. Beiträge zur Geschichte d. antiken Pneumalehre* (Stud. z. Geschichte und Kultur d. Altertums XVIII, 3), Paderborn, 1933, p. 55.

[6] See E. R. Dodds in: *Proclos, The Elements of Theology. Revised Text with translation, introduction and commentary*, Oxford, 1933, Appendix II: *The Astral Body in neo-Platonism*, p. 313.

[7] Marsilius Ficinus, *De Vita Coelitus Comparanda*, lib. III, cap. 3, Venetiis. Aldus. 1516, fol. 153r. To this: D. P. Walker, *Spiritual and Demonic Magic from Ficino to Campanella*, London, The Warburg Institute, 1958, pp. 38 *seq.*

[8] Agrippa a Nettesheym, *De Occulta Philosophia*, lib. I, cap. 14, Lugd. 1550, p. 33.

[9] Verbeke, *loc. cit.*, 1945, p. 364.

[10] In natura quidem intueri nihil aliud est quam esse tale et tale quiddam facere. Ficinus commenting on Plotinus, *Ennead*, III, 8, 1 *et seq.*, Basileae, 1615, pp. 339 *et seq.* In Nature to contemplate is nothing but to be something and to do something.—Nature as a "sleeping spirit": W. R. Inge, *The Philosophy of Plotinus*, London, 1918, vol. I, p. 152, quoting from Schelling.

instantaneous *conversion* of an impulse of the spirit, or will, into material change.

Man, too, is an intermediate being. His body partakes of the divine spark of light. Hence he is a *microcosm*. For in him all constituents of the world are represented: heaven in his spirit and soul, and the dark abyss of the waters of matter in his body. He was created to replace the world of Lucifer and his fellow angels who had sunk into the abyss of matter completely. Through the creation of man the spark of divine light was saved, for it had been possessed by the evil principle who arrogated divinity to himself. In contrast to him, man is eligible for redemption[11].

In man, therefore, that cosmic duality is reflected which is caused by the independence of original matter. This is uncreated and hence coordinated to God. There is, however, a struggle between them, the ultimate outcome of which is redemption, the victory of light over darkness. In this sense the early Platonist Numenius of Apamea (2nd century A.D.) had said that the souls adhere to the original water that is animated by the breath of God[12]. Hence there is traffic between the upper world of the spirit and the lower world of matter—a process with the uniform aim of redemption—redemption that is of the soul from the fetters of matter and of the spiritual spark that can be found hidden in matter everywhere. Thus the *Opus* of the *alchemist* is dedicated to such redemption as the perfection of metals will afford. To be successful, the process in the furnace must be accompanied by a corresponding purification of the soul of the worker. Hence the close relationship between Alchemy, Gnosticism and neo-Platonism, not only in Hellenistic times, but

[11] According to Origen, *De Princip*, III, 5, 4, God created the world in order to ban the fallen spirits into material bodies. See also: F. Ch. Baur, *Die christliche Gnosis oder die christliche Religionsphilosophie in ihrer geschichtlichen Entwickelung*, Tübingen, 1835, pp. 173–175 (Fall of Sophia) and p. 591, with reference to Böhme's *Aurora*, 16, 75; 14, 62; *Drei Principien*, 10, 8; 10, 11.—The idea was poignantly expressed by the Paracelsist Oswald Croll (1580–1609) in the introduction to his *Basilica Chymica* of 1608: "God created man that the number and losse of the rebellious Angells might be made up in the kingdome of Heaven". *Philosophy reformed in four tractates* translated by H. Pinell, London, 1657, p. 54. See W. Pagel, *Paracelsus. Introduction to Philosophical Medicine in the Era of the Renaissance*, Basle and New York, 1958, p. 207. See also: H. J. Sheppard, *Gnosticism and Alchemy, Ambix*, 1957, VI, 86–101 (p. 92: the material world coming into being through the fall and activity of a lesser deity). *Idem, The Redemption Theme and Hellenistic Alchemy, Ibid.*, 1959, VII, 42.

[12] "Prosizanein to hydati tas psychas theopnoi onto" Numenius in Porphyry *Antrum Nympharum* cap. 10. See: M. Joel, *Blicke in die Religionsgeschichte*, Breslau, 1880, vol. I, pp. 164–165.

also throughout the Middle Ages and in the Renaissance[13]. Finally liberation from disease—*medicine*–involves redemption—the conquest of the evil that attacks man in the form of disease seeds and disease demons. These invade the body, breaking up its organic simplicity and coherence by introducing corruption, whereby the parts are forced back into the realm of dead and dark matter.

Alchemy and Medicine thus form two aspects of natural *magic* already in Hellenistic times. The Magus applies the principle of *sympathy*: everywhere like yearns to unite with like. This principle derives from the Platonic correspondences between archetype and image, the world of magisterial and "sophic" models and patterns on the one hand, and that of empirical objects on the other. One technique used by the magus is to shut up a *pneuma* or demoniac or astral force in a cameo (gem, *gamaheu*) or in a ring or in an animal. By capturing a virtue in this way the Magus is able to unite it with a corresponding constituent in his own body and thereby achieves concrete effects in the outside world. In this also lies his *mantic* power of divination. It is due to a traffic between spirits. The "seat" of magic, however, should not be searched for in the Magus, for it lies in Nature in which as by a magic chain everything is interconnected and alive. It is the task of the Magus to adapt himself to Nature so closely that he can influence it by setting, as it were, a sympathetic chord into vibration[14].

By virtue of their spiritual character the effective and active powers in this world are *Logoi*—it is these which persist and assume corporality in the form of the *Semina*. Each living being develops from a hidden seed. It eventually perishes, but not without having formed new seed. Owing to this *cyclic—circular*—process the individual survives by transmitting the specificity of his breed to succeeding generations. The association of seed with *Logos* originates

[13] M. Berthelot, *Introduction à l'étude de la Chimie des Anciens et du Moyen Age*, Paris, 1889, pp. 247 *et seq.*; p. 235. *Idem, Les Origines de l'Alchimie*, Paris, 1885, p. 76; p. 272: "Le but de la philosophie, c'est la dissolution des corps (materiels) et la séparation de l'âme du corps" (with ref. to Stephanus, *De magna et sacra arte*, lib. I, ed. J. L. Ideler, in: *Physici et medici Graeci minores*, vol. II, Berol, 1842, p. 215). *Ibid.*, p. 165; Soul as prime matter of things, *ibid.*, pp. 252, 276. E. O. von Lippmann, *Entstehung und Ausbreitung der Alchemie*, Berlin, 1919, pp. 319, 323, 324, 376, 381. On Gnosticism and Alchemy, pp. 235–247. R. P. Festugière, *La révélation d'Hermes Trismégiste*, I: L'Astrologie et les Sciences Occultes, Paris, 1950, pp. 217–282.

[14] Verbeke, *loc. cit.*, 1945, pp. 326–330, referring to A. Dieterich, *Abraxas*, Leipzig, 1891, p. 58. H. Ritter, *Picatrix, ein. arabisches Handbuch hellenistischer Magie. Vorträge d. Bibliothek Warburg*, 1921–1922, Leipzig u. Berlin, 1923, pp. 94–124 (particularly p. 106). Of older sources see: I. Gaffarel, *Curiositez inovyes sur la sculpture talismanique des Persans, Horoscope des Patriarches, et lecture des estoilles*, Paris, 1629, pp. 94 *et seq.*

in the Stoic concept of the *Logoi Spermatikoi*—the seed-bound rational impulses and directions. This concept reflects the Monism of the Stoic School. The world is the original *Pneuma*, the original *Logos* out of which the individual beings arise—each embodying a *Logos*. This idea was partly accepted by neo-Platonism[15].

Neo-Platonism radically altered the status of *Time* in philosophy. Aristotle had defined it as the number that measures motion—thereby degrading it to the rank of a merely conventional aid for the mind. By contrast Plotinus vindicated Time as a power existing in reality—namely that power which makes motion possible. This he achieved by associating time with soul—the soul of the world as well as the soul of the individual. Time thus becomes the instrument by means of which eternity acquires a hold on the cosmos. Owing to its link with soul, time assumes a *qualitative* character. It is no longer a mere measure of quantity, but is determined by the differences between individual processes and actions[16].

## Neo-Platonic and Gnostic Trends in the speculation of Paracelsus. The Spirit and the Astral Body. The Light of Nature

Are there any traces of these neo-Platonic and Gnostic ideas in Paracelsus, and if so, how did he develop them and what answers did he give to the problems which they raised?

According to Paracelsus man is the lesser world, for in him all things of the greater world are united—they do not, however, enter the organism as bodies, but in the form of "spirits", i.e. as powers and virtues[17].

In this, Paracelsus expresses the idea fundamental to him that what really interests the "philosopher" is the invisible world of the "occult" virtues that are celestial and "astral", the world of the spirit and "Logoi". Unmasking all material beings and actions as the product of spiritual forces, he implements

[15] H. Meyer, *Geschichte der Lehre von den Keimkräften von der Stoa bis zum Ausgang der Patristik*, Bonn, 1914, pp. 13 *et seq.*, p. 64 and *passim.*

[16] H. Leisegang, *Die Begriffe der Zeit und Ewigkeit im späteren Platonismus. Beitr. z. Gesch. d. Philos. d. Mittelalt. ed. C. Baeumker, vol. XIII*, no. 4, Münster, 1913. J. F. Callaghan, *Four Views of Time in Ancient Philsophy*, Cambridge (Mass.), 1948. W. Pagel, *Van Helmont De Tempore and Biological Time, Osiris*, 1949, vol. VIII, pp. 346–417. H. Weiss, *Notes on the Greek Ideas referred to in Van Helmont's De Tempore, Osiris, ibid.*, pp. 419–449. W. Pagel, *The Reaction to Aristotle in XVIIth century Biological Thought. In: Science, Medicine and History*, Oxford, 1953, vol. I, pp. 493–494.

[17] Man a microcosm "not in form and matter, but by possessing all the powers and virtues of the greater world". *Bücher von den unsichtbaren Krankheiten* (1531/32), Ingang des vierten Buches, ed. Sudhoff, vol. IX, pp. 308–309.

one of the basic postulates of neo-Platonism. Indeed, Paracelsus follows this up in detail in his pathology. What is visible as a pathological change in the organs is the product of an interaction between two spirits: the spiritual cause of the disease which enters the body from outside and the spiritual representative of the body or the organ invaded. This is not attacked directly and physically, but in a more subtle way. It is alienated from its normal functional schedule which is controlled by a spiritual "director", the *Archeus*. "The spirits know each other . . . they speak the same language . . . now suffers the body . . . not in a material way, but from the spirit which calls for a spiritual remedy[18]." Diseases are therefore not "*Corpora*, hence spirit should be used against spirit"[19]. Disease is thus seen as a product of the inter-communication of spirits—a feature with which we are familiar from Gnostic and neo-Platonic speculation.

The neo-Platonic emphasis laid on the Invisible and Spiritual leads Paracelsus to take special interest in fugitive and "pneumatic" substances and phenomena in nature. The *Arcana*, the uncreated, divine and miraculously powerful agents, are represented as volatile. They are directed by the *Astra* like "feathers in the wind"[20]. Paracelsus visualizes a spirit in each "essential thing", and hence as many spirits as individuals and objects in nature[21]. It is these spirits that endow things with "life", i.e. form and function. For "life is a spiritual, invisible and impalpable thing"[22]. It is the same spirit which makes inert material chemically reactive which renders it "male" ("*männisch*")[23].

"Spirit" used in this sense by Paracelsus has nothing to do with reason (ratio) and is particularly alien to Aristotelian and formal logic. What he

[18] The spirits know each other . . .: *Volumen Paramirum* (De Ente spirituali), ed. Sudhoff, vol. I, pp. 217–218.

[19] Diseases are not *Corpora* . . .: *Paragranum*, tract. II (Von der Astronomey), ed. Sudhoff, vol. VIII, p. 178.

[20] *Arcana* directed by *Astra* like feathers in the wind: *Paragranum*, tract. III (Von der alchimia), ed. Sudhoff, vol. VIII, p. 185.

[21] A spirit in each "essential thing": *De Natura Rerum*, lib. IV, de vita rer. natur., ed. Sudhoff, vol. XI, pp. 329–330.

[22] "The life of each object is a spiritual, an invisible and incomprehensible being, and a spirit and a spiritual thing". *Die neun Bucher de natura rerum* (Villach, 1537). Lib. IV De Vita rerum natural, ed. Sudhoff, vol. XI, p. 329.

[23] Spirit making inert material active ("*männisch*"): sulphur by ignition, mercury by sublimation and salt by resolution—the latter producing a spirit (vitrioli, tartari, aluminis, nitri) with impetuosity ("*Ungestümikeit*"). *Opus Paramirum*, lib. I, cap. 3, ed. Sudhoff, vol. IX, p. 52.

means are the deeper strata of the personality, the sphere of will and wilful imagination. "What lives according to its will, lives in the spirit; what lives according to reason, lives against the spirit"[24]. Will and imagination are closely linked with what Paracelsus calls the *"Light of Nature"*. This embraces all phenomena and things which—though invisible—are accessible to our search and understanding—unlike things divine which are not. More particularly it is the specific form and function of an individual tending towards a specific goal, its *Entelecheia*, which belongs to the "Light of Nature". This in turn is subjected to the world of the Astra and the soul of the world. The "light of nature is a pupil of the Holy Spirit[25]; man receives its teaching in dreams when nature in him speaks to itself. Here again we encounter the traffic between spirits.

The Paracelsian "spirit" in many respects corresponds to the neo-Platonic chariot or vehicle (*ochema*) or envelope of the soul. It is the *sidereal*, the *astral* body. Through it the stars confer on man "all kind of worldly (perishable) wisdom and art". It is wisdom concerned with nature (*"natürliche Vernunft"*) which is here contrasted with eternal wisdom[26]. But through it man gains some though inadequate access to eternal wisdom, for there is a correspondence between them. It is finally the astral body, and not his coarse and visible material body, that elevates man over the other creatures. God gave it to the star and from it to man[27].

## The Passions of the Soul and Insanity

There is, however, another astral gift which is transferred to man in his astral body: the emotions and passions. Temperament is also an astral gift[28]. It operates not as the ancients believed through the visible humours, but through invisible inclination. It is a spiritual effect that emerges in divination and dreams.

[24] Reason versus spirit: *Volumen Paramirum*, ed. Sudhoff, vol. I, pp. 217–218.

[25] *Light of Nature*—a pupil of the Holy Spirit: *Fragm. de Fundam. Sapientiae*, ed. Sudhoff, vol. XIII, p. 325.

[26] The *astral body* conferring *"natürliche Vernunft"*: *Philosophia sagax*, lib. I, cap. 1, ed. Sudhoff, vol. XII, p. 29.

[27] Astral body elevating man over other creatures: *Philos. sagax*, lib. I, cap. 3, *De Compositione Humana*, ed. Sudhoff, vol. XII, p. 55.

[28] Astral nature of temperament and passions: *Philos. sagax*, lib. I, cap. 10, *Von dem Dono Inclinationis*, ed. Sudhoff, vol. XII, pp. 229 *et seq.*, and *ibid.*, cap. 11, *Von dem Dono Aegrorum*, pp. 258 *et seq.*

If emotions and passions are bound up with the astral body, so is *insanity*[29]. It develops when the divine spirit in man is subjugated by his animal instincts: lust, greed, covetousness. These are stirred up by the stars, each star acting on man like a specific drug, for example hemlock. The mean man has chosen Saturn as his mate—each passion one star.

This idea can be directly traced back to Gnosticism. We mentioned the neo-Platonic view of the astral body as the vehicle (*ochema*) of the soul. Owing to its inclination towards the body, the astral body may drag the soul down into the depth of emotional life, the more so the coarser and more material its texture. Indeed, in line with this, several ochemata had been distinguished in later neo-Platonism: the very fine ethereal ochema being even visualized as immortal. In Gnosticism, the astral body is represented as an attachment—*Prosartema*—to the soul, or else as a mimic and coalescing pneuma (*Antimimon* or *Prosphyes Pneuma*). This impresses on our souls the images of wolves, monkeys, lions and thereby evokes those passions that are peculiar to each of these animals[30].

To Paracelsus the astral body is a "bodily spirit"—i.e. it must be distinguished from the non corporeal divine soul[31]. In this, too, Paracelsus adheres to the neo-Platonic position as opposed to Stoicism,which knew of no difference between soul and a fine material breath (Pneuma).

The astral body is, therefore, according to Paracelsus, accessible to examination in the "*Light of Nature*". Not so the soul, which belongs to the realm of belief and theology. Further distinctions which Paracelsus made concerning the soul and astral body can be correlated with similar distinctions made by neo-Platonists, notably Proclus. Another neo-Platonist, Jamblichus, emphasizes in his treatise *On Mysteries* the difference between reasoning thought and soul, on the one hand, and the secret (*arrheta*) transcendent works and the power of the ineffable symbols that are only understood by the gods, on the other. It is through these works and symbols that the virtues and powers immanent in material bodies achieve union with the gods, whereby theurgy, magical science and divination are made possible[32]. This idea may well be applicable

[29] Insanity and star: *Philosophia Magna* 3 *Liber de Lunaticis*, Tract. III, ed. Sudhoff, vol. XIV, p. 59.

[30] Prosartemata: Baur, *Gnosis*, *loc. cit.*, 1835, pp. 214 *seq.* Bousset, *loc. cit.*, 1907, pp. 361 *et seq.*

[31] Astral body to be distinguished from the divine soul: *Philos. sagax*, lib. I, cap. 3, ed. Sudhoff, vol. XII, pp. 53–54.

[32] Jamblichus, *De Mysteriis liber*, ed. G. Parthey, Berol, 1857, sect. I, 21, p. 65; II, 11, pp. 96–97; IX, 10, pp. 284–285. See also *ibid.*, V, 23, p. 232.

to the Paracelsian Astral Body. As we have seen, this is represented as a "bodily spirit". If, according to Jamblichus, the forces immanent in bodies are capable of union with the gods, rather than our soul, the astral body *qua* bodily spirit could provide a more suitable medium for divine powers than the intellect, and, in particular, its reasoning powers which Paracelsus deprecated as "animal".

### The magisterial position of the Ideas as expressed in sex differentiation—*Iliaster*—*Semina*—*Archei*—*The Tria Prima* (Sulphur, Salt, Mercury)

A principle fundamental to Paracelsus' view of the world and man is that of *sexual duality*. It is a principle that he finds operative even in disease. Epilepsy in the female is a different disease from epilepsy in the male[33]. A drug effective in men, may fail in women[34]. Like the Valentinian Gnostics before him[35], Paracelsus follows in this the Platonic principle of the preformation and actualization of all phenomena in this world in the divine sphere of the ideas and spirit. There is nothing in the lower world of creation that has not its archetype in the upper world of ideas. Hence there must be an equivalent of male-female duality in the latter. In this the female stands for an emergence of the simple One, quiescent in itself, into the realm of duality and activity. It indicates some loss of status—associated as it is with a process of splitting up and action. Thus Paracelsus says: "God became double, two persons in one[36]".

[33] Disease in the male and female: *Opus Paramirum*, lib. IV, *de matrice*, ed. Sudhoff, vol. IX, pp. 194–195; *ibid.*, p. 206.

[34] Drug action and sex: *Op. Paramirum*, lib. IV, *de matrice*, ed. Sudhoff, vol. IX, pp. 202 *et seq.*; see also *ibid.*, pp. 184 *seq.* On sex and disease: P. Diepgen, *Paracelsus und das Problem der Frau. Nova Acta Paracels*, 1957, VIII, pp. 49–54.

[35] Sex differentiation in Valentinian Gnosis: Baur, *Gnosis, loc. cit.*, 1835, pp. 150–154.

[36] God became double: *Liber de Sancta Trinitate*, in Sudhoff, *Paracelsus-Handschriften*, No. 86, Bl.264b–276b, Berlin, 1899, p. 348.—The idea was fully expressed in the theosophic literature of the early seventeenth century, for example in the *Studium Universale* (1618) attributed to Valentin Weigel: "God is the Word, one God, but divided as personality, there is God and His wife, His wisdom, a complete God and creator: just as Adam was made complete man together with his Eve. This heavenly Eve made God in the beginning God and creator, she is the mother of all that is alive, through her all is manifested, without her there would be no God, no creature, only eternity without time. Therefore eternal and incomprehensible divinity emerged from His eternal hiding and manifested Himself through heavenly Eve. She was in the beginning and before all creature. Afterwards through her God emitted the Son to the world, that is God made himself Son through Wisdom, and yet remained the old God unchanged". Cap. 4, Ed. used 1695, s.*l.* (Sam. Müller), sig. B5.

However "heavenly woman" is not endowed with "power", but "fills the place of God the Father and makes Him manifest and complete as a Father". This development was repeated by Adam according to the principle of correspondence. Adam corresponds to God the Father and hence is more intimately connected with the world and the elements than is the woman[37]. Adam carries the "*Limbus*"[38], that is the threshold on which spirit and matter come together in the smallest possible compass to form the seed from which the world and he himself were made. Woman serves to manifest and perfect Adam, just as she served God, and again without acquiring any of his power. The apex of perfection wherever achieved is thus symbolized by a hermaphroditic being. Such is the *Rebis* in Alchemy, the peak obtainable in the process of transmutation, the *Quinta Essentia*, the Salt which, according to Thurneisser[39], is characterized by its dual, acid-alkaline nature. Ficino said that the Indian sages already called the world a hermaphrodite whose male and female parts are kept together by the world soul[40]. From the bi-sexual nature of the whole follows that of the individuals, including the planets. Female air is attracted by male fire, male water by female earth. The action of the magus is that of the ploughman who marries heaven to earth, joining divine life as contained in the seed with matter. The same idea is expressed in the *Hermetic Books*, notably the *Poemander*[41].

The Platonic correspondences between our world and the invisible magisterial worlds above us are reflected in Paracelsus' idea of the *Iliaster*. This embraces in an ideal form all possible beings and events that can occur in reality. Similarly the term *Aquaster* stands for the "sophic" archetype of all that is watery. Paracelsus pays particular attention to the liminal stages which lead from the ideally preformed to the really existing. These threshold objects between the Ideal and the Real, between Spirit and Matter are the *Semina*. From them, Paracelsus says "comes the foundation in all our knowledge and insight"[42]. For all things have a seed, and in the seed all things are

[37] The male (Adam) and the elements: *Labyrinthus Medicorum*, cap. 3, ed. Sudhoff, vol. XI, p. 178.

[38] Limbus: *Opus Paramirum de matrice*, ed. Sudhoff, vol. IX, p. 201.

[39] Thurneisser zum Thurn, Leonhart, *Quinta Essentia, das ist die höchste subtilitet, krafft und wirckung beyder . . . Künsten, der Medicin und Alchemy*, 2nd ed., Leipzig, 1574, p. 162. See also: *Aureum Vellus*, Tract. III, *Splendor Solis*, Rorschach, 1598, p. 191: Von dem Rebis einem Stein.

[40] Ficinus, *De Vita coelitus comparanda*, Lib. III, cap. 26, ed. Aldus, 1516, p. 168.

[41] Hermetis Trismegisti *Poemander* rec. G. Parthey, Berol, 1854, cap. 1, pp. 4–8.

[42] Semina as the foundation in all our knowledge: *Philosophia sagax*, lib. I, cap. 7 (*Probatio partic. in scientiam signatam*), ed. Sudhoff, vol. XII, p. 177.

enclosed. In them we observe nature at work—that nature which Plotinus visualized as a "sleeping spirit" and in which action and being are equivalent to contemplation in the spiritual world. In this we may find the very root of the Paracelsian dictum: "the seed lies in speculation"[43]. He thus tries to express the intimate connection of material effects as emerging from the semina with the sphere of will and imagination. To Paracelsus each seed stands for one idea, one logos that is about to be translated into our reality—this closely approximates the meaning of the *Logoi spermatikoi* of the *Stoa*, as accepted in neo-Platonic speculation. The Hermetic treatise *Poemander* expressed the same thing, identifying God's universal and creative power with that of the sower: in heaven he sows immortality, on earth transmutation, in the universe life and motion[44].

The *semina* are "astral", i.e. they hail from heaven and have a power superior to that of the material elements. In this they are emulated by the three principles *Mercury, Sulphur and Salt*—as long as these have not yet "impregnated matter", i.e. assumed a material cover. In this pre-material form they are "*Simplicia formalia*" that give matter a certain directive. Thus Mercury enlivens the parts, sulphur makes them grow, and salt keeps them together by giving them firmness. This the principles achieve by means of their seminal properties and through the occult vital powers of "*signature*" that account for taste, smell and colour. These are immanent ("*insitae*") to the principles. Both the *semina* and the *principles* are more closely related to spirit than to matter, and hence both form the class of the "formal simples" —as opposed to the traditional elements of fire, water, earth and air, which should be regarded as "material simples" ("*Simplicia materialia*"). They are the passive substratum that is acted upon by the active *principles* and *semina*. The former are visible, the latter not, and they are only recognized by the life, motion and function which they maintain.

It was thus that the foremost French Paracelcist Quercetanus (Duchesne 1544–1609)[45] saw the *semina* and *principles* of Paracelsus in two stages: (*a*) an ideal form—that of the *Simplicia Formalia* which belong to the celestial sphere

[43] Seed and speculation: *Das Buch von der gebärung der empfindlichen dinge in der vernunft*, tract. I, cap. 4, ed. Sudhoff, vol. I, p. 256.

[44] *Poemander*, ed. Parthey, *loc. cit.*, 1854, cap. XIV, 10, pp. 133–134.

[45] Quercetanus, Jos., *Ad veritatem Hermeticae medicinae ex Hippocratis veterumque decretis ac therapeusi: nec non vivae rerum anatomiae exegesi, ipsiusque naturae luce stabiliendam, adversus cujusdam Anonymi phantasmata Responsio*, Lutet. Paris, 1604, p. 162, cap. XIV (De tribus Chimicis principiis, quae in quovis naturali corpore continentur, ipsumque constituunt).

of magisterial forces not yet incorporated in material objects, and (*b*) as directive forces present in the empirical objects of nature. Thus mercury makes itself noticeable by the acidity and penetrating power that it lends to fluids, being an ethereal body of highest subtility, a spirituous substance, the essence and pabulum of life. Sulphur is distinguished by conferring sweetness, viscosity and an oily quality which supports and maintains flames, and by emollient and agglutinating properties. Salt makes a body dry and earthy; it promotes solution, coagulation, cleansing, and evacuation.

The three principles, says Quercetanus, correspond to the *Spiritus, Anima* and *Corpus* of the *Hermetic* literature; the Spirit to Mercury, the Soul to Sulphur and the Body to Salt. Sulphur forms the intermediary joining Spirit to Body. It is the *vinculum animae* that has affinity both to body and spirit—like the astral body of the ancients and Paracelsus. In our elemental sphere air is most akin to mercury: all that is powerful and vital, all "*vis* and *acumen*" in spirit of wine, for example, derives from its aerial parts. Air, together with the mercury adherent to it, either escapes or is converted into a "spiritual" or "mercurial" water which owes its sharp astringent taste to mercury or *sal armoniac*. Air and earth are joined together by water. In the elemental sphere the triad of air, water and earth thus corresponds to the three principles in the astral or celestial sphere. There is no need for a fourth element—fire. For this is identical with "heaven" or "ether"—the *fourth* (formerly called *fifth*) *essence*. This had already been the view of the Hermetic thinkers, Quercetanus says. Heaven, therefore, is a pure ethereal fire endowed with virtues far more subtle, pure and powerful than those of the elements, enabling it to penetrate everywhere and to distribute forms and virtues to each individual object. It impregnates the earth by transferring its *semina* to it through the winds, thus being the primary cause of all form, power and action in every object of the inferior world. These *semina* the heavens received from God; they include the most simple and perfect ones such as the stars and planets and also an infinity of other "*astra*" which confer "vital faculties and complexions" to the host of the inferior elements, which they animate and "inform". In action the lower elements are similar to heaven, but they differ in that heaven is activity pure and simple, whereas the inferior elements also involve corruption and suffering by their action.

It is the celestial—spiritual—essences and forms which the physician and naturalist must study and try to extract, for they alone are productive of miraculous effects. These "formal and spiritual principles" constitute the "universal balsamic medicine" in which all parts are homogeneous, most simple, pure and highly spiritual. It is the true "*quarta essentia*" ("Quintessence") and "celestial stone of the philsophers".

Paracelsus saw working in the *semina* an active force, the *Archeus*. The world is full of such "workmen" or beings intermediate between matter and spirit. Late neo-Platonism had visualized the world split up into innumerable emanations—to which the Paracelsian idea of innumerable *Archei* is comparable. In this field we also find the emphasis laid by neo-Platonic speculation on the traffic between spirits and on the information which we receive about the realm of the spirits—points that were equally emphasized by Paracelsus, who made them the cornerstone of his concept of magic and divination. The *Poemander* too, had expressed these ideas: soul-like principles—demons—can take possession of the soul which they subject to torture and stimulate to evil deeds. There is a communication between souls—the souls of the Gods with human souls and those of man with those of animals[46]. Man occupies an exalted position, for he is possessed of *Nous* and therefore eligible for communication with God who speaks to him through dreams and symbols. It is thus that he acquires the power of divination[47]. Paracelsus' speculations on the traffic between spirits are in many respects reminiscent of those of the Kabbala, notably the later—*Lurian*—trends of the 16th and 17th centuries, including the idea of psychical pregnancy (*Ibbur*) and possession (*Dibkuth*)[48].

The Paracelsian *Archeus* may well be interpreted as the object itself in its pre-formed "astral", magisterial or "sophic" state. As such the *archeus* is a principle responsible for the moulding of an individual with its specific plan of form and function. It is an individualising principle. At the same time it is part of the world soul and as such connected with divinity. Owing to this it confers the gift of life on individual objects. In this we may see a reflection of the Gnostic idea that the *archon* joins the powers of light with matter, whereby the latter is transformed. These powers are the sparks of life that are specific to each individual. The *archon* can join them to matter as well as separate them from it, an activity comparable to the spa-gyric, i.e. separating and

[46] *Poemander*, cap. X, 20–22, ed. Parthey, *loc. cit.*, 1854, pp. 80–82.

[47] *Poemander*, cap. XII, 19, ed. cit., pp. 110–111.

[48] Ibbur and Dibkuth see the loci quoted by Pagel, *Paracelsus*, 1958, pp. 216–217. On possible, but rather doubtful connexions between Paracelsus and the Kabbala see: G. Scholem, *Alchemie und Kabbala. Ein Kapitel aus der Geschichte der Mystik. Monschr. Gesch. u. Wissensch. d. Judent*, 1925, LXIX, 13–30; 95–110. R. Eisler, *Zur Terminologie der jüdischen Alchemie, ibid.*, pp. 364–371 (notably on the term *suspitha*—residual deposits —and its kinship with "*sepsis*"—corruption and fermentation to which also the metals are subject. According to Eisler gold must ferment and corrupt in order to convert metals into their primordial matter—the dark *chaos*—then into red copper, white silver and finally yellow gold.) See also: G. Scholem, *Nachbemerkung* to Eisler, *ibid.*, pp. 371–374. K. Preis, *Die Medizin im Sohar, ibid.*, 1928, LXXII, pp. 167–184, especially p. 170.

combining work of the alchemist[49]. Paracelsus calls the *archeus* (*archon*) the *internal alchemist.* It forms the individual being and directs its vital functions —first and foremost digestion. For this is the main agency through which the body communicates with the outside world. Material belonging to the latter is transmuted into constituents of the individual with its own properties that are specific to it and its species. Their consumption and excretion, i.e. their return to the non-specific state in the outside world, is also governed by the *archeus.*

### THE ELEMENTS—WATER AS ORIGINAL (PRIME) MATTER

*Archei* not only act in man and other beings, but also in the *Elements.* These Paracelsus sees not as the atomic constituents of every object in the ancient sense, but as dwelling places and matrices. Each of the elements thus has its own offspring: water the minerals and metals, earth man and plants. The *archeus* of water forms the minerals, and these bear the "seal" of their mother: water. Though a "fruit" of water, however, the minerals and metals grow in the earth where they are moulded by the terrestrial *Archeus*[50]. Or in symbolic language: Nature generates a tree in water. This grows out into the earth where it brings forth fruit: the earthborn minerals and metals[51]. This is the product of a vital action, i.e. it is specific and cannot be reproduced *in vitro.* Hence the alchemist finds it much easier to transmute than to generate metals[52].

[49] The *archon* works like the alchemist, joining the spark of light to matter whereby the latter is endowed with qualities and virtues—and transformed. These virtues become separated from matter, however, when the pneuma achieves liberation and returns to divine simplicity. Again, this process corresponds to the joining and disjoining (spa-gyric) action of the alchemist and also to the migration and creation of soul. In the Gnostic treatise *Kore Kosmou* the demiurge prepares "un mélange d'animation" for the creation of the soul in the same way as the alchemist prepares the "sophic mercury" destined for the animation of all metals. It forms a foam on the surface, comparable to the foamy spermatic fluid, and is a fiery water and fluid spirit ("water of life"). See: A. J. Festugière, *La création des âmes dans la Kore Kosmou. In: Pisciculi. Studien z. Religion und Kultur des Altertums F. J. Dolger dargeboten,* Münster, 1939, pp. 102–116. The present author is indebted to Professor J. R. Partington for this reference.

[50] Metals, water and earth: *De Natura Rerum,* lib. I, ed. Sudhoff, vol. XI, p. 318.

[51] *Das Buch de Mineralibus,* ed. Sudhoff, vol. III, p. 37. Cf. *Philos. Paracelsica de gener, et fruct. quatt. elementor,* Tract. III, cap. 10: Vom Archeo der Metallen, ed. Sudhoff, vol. XIII, p. 105.

[52] *De Natura Rerum,* lib. I de gener. rer. natur., ed. Sudhoff, vol. XI, p. 318.

Water has a much farther reaching significance, however. In Gnostic and early alchemical speculation, it stood for matter at large. It was the dark abyss, the primeval *chaos*. This was represented as the *uncreated* principle of evil and matter and, in a dualistic view, coordinated to divine light. All matter was water and all transmutation operated by the powers of light, all creation and separation took place in and on water. Paracelsus says: "The water was matrix; for in water there was created heaven and earth and in no other matrix . . . as the world was nothing but a water and the spirit of the Lord was on the water, the water was made into the world[53]". Moreover, water is "the receptacle of the seed from which man grows, which seed is the *limbus*"[54]. Finally: "Man with his angelic body was in heaven, that is the part above his belt; with the other part he was on the water"[55]. In the last resort these ideas go back to the Biblical saying that the spirit of God hovered over the waters. Any possible connection with a succession in time which may have been construed from this—to the effect that water was the first thing to exist—had been rejected already by the early Jewish and Christian commentators. There is no intention in the *Thorah* to fix any chronological order in the narrative of the creation, let alone any implication that God found water as the pre-existing material from which to create the world[56]. Just this, however, is the Gnostic position according to which matter was uncreated and pre-existing. With this several other ideas were connected: the material world was created in connexion with the fall of Lucifer and the angels whereby these were banned into the prison of material bodies. Moreover the material world including man was said to be due to the activity of a fallen deity (*demiurge*). Finally the divine spark was thought to have been transferred from the *demiurge* to man who was destined to replace the world of the fallen deity (Lucifer). Man thus forms a world of his own—a microcosm—which like the cosmos at large is composed of water and divine spirit. Possession of the divine spark makes man eligible for redemption—which is closed to Lucifer and his realm. In and through man the spirit of God returns to God[57].

[53] Water was matrix: *Opus Paramirum*, lib. IV, *de matrice*, ed. Sudhoff, vol. IX, p. 191.

[54] Water receptacle of seed (limbus): *Opus Paramirum de matrice*, ed. Sudhoff, vol. IX, p. 191.

[55] Man in heaven and in water: *Liber Azoth*, ed. Sudhoff, vol. XIV, p. 593.

[56] Raschi to Genesis at several places: No chronological order intended by the report on creation. See also: Hirsch Graetz, *Gnostizismus und Judenthum*, Krotoschin, 1846, pp. 30–35. M. Joel, Blicke i.d. Religionsgesch, *loc. cit.*, pp. 162–166; Excurs II: Die Gnosis.

[57] See above (note 11) the loci from Origen, Baur, Böhme, Croll, Pagel and Sheppard.

The return of the soul to God and of the astral body to the stars was also assumed by Paracelsus[58]. We shall see presently that he also incorporated some of the other Gnostic positions which we mentioned.

### Prime Matter—Creation versus Preformation

First of all we must discuss the position of the primeval waters, the abyss of matter, in the cosmology of Paracelsus. Did he also follow in this the Gnostic doctrines and speculations? Did he also regard original matter as something coordinated to God, a power uncreated and not originally subjected to Him? Indeed passages could be adduced from the Paracelsian *Corpus* which seem to support this. On the other hand, the opposite view could be defended—namely that Paracelsus believed in the creation of matter by God. A final decision in this question is therefore hardly possible, even when the testimony of the Paracelsists is called in. We must content ourselves with reviewing the evidence.

Paracelsus says of God that "He made an element water and from it generates the minerals so that they grow daily for the use of mankind"[59]. Thus water was destined to become the matrix of ores, metals and stones. So far the passage is clear. What follows, however, is less so. Here it says that "the first was with God (*bei Gott*), the beginning, that is *ultima materia*; this *ultima materia* He made into prime matter. As fruit that is to yield other fruit has seed, the seed is in prime matter. Thus ultimate matter of the minerals is made into prime matter that is a seed and the seed is the element of water . . ."[60]. In other words God created water as the mother of minerals. This created water, however, was not primeval matter, which here appears to be called ultimate matter and was "with God". From it God created the "prime matter" of the minerals, i.e. their seed, and this divine seed is the element of water which he created.

[58] Return of astral body to stars: "Through death the elemental body with its spirit goes to the grave, the ethereal is consumed in its firmament, the spirit of the (divine) image goes to Him whose image it is. Hence each dies in that from which he is, and in this he is buried", *Philosophia sagax*, Lib. I, Prolog., ed. Sudhoff, vol. XII, p. 18. "As the first father dies and with his body returns to the elements, and also with his heaven returns to the star, and hence both are consumed in their father, their children are consumed and buried in their father likewise, that is, what is flesh and blood, in the elements, and that where art and senses lie, in the star; also what is martial is buried in Mars, what is venereal in Venus . . .", *ibid.*, Lib. I, cap. 2, pp. 47–48.

[59] He made an element water: *Das Buch de Mineralibus*, ed. Sudhoff, vol. III, p. 33.

[60] The first was with God: *Ibid.*, p. 34.

The significance of this passage in our context is that primeval matter is assumed to exist "with God" ("*bei Gott*").

In another passage God, Prime Matter, Heaven and finally the soul (*Gemüt*) of man are juxtaposed as eternal and imperishable[61]. From this a primary co-existence of matter with God could be deduced. From the context, however, it would appear to be visualized as one aspect of divinity rather than something independent and of equal status.

It is, however, plainly expressed in the Paracelsian *Corpus* that the "*Mysterium Magnum*", i.e. the first "mother of all creatures" was un-created. It was "prepared" (*zubereitet*) and ever since, nothing like it has existed or ever will exist. Hence God is not a creator, but a separator. For the "*Mysterium Magnum*" contains the individual objects, as a block of marble or wood contains the future statue. The generating power which "was at the beginning of all birth-giving" was separation (*Truphat*)—"the greatest miracle of philosophy". The elements, including water, are late derivatives from the "*Mysterium Magnum*" or, as it is usually called, the *Iliaster*[62].

We read this in a treatise that is often regarded as spurious, the *Philosophia ad Athenienses*[63]. There is, however, no doubt that it was popular in Paracelsian circles and expresses genuine Paracelsian thought.

We merely learn from these passages that the original matrix was uncreated. It is not stipulated, however, that it existed beside and outside God, in a dualistic and Gnostic sense. It may be just as well interpreted in Pantheistic terms, visualizing the original matrix as a God from whom everything emanates. This could find support in Paracelsus' idea of the *Arcana* which are direct emanations from divinity—stepping out to provide the spiritual soul-like specific power and virtue to each individual object. This is the teaching of a treatise which has always enjoyed the reputation of authenticity. Here it says: "all natural things flow from God and no other source . . . the things are His, the herb He created, not however the virtue that is in it. For each virtue is uncreated; that is, God is without beginning and not created. Thus all virtues and powers were in God, prior to heaven and earth, and before all things were created, when God was a spirit and hovered

[61] God, Prime Matter, Heaven and Man: *Liber de Imaginibus*, ed. Sudhoff, vol. XIII, p. 383.

[62] *Philos. ad Athenienses*, text II-IX, ed. Sudhoff, vol. XIII, pp. 390–393.

[63] *Phil. ad Athen.*, unauthentic: K. Sudhoff, *Paracelsus Sämtl. Werke*, I. Abt., vol. XIII, München and Berlin, 1931, p. xi. J. Strebel, following Sudhoff in his Paracelsus edition, St. Gallen, 1945, vol. II, p. 428.

on the waters, that is when God's spirit walked over the waters"[64]. The virtues immanent to objects are therefore divine, supernatural, and without beginning and end—returning to their origin when heaven and earth are destroyed. It goes on to say that God at one point created things—stars, the earth, mountains, herbs, water, fire, air, metals, minerals and planets. "After he had created them they came into being, became apprehensible and visible, and from nothing there was matter which we put to use".

Here, then, the creation of "matter" is mentioned, and that in a genuine Paracelsian treatise. However, "matter" in this context does not mean "primary matter", but the material cover of individual objects. It is therefore hardly relevant in our discussion.

In the genuine book *De Meteoris* (*Liber Meteororum*)[65] each of the four elements—the dwelling places and matrices of objects—is said to have its own body that was made from nothing. It was solely made by the word of God: *Fiat*. Each of these four elements has its own "prime matter": "one is *materia prima* of water, another of earth, another of air, another of heaven". Again a comparatively late stage in the creative process is discussed: the production of a material base for the four elemental realms. It is not, however, the general unqualified matter, the *chaos* and *limbus* which embraces all the elements yet unseparated and in a potential form.

Later, in the *Prologue to the Books on Meteors*, we are told that the place occupied by the four elements had originally been the "heaven of Lucifer who was not ejected from it, but the same heaven was made perishable and elemental; this is his punishment that he must stay therein, whereas he could not forsee that God would convert such a heaven, such a bliss into elements"[66]. Here, then, we learn that something preceded the elements at the place where they are found today: namely Satan and his realm. This, before his punishment, was heaven—to be converted into hell by the creation of the elements from nothing. To be relegated to the sphere of the elements was the very punishment that was meted out to Lucifer. What greater retribution could be exacted than confinement to things perishable and the change from the light of heaven to the darkness which is the transitory world? Hence the devil and his henchmen dwell in the elements, some in water, some in fire, some in air and others in earth. It is the perishable world that God has created as a

[64] Virtues uncreated: *De vera influentia rerum*, tract. I, ed. Sudhoff, vol. XIV, p. 215.

[65] De Meteoris, ed. Sudhoff, vol. XIII, p. 134.

[66] Heaven of Lucifer: Prolog. *Konzepte u. Ausarbeitungen zum Liber Meteororum*, ed. Sudhoff, vol. XIII, pp. 253–254.

penalty for the devil, first the element of air that is the *chaos* or heaven and thereafter the other elements.

This expresses the characteristically Gnostic idea that the coming into being of the material world was closely bound up with the fall of Lucifer and his activity. We quoted above the idea expressed by Origen that God created the world in order to ban the fallen spirits into the narrow confinement of material bodies[67]. We may also recall the saying of Poemander that the word of God that was in the elements left them on their downward journey and joined the *Nous* of the creator. Thus the elements of nature, deprived of *logos*, remained and became matter[68].

Again the passages from Paracelsus just quoted show that the creative act of God appertained to the elements and not necessarily to prime matter. It should be added in fairness, however, that the elements are again definitely stated to have been created from nothing ("also ist der anfang der vier elementen aus nichten beschaffen"). Nevertheless further close contacts with Gnostic ideas emerge from these passages. They are still more evident in what Paracelsus called the *Cagastrum*.

This stands for the splitting up of God's simplicity and unity into the infinite multitude of beings, for elemental materiality, and hence for decay and corruption. All this is due to the fall of Lucifer and of man. Paracelsus believed that some diseases are due to cagastric seed which takes possession of the body after invading it from outside—by contrast with hereditary and endogenous disease which is due to "iliastric" seed. Pleurisy, plague and fevers are such "cagastric" diseases[69]. All *spontaneous generation* belongs to the *Cagastrum*, that is any coming into being without proper parents. The seed of an apple, pear or nut has been there for ever. The cagastric seed emerges here and now from corrupting material. Its offspring differs according to the properties of the matrix.

After the fall the flesh of Adam became cagastric, i.e. subject to corruption—before that it had been iliastric, i.e. divine, immortal and truly alive. Now it is mortal, false and a caricature ("*monstrum*") of its archetype[70]. All that is genuine is iliastric, all that is fake—false metal, a false prophet—is cagastric. In short, *cagastrum* is falsehood, the fallacious phantom of the phenomenal world. Yet in it there resides a positive and independent original power—as it

[67] Fall and creation of material world see above (notes 11 and 57).

[68] *Poemander*, I, 10, ed. Parthey, *loc. cit.*, p. 5.

[69] Cagastric diseases: *Labyrinthus Medicorum*, cap. 11, ed, Sudhoff, vol. XI, pp. 215-216.

[70] Cagaster as "monstrum": *Liber. Azoth*, cap. 1, ed. Sudhoff, vol. XIV, p. 549.

was visualized in Gnostic speculation on the original force of the abyss of darkness and evil.

In spite of all the evidence which we have collected in favour of or at least not against, a Paracelsian belief in uncreated original matter, we do have one outspoken piece of testimony for its creation in the Paracelsian *Corpus*: "Thus God the Father created through His word things not in their ultimate state, but He only created *Prima Materia confusa*, that is the matrix, in which all Nature of the whole world was mixed together . . . called abyss and earth or a thing in which all things lie hidden . . . and this *Prima Materia* was the water on which the spirit of the Lord had hovered . . . *Materia prima* made from nothing and hence called *Abyssus* . . .". This is what the *Secretum Magicum de Lapide Philosophorum* tell us[71]. Matter is created; not so the individual object, or only to the extent that it is part of the prime matter from which it emerges as the result of the separating and composing work of the *Archei*.

The *Secretum Magicum*, however, is certainly not normally regarded as a genuine work of Paracelsus. It first appeared in Huser's Folio edition of 1603 under the title: *Von dreyen gebenedeyten Magischen Steinen, Theophrasti Paracelsi, welches auss seiner Handschrift kommen*. It was then reprinted on several occasions, for example in Gottfried Arnold's *Kirchen-und Ketzerhistorie* where it forms one piece of evidence for the piety of Paracelsus[72]. Thus at all events the treatise informs us about the opinion of some *Paracelsists* in this matter. It is worth while to hear what they have to say[73].

A straightforward account of our question is found in the work of Robert Fludd (1574–1637). In his *History of Both Worlds of the Macrocosm and Microcosm*, he raises the question of the origin of prime matter, whether it was created or not. On this question, he says, there is "*ingens dissensio*" among

[71] *Secretum Magicum*, ed. Huser Fol, vol. II, pp. 672–673.

[72] See K. Sudhoff, *Bibliographia Paracelsica*, 1894, Repr. Graz, 1958, p. 445, and the Huser-Folio of 1603.

[73] Among the Paracelsists, Oswald Croll (1580–1609) fails to give a clear-cut answer about the position of prime matter. He seems to take a Pantheistic view: God is the All out of himself and man is All made by God. *Basilica Chymica* (1608), ed. Hartmann, Genevae, 1643, p. 60, Engl. transl. by H. Pinnell, *Philosophy reformed*, London, 1657, pp. 58 *et seq.* Nor can any direct information be obtained from the author of: *Introductio Hominis oder kurtze Anleitung zu eim Christlichen Leben*, in: *Philosophia Mystica. Eilff Theologico-Philosophiscne Tractätlein, auss Theophrasti Paracelsi, zum theil auss Valentini Weigelii* . . ., Newstadt, 1618, pp. 236–237. Here prime matter is said to have come into being (*ihren Anfang bekommen*) before all time and to embrace all four elements unseparated and mixed together.

philosophers. Most of them believe with Artephius that God created Nature and First Matter. Others, however, with Paracelsus and his followers, call matter a *Mysterium Magnum* that was neither created nor resembles any other creature, but was simply "prepared" by God. The Paracelsists argue that the scriptural verse: "In the beginning (*principio*) God created heaven and earth" does not prove the creation of matter. *Principium* need not mean first in time; it could mean first in some order or process or even first at some place. Indeed when creation occurred there was no time. Nor can heaven and earth have been created first without matter already existing, for "heaven and earth" are *principiata*, i.e. something formed from some more primitive material, from a *principium*. Nor can this *principium* really be a place, for the creative word of God is beyond human comprehension and thus not associable with any place in this world. Paracelsus therefore interprets the scriptural verse differently: God created heaven and earth in the *Mysterium Magnum* that was un-created[74]. With this Fludd has recourse to the doctrine of the *Philosophia ad Athenienses*. He himself, however, does not wish to decide the issue, though from indirect evidence we can say that Fludd favoured the orthodox view of Artephius. Finally Fludd invokes St. Augustine, with whom he declares prime matter not to be anything real, but something that our imagination presents as a "nearly nothing", an intermediate stage between the absolute nothing and something created and endowed with form. It merely exists by virtue of its potentiality; it is really a nothing that may, however, become something through endowment with divine form[75].

Among Paracelsists who definitely asserted that God created prime matter, the abyss of the waters, the *Chaos*, from nothing, we quote Heinrich Khunrath (1560–1605) and Quercetanus whom we mentioned above.

Khunrath says[76] that the very first *weltanfängliche* (world-inchoating) *Chaos* was created by the unique tri-une God. From this afterwards the world was built up. It consisted of heaven, earth and water in tri-unity and was impregnated and animated by the spirit of the Lord, who hovered on the

[74] R. Fludd, *Utriusque Cosmi majoris sc. et minoris . . . Historia*, vol. I, Oppenheim J. Th. de Bry, 1617, pp. 23–24.

[75] R. Fludd, *Tomi Secundi Tractatus Secundus De Praeternaturali Utriusque Mundi Historia*, Frankfurt, 1621. Sect. 1, Port. 1, Part II, lib. 1: De primariis naturae elementis. Cap. 5: De scrupulo nonullorum, qui adversus opinionem meam, qua hylem increatam esse statuo, insurgunt, pp. 89–90. The present author is indebted to Mr. Allen Debus for this reference.

[76] Heinr. Khunrath, *Vom hylealischen, das ist Pri-materialischen Catholischen oder Allgemeinen Natürlichen Chaos der naturgemässen Alchymiae und Alchymisten*, Magdeburg, 1597; ed. used: Leipzig, 1786.

water, i.e. the dark watery abyss formed by heaven, earth and water mixed together. God therefore created prime matter—but, Khunrath adds, he did not create Nature. This developed independently through separation and partition of the ground of primary matter tilled and sown by the spirit of God.

Quercetanus said[77] that God created from nothing the *Chaos*, that is the abyss of the waters. These were animated by the spirit of God. There followed the separation of Light or ethereal heaven—a spiritual body of greatest purity, the *Quinta Essentia*, from the darkness of the waters. The latter became subjected to a process of separation in its turn. A more subtle—mercurial and aerial—liquor was separated from an oily-sulphureous one and this finally from a dry residue—the salt. Heaven, that is light as separated from "dark" water, also consists of these three fundamental "principles" without which nothing can exist or generate. However, only the finest and purest "ethereal" mercury, sulphur and salt are brought together to form the crystalline and diamond-like most simple body of heaven. From it the forms and *semina* are infused into the thicker elements for the generation of each individual object. These forms and *semina* are heaven's "fruit" which in essence is similar to the substance of heaven itself. They generate something similar again inside the elements that provide "thick" covers, through vital impression and influx. The ratio of thick to subtle matter determines the durability of the individual object. One that belongs to air is much less subtle than heaven, but still much finer and more durable than the offspring of water and earth. Mercurial fruit—spirits—of the air are the winds; the sulphur of air makes itself perceptible in the comets, its salt in manna, dew and frost.

*In conclusion* we must admit that Paracelsus conceded a position of prominence and independence to Prime Matter (*Mysterium Magnum, Iliaster, Limbus*)—an assignation that is reminiscent of Gnosticism and Platonic dualism. The evidence suggesting that he believed that it was uncreated and co-existed with God is controversial. He may have meant this in a Pantheistic sense, visualizing prime matter and nature as one aspect of divinity. Nevertheless in his view the creation of individual objects from nothing seems to be overshadowed by a process of separation and the demiurgic activity of the *archei* (archons). The more the world is split up into individual objects and beings—and this individuation seems to be the essential process in the coming into being of the world—the more the need for the material and elemental, for intermediate beings, for residues—the products of corruption of more and more independent primary matter, remote from divine simplicity and oneness and the realm of the spirits.

[77] Jos. Quercetanus, *Ad veritatem Hermeticae Medicinae, loc. cit.*, Paris, 1604, p. 184.

## Cagastrum—Tartar—Diseases versus disease

We mentioned the *Cagastrum* as a reminiscence of Gnosticism in Paracelsus. It embraces the splitting up of simplicity owing to the egotistic yearning of individual objects for independence, resulting from their "fall". This process leads to the efflorescence of "fruit" from the smooth surface of an elementary medium or receptacle. This is the pattern of all bodily change that is indicative of disease. The disease "fruit" consists of residual deposits, the products of pathological coagulation which normally are dissolved and thus do not appear. Health is the solution and assimilation of all that finds access to the body from outside. Disease is the failure of the internal "balm", the "mummy" or *archeus* to dissolve and assimilate. Hence the quest for the universal solvent, the *Liquor Alkahest,* which at the same time acts as a universal remedy.

From these ideas the *Tartar* pathology of Paracelsus developed. He compared the pathological changes in the organs with deposits of tartar in wine vats. They also deserve their name because of the hellish pain and suffering they cause, and finally as the visible expression of cagastric—satanic—interference with the dissolving and assimilating forces of the body, the seduction of the *archeus* from the function allotted to it in the commonwealth of the organism. In this doctrine of tartar, attention is focused on the outside origin of the pathogenic agent. There are as many such agents as there are diseases. Disease and agent are the same thing. Each disease therefore really exists as such, forming an organism of its own with its own functional schedule, imposing it on the body like a parasite. This "ontological" view of disease is alien to ancient medicine, in which disease in general was more important than diseases—there were no classifiable diseases as determined by specific exogenous agents and anatomical changes varying accordingly. There was only the sick man, and any differences in symptoms and signs were thought to be due to differences in temperament as the result of a humoral mixture that was characteristic of the individual.

The independent agents that introduce diseases into the human body from outside bring us back to the Semina and Logoi. Each object and each phenomenon in the world of Paracelsus represents something specific and spiritual—so does disease and even more so its specific "seed". Hence not only the seeds from which objects and organisms are generated, but also those that cause illness are connected with the spheres of will and wilful imagination. Thus are explained the intimate psycho-somatic associations, the "conversion" of thought, inclinations, and desires, into symptoms and pathological changes. One such example is the mole on the skin of a fœtus due to the imagination of the mother.

### Air—Life—Combustion—Fire

One reflection of the exalted position granted to spirit in neo-Platonism may be seen in the attention given by Paracelsus and Renaissance philosophers to the *air*. It is the medium that makes life possible—in man as well as the universe. It transmits the influence of the stars including "astral poison" such as the *contagium*. Air is closely associated with the "*Mysterium Magnum*", the "Mother of all Things", the giver of divine life[78]. Life, generally speaking, was to Paracelsus a process of combustion. "If I say it cannot burn, this is as much as if I said it cannot live". "For in the air is the force of all life"[79]. Life is invisible celestial fire, air enclosed in a body, a tinging spirit of salt[80]. Similarly Agrippa[81] had called the air the spirit of life which penetrates all, endowing it with life and support. It is the spirit that binds all, moves all and fills all. Air is the mirror which reflects all and in which all astral powers are concentrated. Air, and all that it contains, enters through the skin, and that includes even the "spirit of a place", explaining the terror we may experience at the site of a murder. The transmission of spiritual images, and traffic between spirits through the air, explains the phenomena of prophecy and the Paracelsian *Chaomantie*[82]. Not only spiritual, but even corporeal images (*idola*) can become detached, condensed in air and through light and motion fall into perception or exert miraculous effects in us, as Plotinus already taught. Many optical phenomena such as mirages and the *Camera obscura* belong to this field. A further source for the significance of the air as the seat of invisible spirits, of demons and heroes can be found in the hermetic *Asclepius*[83].

Two types of *Fire* had been distinguished in Stoic as well as neo-Platonic speculation: the "sophic" fire of the stars, the fire of the soul that nourishes and confers life (*Pyr Noeron*) and ordinary fire that is merely destructive[84]. Later and notably Gnostic sources mention the bright fire that is in the nature of

[78] Paracelsus, *Volumen Paramirum: De Ente Astrorum*, cap. VI, ed. Sudhoff, vol. I, p. 182.

[79] Paracelsus, *Liber Azoth*, ed. Sudhoff, vol. XIV, pp. 549 and 558.

[80] Paracelsus, *De Natura Rerum*, lib. IV, ed. Sudhoff, vol. XI, p. 330.

[81] Agrippa, *De Occulta Philosophia*, lib. I, cap. 6, ed. Lugduni, 1550, pp. 11 *seq.*

[82] Paracelsus, *Philosophia Sagax*, ed. Sudhoff, vol. XII, p. 95.

[83] *Asclepius*, ed. Mars. Ficino, cap. XII, *loc. cit.*, 1516, fol. 131v.–132v.

[84] Fire of the soul: E. Kroll, *Lehre des Hermes Trismegistos*, Münster, 1914, pp, 266, 285, 301. E. O. v. Lippmann, *Alchemie*, *loc. cit.*, 1919, p. 197.

light and the "dark" fire[85]. Similarly Paracelsus distinguishes between "essential" and "material" fire—the former operates by means of its specific "essential" virtues and powers, the latter through its consuming flame[86]. The Paracelsist Heinrich Khunrath (1560–1605) calls the essential fire "*Ignis Magorum*" and devoted a special treatise to it[87].

Fire and air from the upper sphere are the sources of the soul and life of the body, a breath or spirit infused by God into man—thus we are told by the theosophic author of the *Studium Universale*[88].

## Paracelsus' Conception of Time

Paracelsus' ideas on Time present aspects that concur with the new orientation introduced by Plotinus and Proclus. Following in their footsteps, Paracelsus interpreted time in terms of qualitative standards—as opposed to its quantitative-numerical determination in Peripatetic philosophy. Paracelsus' attitude is partly prompted by his criticism of traditional astrology—another point of contact with Plotinus[89]. Yet time, according to Paracelsus, is still closely correlated with the stars, though not in quantitative-numerical terms. The stars are luminous indicators of time, but do not generate time as the measure of their motion. Nor do they govern or direct man and man's actions. On the contrary, the wise will dominate the stars. It was precisely for the desire to appropriate the power of the stars through magic, that Paracelsus was blamed and associated with the heathen doctrines of Pomponatius (1462–1524) by his main adversary Thomas Erastus[90]. In this, however,

[85] Light and "dark" fire: see loci quoted in W. Pagel, *Paracelsus, loc. cit.*, 1958, pp. 212–213.

[86] Essential and material fire: *De Renovatione et Restoratione*, ed. Sudhoff, vol. III, p. 209. The salamander lives in essential fire: *Liber Azoth*, ed. Sudhoff, vol. XIV, p. 577.

[87] H. Khunrath, *De Igne Magorum Philosophorumque secreto externo et visibili, das ist Philosophische Erklärung des geheimen, äusserlichen, sichtbaren Glut und Flammenfeuers der uralten Weisen und andrer wahrer Philosophen*, Strasburg, 1608. Edition used: Leipzig, 1783.

[88] Pseudo-Weigel, *loc. cit.*, cap. 1, sig. A2 recto.

[89] See for the more important loci: Plotinus, *Ennead*, III, lib. 1, cap. 5–6, ed. H. F. Müller, Berlin, Weidmann, 1880, vol. I, pp. 161–163. Paracelsus, *Philosophia Magna; De Vera Influentia Rerum*, ed. Sudhoff, vol. XIV, p. 219. *De Inventione Artium*, *ibid.*, p. 251 *seq.*

[90] Th. Erastus, *Disputat. de Medicina Nova Paracelsi*, I, Basil, 1572, p. 111; see also pp. 117 and 128. Against Paracelsus on the "augural" power of words and "characters," p. 169. Against augurs and the omens derived from the action of birds: pp. 198–199, 221–222. See Pagel, *Paracelsus, loc. cit.*, 1958, p. 317.

Paracelsus had been foreshadowed by Ficino, who taught the scholar how to overcome the adverse influence of "his" star (notably Saturn) on his body[91]. Paracelsus recognizes a close connexion between time and the stars in so far that the latter maintain, as it were, a register or "portrait" of all change and all events on earth and in the life of man. Moreover, the virtues immanent to all objects and man are "astral" and each follows the pattern indicated by its cognate star. Virtue in this sense stands for the course that is specifically followed by the individual in unfolding his own life according to his own specific schedule. This is the "internal knowledge" (scientia) which enables the organism to direct its form and function towards the achievement of its own specific purpose in life, to its own perfection. This internal working of nature towards perfection in the individual, Paracelsus calls the "Light of Nature"—at all events that is one of the principal meanings of this term, whereby it is associated with the stars. For the intrinsic plan of form and function lies with the astral body, the quintessence and spirit of the individual organism—a spirit that is in the last resort derived from the stars. Each individual object reaches its perfection at a certain moment. This climax in the life of the individual, Paracelsus calls its "monarchy". Time, then, is determined by the points at which individual objects achieve perfection. One group of objects comes to such maturity in summer, another in autumn or even in winter; some things reach their monarchy at a quick, others at a slow pace. Time, therefore, is the chain that connects the summits of monarchy experienced by individual objects at certain points. It indicates the relationship between these monarchies. In other words it entirely depends upon the quality and "virtue" of the object. Hence all that matters in time is the present[92]—the moment that is, when perfection is reached. Time is therefore no number, no instrument of counting; it has nothing to do with succession as such, with "empty" time. By contrast, each individual thing has its own time, its own pace and rhythm of life, as intrinsic in its seed and derived from the "astra".

Not only individuals, but also periods and epochs in the life of humanity have their own time. This is the *Zeitgeist* (spirit of time). What is valid today may have lost its reality tomorrow. Ancient medicine had its climax in antiquity; it is of no use today. Paracelsus thus feels his vocation for the creation of a new medicine born out of the specific exigencies of his own time.

[91] Ficinus, *De Vita coelitus comparanda* (1489); see Pagel, *Paracelsus, loc. cit.*, 1958, p. 220.

[92] Importance of the present, the "now": *Die erste Defension* (1537–38), ed. Sudhoff, vol. XI, pp. 127–128. On the Light of Nature and its connexion with the stars: *Philos. sagax*, I, cap. 1, ed. Sudhoff, vol. XII, p. 23. See Pagel, *loc. cit.*, 1958, p. 75.

Before Paracelsus, Arnald of Villanova (1235–1311) had been actuated by similar motives. There are further points of contact between these figures, although Paracelsus himself gives Arnald but limited credit and only for such Franciscan-Joachimite and Chiliastic ideas[93] as were connected with the prophecy of an impending end of the world, the coming of the Anti-Christ and the "Third Kingdom". In the same field we find Paracelsus quoting with approval the prophecies of Hildegard of Bermersheim (commonly called Hildegard of Bingen, 1098–1179)[94].

In associating Time with the specific virtue intrinsic to the object, Paracelsus foreshadowed the biological concept of Time that was to be developed by Joh. Baptista Van Helmont (1579–1644). The latter in turn was inspired in this by neo-Platonic speculation.

## The Principle of Trichotomy and the Tria Prima

One of the principles adhered to by Paracelsus is that of *trichotomy*. Man consists of a divine spirit, an astral body and an elemental body. This division repeats the trichotomous anthropology of Hermetic and Gnostic literature and of neo-Platonism. It was also preceded by mediaeval alchemy in which metals were compared with organic bodies ascribing to them body, soul and spirit. For example the "Philosopher" says: The "dragon" is "live silver" extracted from bodies and possessing body, soul and spirit[95]. Mercury (*Aurum vivum*) is cold, moist and black in virtue of its body, but warm and dry, in virtue of its spirit, and white in virtue of its soul[96].

A further significant example is the *Tria Prima*: Salt, Sulphur and Mercury which are supposed to be the principal constituents of all objects. This trichotomy is largely an original Paracelsian conception[97]. At all events it was Paracelsus who inculcated and applied it in detail. His alchemist predecessors had preferred such dichotomic divisions as male-female, active-passive,

[93] *Opus Paramirum*, I: De Orig. morbor. ex tribus substant. prim., ed. Sudhoff, vol. IX, p. 54. On Paracelsus and Arnald de Villanova see: P. Diepgen, *Die Weltanschauung Arnalds von Villanova und seine Medizin, Scientia Milano*, 1937, p. 41. *Idem*, "Theophrastus von Hohenheim", *Research and Progress*, 1942, VII, 111–112. Pagel, *Paracelsus*, *loc. cit.*, 1958, p. 249 *et seq.*

[94] Paracelsus, *Fragmenta cum libro de fundamento sapientiae congruentia*, ed. Sudhoff, vol. XIII, p. 334. Pagel, *loc. cit.*, 1958, p. 210 *seq.*

[95] *Rosarium Philos.*, ed. Manget, Bibl. Chem., vol. II, p. 94.

[96] Roger Bacon, *De Arte Chymica*, Francof., 1603, p. 46.

[97] See R. Hooykaas, *Chemical Trichotomy before Paracelsus?*, Arch. Internat. d'Hist. des Sciences, 1949, XXVIII, 1063–1074.

Sulphur-Mercury. The *Salia* of metals had been discussed—but not in the Paracelsian sense of a third principle; they rather indicated a state of hardening which called for solution. It is also true that the *Latin Geber* speaks of the *Tria Principia* of metals, namely Sulphur, *Argentum Vivum* and Arsenic—but in this Arsenic occupied no position similar to that of *Sal* in the Paracelsian scheme[98].

No chemical or alchemical predecessor of the Paracelsian scheme is therefore readily demonstrable. There is no doubt, however, that it is in accordance with neo-Platonic and Hermetic tradition. Paracelsus himself referred to Hermes who called the soul the intermediary between Spirit and Body. This soul Paracelsus identified with Sulphur: "the soul is the sulphur which reconciles two opposites and joins them together into one"[99]. Hermes rightly said, Paracelsus adds, that all seven metals, and also the "tinctures" and the Philosophers' Stone derive from three substances which he calls spirit, soul and body. These are indeed the *Three Principles*.

In this context it is of particular interest that Ficino is quoted by the commentator of a late, probably spurious "Hermetic" tract dealing with alchemical problems, which also gives itself a "Hermetic" garb by interpreting the trichotomy of soul, spirit and body in chemical terms. This is the *Tractatus Aureus de Lapidis Physici Secreto*, first coming to light as late as 1600[100]. Here we are told of the conjunction between heaven and earth—the former corresponding to the soul, the latter to the body. For this conjunction there is need for "something third"—this Marsilius Ficinus called something most subtle, no longer body and almost soul and not soul, but almost body[101]. In the physical world heaven corresponds to "useful water" and earth to "useless residue", the "*Faex*". Between these two stands the spirit—endowed with two aspects: that of a physical substance and that of an occult spirit. It is comparable to a subtle smell or fine balm and as it is believed to be combustible presented as sulphur.

Here, then, we find in an alchemical tract composed in the ancient—"Hermetic"—fashion the trichotomy of the Principles: the fluid-airy heaven

[98] Geber, *Summa Perfectionis*, lib. I, cap. 27. In: *De Alchimia*, Nürnberg, Joh. Petreius, 1541, p. 60, also cap. 25, p. 55, and cap. 26, p. 56. See on the position of arsenic in comparison with the Paracelsian Salt: Hooykaas, *loc. cit.*, 1949, p. 1070. W. Ganzenmüller, *Paracelsus und die Alchemie des Mittelalters* in: *Beiträge z. Geschichte d. Technologie und Alchemie*, Weinheim, 1956, p. 306. W. Pagel, *loc. cit.*, 1958, p. 269, note 215 and p. 270.

[99] Paracelsus, *De Natura Rerum*, lib. I, ed. Sudhoff, vol. XI, p. 318.

[100] In: Manget, *Bibliotheca Chemica et Curiosa*, Genevae, 1702, vol. I, pp. 400–445 (notably pp. 422 *et seq.*).

[101] See above, note 7.

animating the universe and corresponding to Paracelsian Mercury, earth representing dead "*faex*"—the Paracelsian *Sal*, and as the intermediary bridging the contrast a combustible subtly corporeal spirit or smell—the Paracelsian Sulphur.

Neo-Platonic trichotomy could not fail to appeal to Paracelsus also because of its connotation with the Christian-religious trichotomy.

## The Symbol of the Circle

Traces and reflections of neo-Platonic circle symbolism can also be found in Paracelsus. He visualizes the *Iliaster* and *Idechtrum*, the ideal world in which all possible events and creatures are preformed, as a Globule[102]. "Sphaera-globule" is the term commonly used for heaven and universe[103]. Man, an offspring partly of the star and partly of the earth, is microcosm and quintessence of the whole "machina mundi", he is the *centre* into which all *spheres* "infuse" their rays. Man is in the centre of all creatures and of the whole "machina mundi". Indeed the latter was created because of and for the centre. All that is external to man, converges upon him and he as the centre receives it[104].

More explicitly the symbol of the circle was used by some Paracelsists, notably Croll, Severinus and Michael Maier.

It is the centre of all circles which we must approach in our investigation of nature—as against the circulatory motions of the elements which were the subject of ancient philosophy. God's work is circular in that all that was made tends back to Him in "circular rotation". Hence the work is perfect. God is the centre—for all derives from Him. He is the circle—for he embraces all. This we are told by Oswald Croll (1580–1609)[105] the Paracelsist. He also connects the spheres which compose the world, each with a specific seed. In this again we find traces of circular symbolism, for all comes from and returns to seed—as we witness in plants and trees. Hence prime matter is the seed of the whole world and the latter the seed of Adam.

[102] Paracelsus, *Fragmenta Anatomiae Theophrasti*, ed. Huser Fol., vol. II, p. 21; ed. Sudhoff, vol. III, p. 465. *Secretum Magicum von dreyen Gebenedeyten Magischen Steinen*, ed. Huser Fol, vol. II, p. 671. K. Goldammer, *Paracelsus. Natur und Offenbarung*, Hannover, 1953, p. 35 (quoting from *Psalmenkommentar* to Ps. 150, 22).

[103] See M. Müller's *Registerband zu Sudhoff's Paracelsus-Gesamtausgabe*, Nova Acta Paracels. Einsiedeln. Supplementum, 1960, p. 101, sub: *globul.*

[104] *Entwürfe zur Astronomia Magna*, De Compos. humanae generat, ed. Sudhoff, vol. XII, p. 454.

[105] O. Croll, *Basilica Chymica*, ed. Hartmann, *loc. cit.*, 1643, p. 57 *seq.*

The seed—owing to its intimate blending of body and spirit—is a true *Ens*. Developing into the corruptible object it becomes *Non-Ens*. Before perishing, however, this has developed further seed, and thus regenerated its seminal *Ens*—a cycle that is ever repeated. This "circular perfection" of the seeds makes the continuity of the world possible. Thus we are told by another Paracelsist, some thirty years prior to Croll: Peter Severinus (1542–1602)[106]. He also saw in the seed the carrier of internal wisdom—a *scientia* that can neither be taught nor learned. It is that intrinsic awareness that enables things to realize their specific life-aims within their own time. With all this Severinus felt himself to speculate on Platonic lines.

Finally we may refer to the "physical circle" which the Rosicrucian and Alchemist Michael Maier (1568–1622) believed himself to recognize in gold[107]. It indicates the perfect equality of all its constituents—an equality that is also found in the sun, the king of the planets, and in the human heart. Gold, sun and heart make harmony in the world possible. In this a circulation is operative: Divine strength flows into the sun, from there into the gold harboured by the earth and from the latter into the heart. It is by rotatory movement that the "circle of gold" achieves simplicity and homogeneity—the squaring of the circle.

### Magia Naturalis—Gamaheu—Engraved Images

Mighty power is wrought in Words, Plants and Stones. According to neo-Platonic as well as Paracelsian speculation, the *magus* transfers the powers of the stars to plants and in particular to gems—these are the *Gamaheu* of Paracelsus and may be regarded as the successor of the Gnostic and Abraxas gems with their characteristic graven images. Paracelsus believed in the natural occurrence of such images as are found on rocks and in caves and secret passages. They appeared at God's command, carrying a secret message that is understood by magicians and chiromancers[108]. With this Paracelsus took sides in a controversy that had stirred up mediaeval opinion. Consciously or unconsciously he supported the view of Konrad von Megenberg (1309–1374) whose *Buch der Natur* he is likely to have known. This was largely, but not entirely, a German version of the Encyclopedia written in Latin by Thomas of Chantimpre (*c.* 1201–1270). One of the points in which Konrad disagrees

[106] Peter Severinus, *Idea Medicinae Philosophicae*, Basel, 1571, pp. 89–90. See W. Pagel, *William Harvey and the Purpose of Circulation*. *Isis*, 1951, XLII, p. 34.

[107] Mich. Maier, *De Circulo Physico Quadrato*, Oppenheim, 1616. See W. Pagel, *Isis*, *loc. cit.*, 1951, XLII, 36.

[108] Paracelsus, *De Imaginibus*, ed. Sudhoff, vol. XIII, pp. 373–375.

with the master is precisely the natural occurrence of the images: Thomas had denied, Konrad asserted it[109]. The latter referred to the consonant opinion of Techel the Jew (Thetel, Zahel), in almost the same laudatory terms as the author of the Paracelsian treatise *Liber Principiorum Paracelsi*, the so called *Schlangen—und Spinnenbuch*[110]. Here Techellus, the author of a lapidary, translated and incorporated in Thomas' encyclopedia, is praised both by Konrad and by the *Liber Principiorum* as a great master in Israel. It is true that this Paracelsian treatise, although admittedly based on genuine Paracelsian sentiments, is commonly regarded as spurious[111]. However, the same support is given to Konrad's opinion in *De Imaginibus*, a treatise of the Paracelsian *Corpus* which has always enjoyed the reputation of authenticity[112].

## Possible Patristic, Mediaeval and Renaissance Sources for neo-Platonic trends in the speculation of Paracelsus
### Light of Nature—Chaos—Semina

The frequency and significance of neo-Platonic ideas in the work of Paracelsus are not surprising. For it was in Renaissance neo-Platonism that he could find the sources and traditions that led to the uncovering of the Occult and Invisible in Nature. These *Magnalia Naturae* were to Paracelsus the *Magnalia Dei*; to search for and acquire knowledge of them fulfils divine will and human destiny. Hence this is the way to truth—it is given to the layman, the simple and unlearned, the observer of nature, unprejudiced by complacent human reasoning, formal logic and book learning. It comes to the chosen in their sleep, in dreams and visions and in the constraining reality of signs and symbols that reveal the truth at once. "*Scientia*" is primarily in the object, and we acquire it as the result of a union of the observer with the object. This he can attain by virtue of being a microcosm in which all components of the greater world are represented. As like unites with like, such a union can take place in him, supported by the action of the world soul. This is the way that will confer power over the stars, it is the royal road of natural science and medicine: all that may be briefly summarised in the term *Magia Naturalis*—the art of marrying heaven with earth, as Pico della Mirandola (1463–1494) had defined it.

[109] Konrad von Megenberg, *Das Buch der Natur*, ed. Fr. Pfeiffer, Stuttgart, 1861, Lib. VI, 84, Von dem Tethelspuechl, p. 469.

[110] Paracelsus, *Liber Principiorum*, cap. 5, ed. Sudhoff, vol. XIV, p. 503.

[111] E. Schubert and K. Sudhoff, *Paracelsus-Forschungen*, vol. II, Frankfurt, 1889, p. 137, note.

[112] See for a detailed discussion: W. Pagel, *Paracelsus and Techellus the Jew*, *Bullet. Hist. Med.*, 1960, XXXIV, pp. 274–277.

We mentioned in several places Marsilio Ficino and Agrippa of Nettesheym. Both these can be safely regarded as fixed points in the literary sources through which neo-Platonic and magic tradition came to Paracelsus. There are, however, other probable sources of inspiration, notably Trithemius (1462–1516), one of the learned ecclesiastic teachers of Paracelsus, and the large library which he is known to have possessed and continually enriched with alchemical and "pansophic" treatises[113]. There was also contemporary alchemical literature such as Brunschwig's *Destillirbuch*. For leading philosophical ideas such as the rejection of scholastic and book-learning in favour of the simple experience that leads the mind of the apparently ignorant to truth, Paracelsus could have found a number of predecessors since the days of Petrarch (1304–74), notably in Nicolaus Cusanus (1401–64). It was here that the layman—*Idiota*— was introduced in a dialogue with the learned philosopher whom he has no difficulty to confound, and it is here that we find the first recommendation of the use of the balance in biology and medicine as a means of uncovering the occult laws and rules inherent in vital functions[114].

In propounding his anthropocentric philosophy and basing it on neo-Platonic speculation, Paracelsus is rightly regarded as an exponent of the Renaissance. It must be borne in mind, however, that there is much that is mediaeval in his speculations. In this he can be seen in contact with those trends in mediaeval philosophy that brought about a revival of Platonism. It is not accidental that through this neo-Platonic aspect, and its reception of Stoic elements, mediaeval philosophy inspired naturalism. Thus the symbolism connected with light as a direct divine force in the cosmos greatly advanced the study of optics. This neo-Platonism was as close to mysticism as to natural science[115].

Paracelsus throughout the phases of his literary activity used the term *Light of Nature* to indicate a concept of considerable importance in his speculations on man and his position in the cosmos. He regarded nature as the totality

[113] On Trithemius and the alchemical tracts of his "pansophic" library: W.-E. Peuckert, *Die grosse Wende*, 1948, pp. 430–431. See also K. Goldammer, *Die bischöflichen Lehrer des Paracelsus*, *Arch. f. Gesch. d. Med.*, 1953, XXXVII, 234; *idem*, *Paracelsus-Studien*, Klagenfurt, 1954, pp. 35 *et seq.; idem*, *Lichtsymbolik in philosophischer Weltanschauung, Mystik und Theosophie vom* 15.-17. *Jahrhundert. Stud. Gen.*, 1960, XIII, 670–682 (p. 674).

[114] On Nic. Cusanus see literature quoted by W. Pagel, *Paracelsus*, 1958, *loc. cit.*, p. 199 and pp. 279–284.

[115] See, for example, on Petrus Hispanus in this connexion: H. Schipperges, *Medizinischer Unterricht im Mittelalter*, *Deut. Med. Wochschr.*, 1960, LXXXV, pp. 856–861. *Idem*, *Makrobiotik bei Petrus Hispanus*, *Arch. f. Gesch. d. Med.*, 1960, XLIV, pp. 129–155. On the mediaeval and Renaissance tradition, see also: W. Pagel, *Religious Motives in the Medical Biology of the XVIIth century*, *Bullet. Hist. Med.*, 1935, III, 97–312 (p. 220 on Patrizzi and light-symbolism).

of active impulses that are specific to each living being and notably man. In it he believed the same *Logos* to be operative as the cosmic—astral—force that "illuminates" the mind. It is a light immanent in cosmic life of which individual objects partake. Paracelsus consistently emphasized the superiority of the divine Light of the Spirit over the Light of Nature. Yet he could not avoid giving the latter a theological meaning, and finding in it, too, a divine gift—at all events at some periods in his life[116]. We mentioned above Paracelsus' use of the concept to illustrate the perfection that is reached by the individual in his own time and in connexion with the Astra (see above, note 92). The various phases and versions of the Light of Nature in the work of Paracelsus have recently been fully investigated by Goldammer[117].

The influence of mediaeval neo-Platonism may have reached Paracelsus in various ways. He knew Arnald of Villanova and Hildegard of Bermersheim, as we mentioned above[118]. He also knew the alchemical Lullists and John of Rupescissa. Miss Yates has shown recently how much of John Scotus Eriugena (9th century) can be found in Lull (1234–1315)[119]. Some of John's positions can be correlated to Paracelsian ideas. To explain the coming into being of our phenomenal world, John tried to reconcile the neo-Platonic and the Christian point of view—with the result that the former prevailed. The world is seen

[116] The interdependence of the Light of Nature and the Light of Grace is well expressed in Pseudo-Weigel, *Studium Universale*, cap. 1, ed. 1695, *loc. cit.*, sig. A2 verso and A3 recto: Our physical body is maintained by the earth. The firmament gives us all earthly wisdom, arts, languages, faculties (except Theology), offices and crafts. The spirit of God teaches us true theology, and through theology we learn astrology, magic, philosophy, physics, alchemy, arts and crafts . . . and although such things derive from the star, the Light of Nature must be kindled by the Light of Grace, that is by Christ, the Word of God, the Spirit of God that is in all things. The light of Nature is briefly called: *Astrologia* and that of Grace: *Theologia* (cap. 2). Similarly Simeon Partlicius of Spitzberg invoked both these lights as the way to knowledge and learning in chemistry. The sidereal spirit "attracts" all human wisdom, sciences and arts and crafts through the rays of the upper stars, whereby heaven is the father and teacher of all knowledge except theology which is taught by the Holy Spirit. The Light of Grace makes the true theologian, not however without philosophy. The Light of Nature makes the true philosopher, not however without theology which is the fundament of true wisdom. *Medici Systematis Harmonici . . . Prodromus*, Francof, 1625, p. 70.

[117] K. Goldammer, *Lichtsymbolik in philosophischer Weltanschauung, Mystik und Theosophie vom* 15. *bis zum* 17. *Jahrhundert, loc. cit., Studium Generale*, 1960, XIII, pp. 670–682. This also contains a detailed account of Nic. Cusanus, Agrippa, Seb. Franck, Weigel and Boehme.

[118] See above, notes 93 and 94.

[119] F. A. Yates, *Ramon Lull and John Scotus Erigena, J. Warburg and Courtauld Inst.*, 1960, XXIII, pp. 1–44.

as a process of emanation in which necessity seems to override free divine disposition. God is made to "descend" to the primordial causes and hence to the lower products of their *creative* activity[120]. In order to explain how the immaterial God was able to effect material creation, John followed Gregory of Nyssa. The latter had regarded corporeal quality as primarily spiritual and only becoming perceptible through a secondary modification[121]. Finally John strove to demonstrate the *microcosmic* nature of man. The latter embraces all stages of created being, for he knows intuitively like an angel, reasons like man, perceives like an animal, is alive like a plant and exists with a body as well as a soul[122]. This position of man is closely associated with the idea of redemption. Man is eligible to it, as he represents the whole creation returning eventually to God[123]. In this connexion we may recall the Gnostic view of microcosmic man created to replace another world—that of fallen Lucifer and his angels. In contrast to the latter man *qua* microcosm is accessible to redemption. Similar ideas can be found in Paracelsus and such Paracelsists as Croll and Böhme[124].

We mention these ideas as characteristic of mediaeval neo-Platonism in general. We have no evidence that they influenced Paracelsus directly. However, as Miss Yates puts it: Scotus Eriugena was "hidden in Lullism" and the latter was a strong source of inspiration for the Renaissance. Its influence on alchemy has always been obvious through the Pseudo-Lullians who correctly searched in Lull for "systems for calculating elemental influences which they proceeded to use and to adapt for their own purposes"[125]. Moreover, in formulating his conception of *Chaos*, Lull shows striking similarities to John Scotus' ideas. In creating the elements the attributes, the "names" of God are instrumental: the elements are visualized as essences without bodily form. As *Igneitas, Aeritas, Aqueitas, Terreitas* they constitute the *Chaos*. Similarly John Scotus Eriugena had developed the late-Platonic idea that bodily qualities such as colour, gravity, consistency, quantity, size and form are spiritual determinations, not unlike the Aristotelian categories, belonging to the

[120] A. Schneider, *Die Erkenntnislehre des Johannes Eriugena im Rahmen ihrer metaphysischen und anthropologischen Voraussetzungen*, Berlin u. Leipzig, 1921–1923 (Part I), p. 15.

[121] Schneider, *loc. cit.*, p. 17.

[122] Schneider, *loc. cit.* (Part II), p. 74.

[123] Yates, *loc. cit.*, pp. 5 and 12.

[124] See the loci quoted in W. Pagel, *Paracelsus, loc. cit.*, pp. 205–207.

[125] Yates, *loc. cit.*, 1960, p. 41.

divine intellect[126]. All this may remind us of the Paracelsian *Iliaster* and *Aquaster*—the ideal prelude of the created world. It is from the *Primordial Causes*, the *Logos*, that the *Chaos* of John Scotus emerges—the *Materia Informis* that also embraces space and time to give rise in turn to the four elements. At the top of the ladder we have God, the source of all, creating and not created, who is only definable by negative statements. He is followed by the attributes ("names") of God: Bonitas, Essentia, Vita, Sapientia, Ratio and others. These constitute the *Primordial Causes*, the *Logos*. Though *created* themselves, they are *creative* in their turn. There follows the *Chaos* with space, time and the elements—created and not creating—and finally, again God to whom the All returns through redemption. This is the Scotist scheme of the four *Divisions* of *Nature* and essentially the platform from which the Lullian "tree of the elements" arises[127]. Paracelsus' speculation on Prime Matter which we followed up in detail, as an important part of his cosmology and natural philosophy, offers certain comparable aspects, for example the creation of the elements in prime matter (*Chaos*) as the first act through which heaven and earth are formed (see above, p. 144). On the other hand the term *Chaos* is introduced by Paracelsus in various meanings that are more remote from the conception of prime matter. Generally speaking *Chaos* stands for any medium or habitation from which an object derives its means of subsistence or certain qualities. There is for example a *chaos mineralis* that "leads and feeds immovable things"[128]. It is from its *chaos* that urine derives its colour[129]. Most consistently the term is used in connexion with air as the atmosphere surrounding the living being and providing the source of its life. It is the "*medium interstitium*" between heaven and earth, of a greenish transparency, almost invisible and of "miraculous clarity". Fire, the globe of the earth, and water are suspended in it—"as yolk in the egg is held by the white". It also feeds them, however; for example it feeds fire that may "hang" in the air[130]. Such *chaos* is not only *on* the earth, but also *in* the earth, notably in mines where it may poison the miner by causing "*Bergsucht*"—miners' disease[131]. Similarly it is found *in* the human body—it is the air that is dispersed throughout it, causing epilepsy when moved

[126] Yates, *loc. cit.*, p. 19.

[127] Yates, *loc. cit.*, p. 41.

[128] *Chaos mineralis: De modo pharmacandi*, lib. I, tr. 2, ed. Sudhoff, vol. IV, p. 448, and *Fragm. de modo pharmacandi*, lib. I, tr. 1, ed. Sudhoff, vol. IV, p. 473.

[129] *Kurtzes Büchlein de Urinis*, ed. Sudhoff, vol. IV, p. 623.

[130] Paracelsus, *Philosophia de generationibus et fructibus quattoor elementorum*, lib. I de elemento aeris cap. 10, ed. Sudhoff, vol. XIII, p. 16.

[131] Paracelsus, *Von der Bergsucht*, lib. I, tr. 1, cap. 2, ed. Sudhoff, vol. IX, p. 465.

violently, or fever when impeded in its movements[132]. It "feeds" the body being drawn from the air which is the specific "food" of the lung[133]. Lying between heaven and earth it is governed by the stars and varies in its composition according to their will. Hence the seasonal changes of the chaos and its "fruit", for example dew (*tereniabin*), or skin pustules (as "fruit" of the inner chaos inside the body)[134]. As a reflection on their astral origin Paracelsus also calls the *Arcana*—the original divine uncreated forces in nature—*Chaos. Arcanum,* he says, is a "*chaos* and can be directed by the *astra* like a feather by the wind" or "*arcana* that are virtue and power and hence are volatile and have no bodies and are chaos and are clear and transparent and subject to the star"[135]. Perhaps it is only in this connexion with the arcana that reminiscences of the prime matter as an ideal prelude to creation can be found. For the arcana are presented as essentially spiritual—life giving—forces and magisterial ideas that direct the formation and function of concrete objects. The same could be said of the Three Principles—Salt, Sulphur and Mercury—which are in the first place such directing powers and only in a very late development finally become as it were crystallized or coagulated into the chemical substance with which we deal in the laboratory or household. We refer in this respect to the ideas of Quercetanus about the *Formal Simples* which we have discussed above (p. 137).

Among the *patristic* sources from which neo-Platonic speculation entered mediaeval philosophy, including John Scotus and Lull, St. Augustine stands in the first rank. It is tempting to find in him a source for Paracelsus, too. The latter mentions him once as the author of voluminous works[136]. This is not much and we should not overrate the inclination and time for actual Augustinian studies which an itinerant physician and lay-theologian of Paracelsus' stamp would have. Nevertheless a few points of contact with Augustinian ideas must be mentioned. In the world of St. Augustine matter is formed according to a preceding ideal creation which is all and at once, and serves as the directive pattern for the concrete world that unfolds itself in time and space. Here

[132] Paracelsus, *Scholia in lib. Paragraphorum,* De Caducis comment. in cap. 2, ed. Sudhoff, vol. V, p. 290. *Theoricae figurae univers. morbor.*, Tab. IX de febribus. Febres ex aere (cc) Oppilatum, ed. Sudhoff, vol. III, p. 453.

[133] Paracelsus, *Ursprung der frantzosen,* lib. II, cap. 2, ed. Sudhoff, vol. VII, p. 211.

[134] Paracelsus, *Blatern, leme, beulen . . . der frantzosen,* lib. III, cap. 8, ed. Sudhoff vol. VI, p. 364. Chaos under astral influence: *Bergsucht,* lib. I, cap. 2, ed. Sudhoff, vol. IX, p. 465.

[135] Paracelsus on Arcana: *Paragranum,* tr. III von der alchimia, ed. Sudhoff, vol. VIII, p. 185. *Ibid.*, p. 186.

[136] Paracelsus, *Auslegung der Papstbilder,* ed. Sudhoff, vol. XII, p. 576 (to fig. XXVI).

again we meet the ideal *chaos*—the "seed of heaven and earth", the receiving "womb" *in* which (rather than *out of* which) things are made[137]. Paracelsus elaborated the idea of the elements as "wombs" and "mothers" in great detail, modifying the original Platonic and Augustinian idea in his own way. Prime matter is represented as the "seed of heaven and earth" by such Paracelsists as Croll and Quercetanus (see above, p. 148). We referred to the significance of the *Semina* in the whole doctrine of Paracelsus at some length (see above, p. 136). Indeed we are justified in speaking here of Augustinian motives. For it was St. Augustine who conceived of "seeds hidden in the corporeal elements of this world of all things that are bodily and visibly born"[138]. These are "causal" and "primordial reasons" laid by God into the earth. Preformed and encompassed by these "seeds" all future denizens of the earth—plants, animals and men—wait to be called out in the course of time. Thus the earth is the mother of all living beings, the receptacle of its germinal forms, and the world is pregnant with the causes of all beings; it is like a grain of seed[139]. The "seminal reasons" (*logoi*) watch over the objects stepping out from seminal potentiality into the actuality of the concrete object.

In these speculations St. Augustine is indebted to neo-Platonism and the idealistic version that it gave to the Stoic idea of the Pneuma as a "breath" of finest—ethereal—corporality[140].

The same neo-Platonic influences are operative in Hellenistic and mediaeval alchemy and the latter may well be more intimately related to the world of Paracelsus than any of the original sources including St. Augustine. Indeed, Cumont's *Disciples infidèles de Plotin* are the direct ancestors of Paracelsus[141].

## Epilogue: The significance of neo-Platonic and Gnostic Ideas in the work of Paracelsus and its limitation

The affiliation of Paracelsian speculation to neo-Platonism has often been mentioned in the many essays written on all aspects of Paracelsus' life and work. This, however, is usually couched in general terms and without a detailed

[137] *De gen. c. Manich*, I, 7, 11. See: H. Meyer, *Geschichte der Lehre von den Keimkräften*, Bonn, 1914, pp. 145–150. For the *Platonic* original of *womb-symbolism* in connexion with the *Chaos:* Timaeus 49A and 51A. F. M. Cornford, *Plato's Cosmology. The Timaeus of Plato translated with running commentary*, London, 1937, pp. 177, 181.

[138] De Trinitate, III, 7, 13. Meyer, *loc. cit.*, p. 163.

[139] *Ibid.*, III, 9, 16. Meyer, *loc. cit.*, p. 171.

[140] See Meyer, *loc. cit.*, p. 212 *et seq.*

[141] E. Wind, *Pagan Mysteries in the Renaissance*, London, 1958, p. 174.

account of the actual ideas that are consonant in both. More recently healthy warnings against overrating the contacts and parallels have been given, especially by Goldammer[142]. "Paracelsus is no dualist, hence he is no neo-Platonist". He saw spirit and matter united rather than separated by the gulf between good and evil, spirit and body, that Platonism and Gnosticism had erected. Again, Paracelsus insisted on the sharp division between God the creator, and the world—a division which was blurred in the emanative cosmos envisaged by neo-Platonism. Finally, the neo-Platonic vision of many worlds returning in succession to their origin, could not appeal to Paracelsus to whom the world was unique and single.

Further limitations have been suggested by Peuckert[143]. He refers to the neo-Platonic catalogue of demons as elaborated by Trithemius and Agrippa, as against Paracelsus who reduced their multitudes to the comparatively short list of the Elemental Spirits (*Elementar-Geister*). However, just this belief in the elemental spirits has been made a cornerstone in the demonstration of Paracelsus' dependence upon his master Trithemius, by Jaques Gohory whose work was published in 1567[144]. He was in no way prejudiced against Paracelsus. On the contrary, he was intent on propagating Paracelsism. What is more, he belonged to the first generation of Paracelsists, removed from the era of the master by no more than two decades. His testimony must therefore be taken seriously and regarded as closer to reality than anything we can say today.

Even so, we have no intention of disputing the originality of Paracelsus where he deviates from the neo-Platonic, Gnostic and alchemical tradition. The strong influence of the latter remains, however, and has been recognized by Goldammer as well as by Peuckert. We would add that Paracelsus elaborates Ficino's and Agrippa's ideas through observation and research into the working of nature. This appears to us as an extension of an existing tradition rather than as an embarcation on a new venture—a first attempt at "technical thinking", as Peuckert sees it. Contacts with Ficino go into "technical" detail in the work of Paracelsus, for example in his ideas on the plague[145]. Like Ficino, Paracelsus enjoins us to find the ways of overcoming the evil influences of the stars by wisdom and moderation, especially in our emotional life, which is largely directed by the stars. To both—Ficino and

[142] Goldammer, *Paracelsus. Natur und Offenbarung*, Hannover, 1953, pp. 33–35, 61–63.

[143] W.-E. Peuckert, *Pansophie. Ein Versuch zur Geschichte der weissen und schwarzen Magie*, 2nd ed., Berlin, 1956, pp. 200–206, 207–213 and *passim*. *Idem, Die grosse Wende—das apokalyptische Saeculum und Luther*, Hamburg, 1948, pp. 60, 426 *et seq*.

[144] *Paracelsi Compendium Leone Suavio auctore*, 2nd ed., Basileae, 1568, pp. 218–225.

[145] W. Pagel, *Paracelsus, loc. cit.*, 1958, pp. 176–178.

Paracelsus—the work of the physician belongs to the realm of "natural magic". Beyond Paracelsus, this part of Ficino's doctrine has deeply influenced medical theory—for example Fracastor's ideas on the *contagium*. Ficino had defined infection as an attraction of like by like—a special case of that sympathy which rules throughout the cosmos, comparable to the response of a cord to the striking of another cord consonant with it[146]. These contacts and parallels between Ficino and Paracelsus remain impressive, even if we find with Walker[147] that the tenor of Ficino's "magic" is "whiter", i.e. more spiritual than the "demonic" brand chosen by Trithemius, Agrippa and Paracelsus.

Moreover, Paracelsus was no systematic thinker, as Goldammer himself has pointed out. Hence we may hit upon Unitarian (monistic) as well as dualist, Theist as well as Pantheist, Christian as well as Heathen, materialist Stoic, as well as spiritualist, neo-Platonic, and Gnostic tendencies, in the work of Paracelsus. We refer to our discussion of the *Prima Materia*, the *Arcana* and related subjects.

Even this very combination of monist and dualist views may remind us of the neo-Platonic attempt at bridging the gulf between them.

Indeed it was *Platonicae Doctrinae* that inspired and informed Paracelsus. It was the *Prisca Philosophia*—the wisdom of the Magi of old, the Rabbis, the Kabbalists and Platonists, given to Adam by God Himself and on His command kept secret and transmitted orally in myths, fables and allegories. Thus we are told by the best of Paracelsian commentators: Peter Severinus (1542–1602) and the latter's admirer William Davison the Scot (1593–ca. 1669). It is the *Hermetic* Doctrine which embraces "*Pyrotechnia*—the chemical art that operates by the aid of fire and makes the physician"[148].

Ever since the days of Erastus, Paracelsus has been accused of Gnostic heresy[149]. This appertained not only to his cosmology and anthropology, but stigmatized even his ideas on disease, and such detailed views as the postulate of independent disease semina which invade man from outside. Other such views which we have mentioned refer to the *Cagastrum*—the deposits caused by coagulation of excretory matter, the products of corruption and spontaneous generation, the fruit of matter and evil prevailing over spirit and good.

[146] *Idem, ibid.*, pp. 182–183, note 153.

[147] D. P. Walker, *Spiritual and Demonic Magic from Ficino to Campanella*, London, The Warburg Institute, 1958, pp. 41, 104 and *passim*.

[148] W. Davisson, *Commentariorum in sublimis Philosophi . . . Petri Severini Dani Ideam Medicinae Philosophicae propediem prodituorum Prodromus*, Hagae Comitis, 1660, p. 31.

[149] Pagel, *Paracelsus*, 1958, *loc. cit.*, pp. 42–43, 204, 315.

There is, however, redemption from evil—liberation from disease as afforded by medicine, liberation from crude matter as provided by the chemist for the soul hidden in minerals and metals, succour and redemption brought to the human soul by "pneumatic man", the *Magus* of the Gnosis, against the threatening *archons* that impede the ascent and reunion of the soul with its divine origin.

In the last resort, this liberating and redeeming act operates through a synthesis of the realms above with those below—and it was Paracelsus who attempted such a synthesis throughout all realms of Nature. In this we are inclined to see his uniqueness and originality. Taken as a whole this attempt is non-scientific and indeed a fruit of "Hermetic", neo-Platonic and Gnostic speculation and practical work, the struggle of the Gnostic *magus* and Ficino's priest-physician for the liberation of body and soul.

ACKNOWLEDGMENTS

The author's thanks are due to the Wellcome Trust for encouragement and support of his work. He is also indebted to Professor J. R. Partington, Dr. F. N. L. Poynter, Mr. Allen Debus, Dr. Joseph Needham, F.R.S., Dr. O. Kurz and Dr. Frances A. Yates for most helpful suggestions.

# VII

## THE PRIME MATTER OF PARACELSUS

No Paracelsian concept stirred up the minds of the Paracelsians and their adversaries as much as that of *Prime Matter*. It is still one of the main stumbling blocks to our understanding of Paracelsian ideas. In a previous paper[1] we discussed some of these difficulties and the inconsistencies which appeared to result from them in Paracelsus' *Hermetic* philosophy and cosmology. In this respect we considered the question as to whether Paracelsus (1493–1541) believed in *creation* or in *preformation* of matter without, however, arriving at a clear-cut answer. It still remains to attempt a more detailed examination of Paracelsus' concept of *Prime Matter*—in the hope of clearing up some of the contradictions and thereby of deepening our understanding of his ideas.

[1] W. Pagel, *Paracelsus and the neo-Platonic and Gnostic Tradition*, *Ambix*, 1960, **8**, 125–166.

## I

### Prime Matter of the World

*What is the Prime Matter of Paracelsus?* To answer this question it may be expedient to present two passages which appear to be of first importance:

The first comes from one of the main works—the *Opus Paramirum* of 1531. In this we are given a cross section through Paracelsus' philosophy and medicine, conceived and matured during his best years. Here it says: "since the *prime matter of the world was the* Fiat, who will dare to explain the *Fiat*? We have, however, some foothold through the fire of *Vulcan* whereby we can explain the *Three Principles* . . ." ("dieweil aber prima materia mundi fiat ist gewesen, wer wil sich unterstehen das fiat zu erklären? nun aber etwas haben wir durch das feur vulcani, dadurch wir die drei ersten erklären . . .")[2].

The second passage is also derived from one of the most incisive and genuine works although this belongs to a late period and is aphoristic rather than systematic in scope—the *Labyrinthus Medicorum* of 1537–38. Here it says in the fifth chapter on chemistry (*alchimei*) and its necessity for the physician: "God created all things, something from nothing. This something is a seed; the seed contains the end of its predestination and office. And . . . there is nothing that is created in its final form, but *vulcan* must complete it . . . all things are created as *prime matter* and after that the *vulcan* follows and turns them into *ultimate matter* through the art of alchemy" ("got alle ding beschaffen hat, aus nichts etwas—das etwas ist ein sam, der sam gibt das end seiner predestination und seines officii, und wie von nichts bis zum end alle ding beschaffen seind, so ist doch nichts do, das auf das end gar sei, das ist, bis auf das ende . . . sonder der vulcanus muss es vollenden . . . das nichts gar beschaffen ist in die ultimam materiam, aber alle ding werden zu prima materia beschaffen, und über das folgt der vulcanus hernach, der machts in ultimam materiam durch die kunst alchimiae . . .")[3].

In these two passages the term *Prime Matter* is used in *different meanings*. The first speaks of the *Prime Matter of the World* and the second of the *Prime Matter of Individual Objects*.

[2] *Prima Materia Mundi* was *Fiat: Opus Paramirum*, I, cap. 2, ed. Sudhoff, vol. IX, p. 48.

[3] All things created from nothing: *Labyrinthus Medicorum*, cap. 5, ed. Sudhoff, vol. XI, p. 187. Compare the relevant passages cited by Pagel, *loc. cit.* (in footnotes 59, 64, 67), pp. 142–145.

It may be noted in passing that this passage from the *Labyrinthus Medicorum* belongs to the Paracelsian sayings collected by the young Goethe in his *Ephemerides* (*Gesammelte Werke*, Grossherzog Wilhelm Ernst Ausgabe, vol. XII: Aufsätze zur Kultur-, Theater- und Literaturgeschichte, I, Leipzig, 1920, pp. 7 *et seq.* (1770): "Paracelsus sagt, Gott habe alle Dinge aus nichts erschaffen in Labyrintho Med., cap. 5").

The *Prime Matter* of the *World as a whole* is the *word*: *Fiat*. It is therefore not matter in the modern sense—at all events not to begin with. The idea of founding the world on the *word* is reminiscent of the *Prologue* to the *Fourth Gospel*: In the Beginning was the Word. This allusion is strengthened by a further passage from the *Book on Minerals*, an early work, which we give in full: "the first was *with God*, the beginning, that is *ultima materia*; this *ultima materia* He made into *prime matter*. As fruit that is to yield other fruit has seed, the seed is in *prime matter*. Thus *ultimate* matter of the minerals is made into *prime matter* that is a seed and the seed is the element of water" ("Nun ist das erst gewesen bei got, der anfang, das ist ultima materia, die selbige ultimam materiam hat er gemacht in primam materiam. als ein frucht, die ein ander frucht sol geben, die selbige hat ein semen: der sam ist in prima materia also ist nun der mineralium ultima materia in ein primam materiam gemachet, das ist in ein sam und der samen ist elementum aquae . . .")[4]. The object of this passage is to convey that God created water as the *matrix* ("mother") or *seed* of minerals and metals. This created water, however, was not primeval matter. This is here called *ultimate matter* and "was with God".

Again the allusion to the Fourth Gospel is obvious. What is said in the latter about the *Logos*, namely that it was in the beginning and *with God*, is here said about *Prime Matter*. Primeval matter from which the world was built indeed corresponds to the Logos of the Fourth Gospel—this seems to be an idea advocated by Paracelsus at least in the two passages given. It serves to emphasize that *prime matter* is no matter in the ordinary sense, but a Logos, i.e. an immaterial spirit that existed by itself—substantially—in the beginning.

The passage from the *Book on Minerals* is also significant for the explicit distinction made between *primeval matter*—here called *ultimate matter*—and the *prime matter* of individual objects, in this case of minerals and metals. Indeed the world began with *ultimate matter* and it is the latter into which material objects will be dissolved in the end.

*Qua Word*, primeval matter is *not* represented as *created*, but it steps out from God as the initiation of Creation, or as it is expressed in a reputedly spurious work, only thereafter was "the word *Fiat* made material, apprehensible, and a body in which there lies and is hidden all that is predestined". It is out of *first matter* as an *Iliastrum* that the *Three Principles*: Salt, Sulphur and Mercury, emerged[5].

[4] The first was *with God*: *Das Buch De Mineralibus*, ed. Sudhoff, vol. III, p. 34. See also: Pagel, *loc. cit.* (footnote 60), p. 142.

[5] The *Word Fiat* made material: *Liber Azoth*, cap. 1, ed. Sudhoff, vol. XIV, p. 549.

The *Iliastrum*, then, is *Logos* and the meanings which have been attributed to the *Logos* of the Gospel should appertain to it[6]. Thus the divine *Logos* is not simply the uttered word. It is a "rational content of thought corresponding to the ultimate reality of the universe" (Dodd) and in a certain sense connotes *Law in Nature*[7]. As such the *Word was*, i.e. existed substantially and not merely was spoken. It so exists as a hypostasis distinguishable from God and yet it remained with Him[8].

The next stage, according to the gospel, is the manifestation of God's word in Life and Light, followed by the *Logos* becoming flesh. Similarly Paracelsus visualizes the materialization of the pure spirit as the next stage—"how the word Fiat became material". This was through the emergence, in the—spiritual—Iliastrum, of the *Three Principles* (*Tria Prima*)—Salt, Sulphur and Mercury[9].

[6] For this the dissertation on *Logos* in C. H. Dodd, *The Interpretation of the Fourth Gospel*, Cambridge, 1953, part II, cap. 12, pp. 263–285, should be consulted.

[7] *Logos*: Law in Nature, see Dodd, *loc. cit.* (footnote 6), p. 263. *Logos* as the ultimate reality of the universe, *ibid.*, p. 267.

[8] *Logos* as hypostasis: Dodd, *loc. cit.*, pp. 264 *et seq.* (p. 269).

[9] *Fiat—Iliastrum—Three Principles: Liber Azoth*, cap. 1, ed. Sudhoff, vol. XIV, p. 549. The idea that the *Three Principles* emerge from the spiritual *Iliastrum* as *Prime Matter* was attributed by Andreas Libavius (ab. 1540–1616), in *De Universitate et Originibus Rerum Conditarum*, Francof. a. M., 1610, pp. 76–78 to the *Archidoxis Magica*, a Paracelsian treatise which "deserves not the light of the sun, but that of eternal fire". In it the *Iliastrum* is said to be the prime matter from which sulphur, salt and mercury were created. We are thus to understand how the word *Fiat* was made material, apprehensible, and a body in which all things are predestined and hidden and then brought out—from the *Iliastrum* through the activity of the *Cagastrum*. This, according to Libavius, means that when God said *Fiat* this word was converted into prime matter, as it were the "demon or spirit of matter". It contains the essential principles of all things each of which assumes at its time appointed by God (divina praefinitione) the *ratio et proportio* of its nature, i.e. is generated and in the beginning created. The *Cagastrum* is also called *Cogastrum*, an *astral* power that *forces* the things that are preformed in an ideal image to step out as natural objects—just as bodies dissolved in water are condensed and solidified by the action of heat and an astral force specific to each object. In Libavius' opinion this doctrine of preformation amounts to a denial of creation—which would merely mean *in yliastro praedestinatum pridem, ex eodem proferre* and that with the assistance of a *Cogastrum*. It is ridiculous that the word *Fiat* should have become "that material and apprehensible body". Why is this not immediately stated where it says that God made heaven, earth, air, water and darkness? To connect this *Fiat* with the mystery of God's son who was begotten from eternity and thus to explain his incarnation is a capital crime, insinuating an analogy between generation through the eternal word and the creation and generation of nature.

These latter are also spiritual rather than material in the common sense—they are the spiritual directors of matter towards the fluid-smoky state (mercury), the inflammable-fatty state (sulphur) and the solid-crystalline state (salt). In this triade sulphur performs the function of the principle uniting two opposites, the "soul" that joins spirit (mercury) to matter (salt)[10].

The materialization of the *Fiat* is thus described in the *Liber Azoth*, a treatise not normally recognized as genuine—probably because of its high-flown speculative and difficult contents. Here we are also told that the spirit of God hovered on the water and carried the Word of God on to it. Thus this water became a matrix—*living* water that is, not *visible* water, but the Word of God that is invisible to the *cagastric*, i.e. bodily eye (in contrast to the internal eye). Or more explicitly, the Word of God became flesh and was *heavenly flesh*. The *Word* of God also brought about the *Fiat* and endowed the soul of the greater world with imagination. Hence the watery matrix and soul became pregnant and gave birth to *earthly flesh*, i.e. matter in the modern sense[11].

In *De Pestilitate*—a treatise often bracketed together with the *Liber Azoth*—the story of the materialization of the word *Fiat* is taken further: Through the *Fiat* first water was created and then from water all other creatures. Water was also the matrix of the *Tria Prima*—which are properly called Sulphur, Mercury and Salt and which are the origin of the elements and the true *materia* from which all animals and mankind were created[12]. This is also found in the *Great Surgery* of 1536 where it is written that "the three things are the prime

[10] *Three Principles*—spiritual: see W. Pagel, *Paracelsus: An Introduction to Philosophical Medicine in the Era of the Renaissance*, Basle & New York, 1958, p. 86; and *Ambix*, 1960, *loc. cit.* (footnote 99), p. 154.

[11] *Word* was *heavenly flesh: Liber Azoth*, ed. Sudhoff, vol. XIV, p. 570; *ibid.*, cap. 2 (De Manna. Vom Engelbrot), p. 589.

The Paracelsian distinction between *living* water and *visible* water as given in the *Liber Azoth* invites comparison with the *male*—active—waters and the *female*—receiving—waters as distinguished by the *Kabbala* and used as designation for the waters which were above and under the firmament (Gen. I, 6 and 7). The former are called *Elohim* and the latter *Adonaj* "and thus the name *Elohim* spread over all things, as the male waters (the active powers) were consummated in the female waters (the receiving powers)". *Die Geheimnisse der Schöpfung. Ein Kapitel aus dem Sohar*, von G. Scholem, Berlin, 1935, p. 64.

On the emergence of the gnostic idea of the "heavenly flesh of Christ" in the work of Paracelsus, Sebastian Franck, Michael Servetus and others, see: H. J. Schoeps, *Vom Himmlischen Fleisch Christi*, Eine dogmengeschichtliche Untersuchung, Tübingen, Mohr, 1951, pp. 54–56.

[12] Through *Fiat*-water created; water as *matrix* of the *Tria Prima*, i.e. the true *materia* from which elements, animals and mankind were created: *De Pestilitate* (sub: Cabala), ed. Sudhoff, vol. XIV, p. 601.

matter of all creatures, also their ultimate matter, the beginning, middle and end of each body"[13].

The word *Fiat,* however, is not limited in its activity to the first creation. It is still alive to-day. It is the *Fiat* which is still present in all things, for the Word of the Lord is the Kingdom of God. Thus it forms the *food* of the "aquastric body", i.e. the ideal pattern of an individual body. It comes to the material body—the "cagastric homunculus"—through the "Mercury of Life"—for this contains the Word of God which once went from His mouth and still issues from it. Accordingly, the Body of Christ—the "heavenly Aquaster" —is called "celestial manna", i.e. the food of the soul[14].

*Looking back* to what we have said we would *conclude* that in the Paracelsian view

(1) *Prime Matter of the world* as a whole must be distinguished from the *Prime Matter of the individual objects.*

(2) *Prime Matter* of the world is not matter, but spirit—in fact it is the Word *Fiat,* the *Logos* of the Fourth Gospel, the Platonic archetype and ideal pattern of the world that is to become a material creation.

(3) As such it is also called *Ultimate Matter,* reserving the term *Prime Matter* for the individual objects in their original state.

## II

### Prime Matter of the Individual Objects

What, then, is the position of *individual objects?* Paracelsus emphasizes that they were created by God[15]. This creative act appertained, however, only to their original state. They were then left to be developed by their immanent "blacksmiths"—the vulcans and archei—each developing at the appointed

[13] Zweites Buch der *Grossen Wundarznei* (1536), tract. II, cap. 3, ed. Sudhoff, vol. X, p. 292—*Tria Prima* are *prime* and *ultimate matter* of all creatures.

[14] *Fiat* permanently active: *Liber Azoth,* cap. 2, ed. Sudhoff, vol. XIV, pp. 557–560 and 568–569.

[15] In Paracelsus' view *creation from nothing does not apply to man.* He says: "first that God created all things from nothing, merely through the *Word;* not, however, man whom He made from something, i.e. from a *massa* which had been a body, a substance and something . . . an extract from all creatures in heaven and earth . . . all elements and all stars . . . that which had been the most subtle and best . . . whence it follows that man is the lesser world . . . earth being man's flesh, water his blood, fire his warmth, air his balm"—*Ein Mantischer Entwurf* (?1536, Munich), ed. Sudhoff, vol. X, p. 648. The idea is reminiscent of *Raschi* to *Genesis* I, 27 ("so God created man in His own image"): "sch'hakol nivra

time, when it is destined to reach its "monarchy" and then involuting and returning to *ultimate matter*.

The original state of the individual object, the state in which it was created, is its *prime matter*. We are told that this is its *seed*[16].

Finally the term *prime matter* loses much of its original meaning and simply denotes any raw material which is converted into a finished product ready for human consumption through the offices of a craftsman, artisan or chemist. Thus grains of wheat are the *prime matter* of bread, made into secondary matter by the baker and becoming ultimate matter when eaten and converted into flesh[17].

[16] *Seed*—the *prime matter* of individual objects: *Labyrinthus Medicorum*, cap. 5, ed Sudhoff, vol. XI, p. 187. *Das Buch De Mineralibus*, ed. Sudhoff, vol. III, pp. 33–34.

[17] *Prime* and *ultimate matter* of bread: *Labyrinthus Medicorum*, cap. 5, ed. Sudhoff, vol. XI, p. 188. See also: *Paragranum*, tract. III, ed. Sudhoff, vol. VIII, p. 181.

---

[15] *continued.*

b'maamar w'hu nivra b'jadajim"—as everything was created by the mere word, man, however, by hands—with reference to Psalm 139, v. 5: "wathascheth alaj cappechah"—Thou hast laid Thy hand upon me. On this the present author is indebted to Mr. Raphael Loewe for the following note: "The source is: Alphabeth of R. Akiba, 2nd Recensio, ed. A. Jellinek, *Beth ha-Midrasch*, part III, p. 59. L. Ginzberg, *The Legends of the Jews*, V, p. 63, n. 3, cites no other Rabbinic sources but very many Christian ones, from the Clementine *Homilies*, Tertullian, etc., onwards. He concludes: The statement which emphasizes the fact that man is the creation of God's hands is probably directed against the doctrine of Philo and the Gnostics who maintain that Adam was partly or wholly created by the angels; comp. n. 14. It is noteworthy that Philo de Somn. 1, 36, emphatically asserts that 'man was not made by hand, but is the work of invisible nature' ".

In a personal communication to the present author Professor G. Scholem mentioned the following implicitly additional Rabbinical sources: *Bereshith Rabba*, Parascha 24, Parag. 5; *Pesikta Rabbathi* 47, ed. Buber 190a and *Zohar*, II, 75b.

For the connexion of the creation of man with his *microcosmic* nature a passage from the *Hermetic Corpus* (XIII, De Regeneratione, 11, ed. Nock and Festugière, vol. II, p. 205) may be mentioned. Here the divine "powers" (*dynameis*), i.e. the divine *logos*, are said to be imparted on regenerated man—expressing intimate unity with God in terms of metaphysical pantheism. Thus regenerated man feels the universe to be in himself and himself to be in heaven, on earth, in water, in air, in animals, in plants (see also XI, 20, *loc. cit.*, vol. I, p. 155, and C. H. Dodd, *The Interpretation of the Fourth Gospel*, Cambridge, 1953, p. 190). Union with the Universe that is in God—a rebirth of man *qua* microcosm—was one of the essential motives in Paracelsian metaphysical pragmatism, recognizable for example in his treatises on *Long Life*.

## III

## Was Prime Matter Created? The Views of R. B. (Robert Bostocke, 1585)

Paracelsus' reputed belief in either the creation or the pre-existence of *prime matter* agitated the minds of the Paracelsians and their adversaries. Among the latter, Erastus in particular hurled ferocious invectives at Paracelsus, whom he accused of having revived Gnostic heresy in this field.

Can we derive any information relevant to this question from our discussion?

First it would appear that Paracelsian *Prime Matter* should not be confused with the "dark abyss" of primeval waters which according to *Hermetic* and *Gnostic tradition* were visualized as the embodiment of uncreated evil separate from and opposing divine goodness, as it were, from outside. It will be shown below that this difference implies no exclusion of an ideological connexion of the Paracelsian *Prime Matter* with *Gnosticism at large* (*vide infra*, in *Epilogue*). Here it may suffice to say that Paracelsus, too, believed in water as the universal *matrix*. This was the receptacle of the *semina*[18]. The latter derive not from water, but from the *Iliaster* (*Limbus, Mysterium Magnum*) which is not material but the ideal archetype of the world and hence something spiritual. Indeed it corresponds to *Logos* and dwells *with God*. Admittedly, like *Logos* it was not created—it rather formed an aspect of divinity though at the same time assuming a substantial existence distinguishable from God. In some ways this may be regarded as reminiscent of the Gnostic view that *prime matter* is uncreated, but still remains removed from the idea of *prime matter* pre-existing outside and separate from God, as represented in some Gnostic philosophies.

If, in Paracelsus' view, *Prime Matter* forms part of divinity this is not incompatible with its pantheistic interpretation in the *Philosophia ad Athenienses*. This treatise has been regarded as an unauthentic document expressing heretical thoughts and it provided the enemies of Paracelsus with much of the evidence against him[19]. In it the "*Mysterium*" or "*Mother*" (*Matrix*) assumes a position of central importance, as in it all objects of nature are generated. This *mysterium* is *uncreated* and *separation* rather than *creation* provides the fundamental pattern of all birth and generation. The

[18] Water—the receptacle of the *semina: Opus Paramirum*, lib. IV, *De Matrice*, ed. Sudhoff, vol. IX, p. 194. Compare the characteristic spiritualist version of the idea that water is matrix in the *Liber Azoth* (ed. Sudhoff, vol. XIV, p. 570 and 589) and its kabbalistic parallel as quoted in footnote 11 above.

[19] *Philosophia ad Athenienses:* see W. Pagel, *Paracelsus*, 1958, *loc. cit.* (note 10), pp. 89 *et seq.*

*Mysterium* of the *Athenienses* may well be compared with the uncreated *Word Fiat* of the *Opus Paramirum*—both representing the *Prime Matter of the World* and both striking the searching mind as an unapproachable secret. Hence the name of *mystery*, prominently used in the *Philosophia ad Athenienses*, though the emphasis laid on separation rather than creation seems to be at variance with some of the classical loci that deal with the coming into being of individual objects.

The view concerning the original ideal pattern of the world, the *Iliastrum*, follows, then, a pantheist rather than a dualist trend. In this it is consistent with Paracelsus' idea of the *Arcana*. These are the virtues immanent in individual objects, carrying the specific power of each. As such they are immediately divine, *uncreated*, prior to all things created including heaven and earth and stepping out from divinity at a time when God was a spirit and hovered on the waters[20]. It is tempting to see the origin of this concept in the *Hermetic Poimandres*. Here the ideal archetypal world preceding the sensible world is the luminous realm of the powers—*dynameis*, the product of the organization of aboriginal *Light*[21]. The emergence of the latter is the first phase in the formation of the world in the original *Nous*. The *dynameis* are represented as radiations of light and the cosmic forces through which God creates the world—just as the *Logos* is the sum of emanations from the eternal *Nous*. These forces are imparted to man in the form of ethical qualities—just as the *Logos* in man is the expression of *Nous* in him.

Interpreting the *Prime Matter* of Paracelsus as the uncreated Logos we find ourselves at variance with two loci in the Paracelsian Corpus[22], albeit regarded as unauthentic, in which the view is expressed that God *created* the "Prima Materia Confusa" of the world, and also with the opinion given by a number of

[20] *Arcana* uncreated: *De Vera Influentia Rerum*, tract. I, ed. Sudhoff, vol. XIV., p. 215.

[21] *Dynameis* forming the luminous world, the ideal archetype of the sensible world: *Poimandres* 7 and 26. *Corpus Hermeticum*, ed. A. D. Nock and A.-J. Festugière, 2nd ed., Paris, 1960, vol. I, pp. 9 and 16; note 65 on p. 25 on "puissances qui constituent la lumière archétype". See also *ibidem*, note 68, on the "power" imparted by Poimandres—"cette dynamis peut impliquer des pouvoirs magiques qui permettent à l'âme de vaincre les archontes dans sa remontée vers l'Ogdoade". *Cf.* Hippolytus *Refutatio Omnium Haeresium*, VII, 32 (Carpocrates), ed. L. Duncker et F. G. Schneidewin, Gottingae, 1859, p. 402.

[22] *De Secretis Creationis*, Die Erste Würckung Gottes, Appendix to: *Chirurgische Bücher und Schrifften*, Strassburg, Zetzner, 1605, p. 106: "Die Fontein des Ursprungs der ewigen Weissheit . . . hat den obersten Thron des Himmels, die Engel in der ersten Materia durch sein ewig Wort geschaffen . . . aus der prima Materia . . . die Gott der Allmächtig aus nichts geschaffen hatte . . . "and: *Secretum Magicum de Lapide Philosophorum*, ed. Huser, Fol. Edit., vol. II, pp. 672–673 (as quoted by Pagel, *Ambix*, 1960, *loc. cit.*, in note 71, p. 146).

Paracelsians including Quercetanus (1544–1609), Khunrath (1560–1605) and—of the older generation—of Adam von Bodenstein (1528–1577) and Dorn (16th century second half)[23].

The question was perhaps dealt with more thoroughly by the unknown early English Paracelsian "R.B." than by anybody else. This author was identified with one Robert Bostocke as early as 1595, ten years after the appearance of his book: *"The difference betwene the auncient Phisicke, first taught by the godly forefathers, consisting in vnitie, peace and concord: and the latter Phisicke proceding from Idolaters, Ethnickes, and Heathen: as Gallen, and such other consisting in dualitie, discorde and contrarietie . . .".* Some aspects of his book have been recently discussed, and its author called the only English writer in the 16th century who was more interested in Paracelsian theory than its practice[24].

For all these reasons a perusal of his book promises important information on the questions raised in the present paper. His twenty-first chapter is devoted to: *"Haw materia prima and misceria magna was the beginnying of all things according to Paracelsus his meanyng: and how all create were at one time in the increate"*

This is what Bostocke has to say: "One other great falt doeth Erastus finde with Paracelsus, for that he saiethe that prima materia and Misterium magnum was the beginnig of al thinges by separation. And this misterie he saieth to be increate hereof doeth Erastus conclude, that accordyng to Paracelsus creation, is nothyng but seperation. Though in this place and many other places of the same booke ad Athenienses he doth treate of the influences which proceed from God (as in the first entery of the same booke he plainly confesseth) and of in warde generations, and fruits, and of inward seperations (for deepe and secrete purpose) yet if Erastus had delte indifferently wyth hym, he myght easely perceive his meanyng in other of his workes, and also in this, where he findeth this horible herecie, concernyng the creation of vizible bodies to be according to Gods worde. For in his booke intituled Paramirum lib. I. cap. 2. he confesseth accordyng to Gods holy worde that Prima materia mundi was Fiat:

[23] Jos. Quercetanus, *Ad veritatem Hermeticae Medicinae*, Paris, 1604, p. 184; Heinrich Khunrath, *Vom hylealischen . . . natürlichen Chaos der naturgemaessen Alchymiae und Alchymisten*, Magdeburg, 1597, ed. used: Leipzig, 1786, pp. 20–21. Adam von Bodenstein, Epistola Commendatoria to Paracelsi *De Vita Longa* Basileae ap. P. Pernam (1562), sig. b6 *seq.* Ger. Dorneus, Physica Genesis in: *Clavis Totius Philosophiae Chimisticae. Theatrum Chemicum*, Argentor, 1613, vol. I, p. 368.

[24] A. G. Debus, *The Paracelsian Compromise in Elizabethan England, Ambix*, 1960, vol. 8, pp. 71–97 (pp. 77–84). The present author is indebted to Dr. Debus for having drawn his attention to Bostocke.

Aud in the same booke to the Athenians he saieth that Materia prima can not be perceiued by senses. Also in that booke Lib. I. cap. primo he plainely affirmeth that the vizible matter of ech thing was create, for thei were not with God at the beginning. For God created them of nothing, and inspired into them life and vertue"[25].

Bostocke defends Paracelsus against the accusations of impiety and Gnostic heresy made by Erastus some thirteen years before. These accusations had been mainly based on the *Philosophia ad Athenienses*. Against this Bostocke refers to other Paracelsian works in which creation of "each thing" had been given prominence and in particular to the passage from the *Opus Paramirum* in which the *Prima Materia Mundi* had been said to be the *Fiat* of God—the passage which we have discussed at length in the present paper. Indeed, according to Bostocke, the Paracelsian God is in the first place a Creator and not merely the separator of a pre-existing "chaos", as Erastus had inferred. Bostocke even goes so far as to declare that the *Prima Materia* of the world "was made, confused and without forme, out of whych all thynges were made . . . for though all thynges were made of that prima materia, yet that was made of nothyng"[26]. In other words the prime matter of the world—the *Fiat*—is here interpreted as an act of creation and Bostocke goes on to say that it was called *Coelum et Terra*—not because it was made as such, but made so *potentia*, "as it were the seede of heaven and earth"[27]. With this Bostocke has recourse to St. Augustine, who, in the twelfth book of the *Confessions*, views the world as made by God from *informis materia* that was made of nothing. He also refers to an ancient chemist who had said of the *simple substance* or the elements which are the matter of nature that they were "created *with* divine *separation*" ("creata *cum* divina *separatione*")[28]. In Bostocke's view there is thus no contradiction between the *Philosophia ad Athenienses* and the other books in which Paracelsus asserts the creative act of God. For the former does treat of the divine influences that reach and govern creatures and are embodied in the *arcana* and *semina*—the powers and virtues that immediately emerge from God and hence are "increate because God is without beginnyng increate"[29].

[25] Bostocke, "*The Difference . . .*" (title as quoted in text above), cap. 21, London, 1585, sig. kl verso to k2 recto.

[26] *Prima materia* made of nothing—Bostocke, *loc. cit.*, cap. 22, sig. kVII verso.

[27] *Fiat*—creation—heaven and earth: Bostocke, *loc. cit.*, *ibidem*.

[28] World made of nothing according to St. Augustine; divina separatio: Bostocke, *loc. cit.*, *ibidem*.

[29] Power and virtue increate: Bostocke, *loc. cit.*, cap. 20. sig. I3 verso *et seq.*

They were in "God of heaven and earth, when the spirit of God was carried upon the waters[30], even so likewise when the heaven and earthe shall perishe, all vertues shall returne to God againe, because they had no beginning". These are the true divine influences which St. Augustine distinguished from those which come to us from heaven or spirits. Indeed, according to Bostocke, it was Paracelsus' opinion that these divine virtues were originally united in God, but "after that by the vertue of the spirite, whiche was caryed upon the waters, they were commanded to doe their offices in the worldly ministration, they were seperated and diuided in offices, life, essenties and beyings". There is therefore no need to let these proceed from a *chaos*, but as treasures of divine wisdom they should be visualized as latent in individual objects, divided and separated in "just and true order, proportion, forme, figure and qualitie" in order to bring the individual to maturation and perfection at the appointed time. Yet there is no idea that the objects of nature are consequently the component parts of divinity in a pantheist sense. It is rather a pan-entheist view that is taken by Bostocke: "as the beames of the Sunne be in those whereupon it shineth, yet the substance of the Sunne is not in them, neither is God in part any where but in singulis totus and in omnibus omnis. . . . The true meanyng of Paracelsus herein is that euery creature maie justly bee saide to be in God, because without God there is nothyng: but yet they be not so in God, that they be of his substance, or parte of hym: For it followeth not, that the thyng that is in an other, is that thyng in which it is. For wine is in the bottle, yet the wine is not the botle . . .". Here again Bostocke invokes St. Augustine who taught "by expresse wordes, that euery creature is in the creator, and God is in euery creature"[31].

Bostocke would thus appear to favour the idea that *Prime Matter* was created and to side with the two passages from *De Secretis Creationis* and the *Secretum Magicum* respectively which we mentioned above and with Quercetanus and Khunrath. Bostocke speaks about Being ("On") and "Logos" as the kernel of *Life* which is immortal and immanent to all objects of nature[32], but does not interpret the prime matter of the world in terms of the uncreated Logos that was *with God* in the sense of the Fourth Gospel. He does say, however, that Paracelsus attributed the beginning of things to prime matter which is *fiat* ("which I judge to be the divine will") as well as to "the first councell of the spiritual motion, as to Misterium magnum, which he meaneth

[30] Arcana in God: Bostocke, *loc. cit.*, *ibidem* with ref. to Paracelsus' *De Vera influentia Rerum*, tract. I, ed. Sudhoff, vol. XIV, p. 215.

[31] Panentheistic view: Bostocke, *loc. cit.*, cap. 21, sig. kV verso to kVI.

[32] Being and *Logos*: Bostocke, *loc. cit.*, cap. 20, sig. kI recto.

to be Christ . . ."[33]. He then argues on both lines: (*a*) the origin of all things is in prime matter which is the—created—*Fiat* and (*b*) it is also in Christ that is to say God's wisdom, word and virtue. "In this sorte Christ that great mistery was the beginnying of all thynges"[34]. This is the *Mysterium magnum* from which not the things themselves (as Erastus erroneously maintains), but each individual "mystery" namely each arcanum or virtue emerged. Bostocke also emphasizes the presence everywhere in natural objects of these uncreated *arcana* and virtues, although he militates against their interpretation in a pantheist sense.

*Taken as a whole* Bostocke's views support the interpretation of *Prime Matter* and the *Mysterium Magnum* as the uncreated divine spirit which assumes a position comparable to the *Logos* of the Fourth Gospel which was *with God* and became *flesh.* Bostocke's plea that Paracelsus' view was that of Pan-entheism and not of Pantheism is debatable. The Paracelsian *Arcana* are immediate divine powers and virtues and as such the only part in objects of nature which have a claim to be real and essential. On the other hand Paracelsus did insist that the *arcana qua* divine are not "natural", for "how can God be natural?" Moreover Paracelsus says that all "virtues and powers were *in* God before heaven and earth"[35]—a passage which may be adduced in support of Bostocke's pan-entheist view. We will certainly agree with Bostocke, however, that the ideological source for the *Semina* of Paracelsus is St. Augustine, although we have no direct evidence that Paracelsus was acquainted with the latter's works in detail[36].

## IV

## Epilogue: Paracelsian Prime Matter and Gnostic Speculation

To *sum up*: The *Prime Matter* of Paracelsus is not matter in the usual sense, but the ideal pattern and spiritual prelude to the material world. It thus approximates to the *Logos* of the Fourth Gospel. Like this it is *uncreated,* as it is a direct emanation from divinity. It is said to be *with God* and just as the *word* becomes *flesh,* so *prime matter* is converted into the *visible and material world.*

[33] Paracelsian *prima materia mundi* was *Fiat*: Bostocke, *loc. cit.*, cap. 21, sig. kII recto.

[34] Christ the beginning of all things: Bostocke, *loc. cit.*, cap. 21, sig. kV recto.

[35] *De Vera Influentia Rerum,* tract. I, ed. Sudhoff, vol. XIV, p. 215.

[36] Paracelsus and St. Augustine: see Pagel, *loc. cit.*, *Ambix*, 1960 (notes 136–140), pp. 162–163. On the *Semina* in the doctrine of Paracelsus: Pagel, *ibid.*, 1960, p. 136.

This *prime matter of the world* must be distinguished from the *prime matter of individual objects*, the *semina*, which are *created from nothing*. From these the objects step out at appointed times and become *ultimate matter* in the form of fully developed individuals. This *ultimate matter of individual objects* must again be distinguished from the *ultimate matter of the world*—a designation of the *prime matter of the world*, occasionally introduced by Paracelsus in order to avoid confusion with the *prime matter of individual objects*.

The Paracelsian prime matter of the world shares with St. John's *Logos* a specific Hermetic, Gnostic, Hellenistic and Rabbinical background[37]. It is unlikely that Paracelsus was aware of this in any detail—however much other Paracelsian doctrines were affiliated to Hellenistic philosophy, Gnosticism and Hermeticism.

At first sight, indeed, Paracelsus' concept of *Prime Matter* does not seem to be informed by what is generally regarded as the basic idea of Gnosticism—the polarity and contrast between divine spirit on the one hand and the dark abyss of matter uncreated and co-existing with God on the other. For, as we have seen, Paracelsian *Prime Matter* is divine spirit and not matter in the usual sense. However, Gnosticism was fundamentally concerned with the origin of the world as the embodiment of evil and the latter was not necessarily conceived as a principle *outside* and separate from God, nor as something substantial. It was indeed meant as a pure principle and as such could be visualized as a part of divinity itself. This *negative principle intrinsic in divinity* would act as a factor limiting and determining God's infinite perfection and indeterminateness, and would do so as soon as God manifested Himself through activity and creation[38]. Even so, however, the contrast between spirit and matter remains the same, although it indicates a rift within divinity rather than two opponents meeting each other. Instead the antagonist arises in God as an inexplicable urge to step out and manifest Himself in a world in which the

[37] See C. H. Dodd, *Interpretation of the Fourth Gospel, loc. cit.*, Cambridge, 1953, Hermetic Literature, pp. 10 *et seq.*; Hellenistic Judaism: Philo of Alexandria, p. 54 *et seq.*; Rabbinic Judaism, pp. 74 *et seq.*; Gnosticism, pp. 97 *et seq.*; Mandaism, pp. 115 *et seq.*

[38] Ferd. Chr. Baur, *Die Christliche Gnosis oder die Christliche Religions-Philosophie in ihrer geschichtlichen Entwicklung*, Tübingen, 1835, p. 23: "Die Materie kann zwar in einem verschiedenen Verhältnis zu Gott stehen, sie wird entweder ausser Gott als ein ihm gleich ewiges Prinzip gedacht, oder in das göttliche Wesen selbst gesetzt, oder sie ist nichts wirklich Substanzielles, sondern nur das Prinzip des Negativen, das sobald die Gottheit sich offenbart, und der Gegensaz des Unendlichen und Endlichen entsteht, von der endlichen Welt, in welcher die Gottheit sich offenbart, als das die Vollkommenheit des göttlichen Wesens beschränkende und begrenzende nicht getrennt werden kann . . .".

perfection of divinity can only exist in a limited and finite form[39]. This internal urge by which God appears bound, as it were, could only be imposed upon Him by matter—the negative principle in Him that denies the absoluteness of divinity. Eventually this principle is subject to negation in its turn and is overcome by redemption—the return of the finite to God. Spirit—absorbed and captured by matter—must be liberated, whereby divine manifestation returns to its point of departure and becomes conscious of its absolute power, i.e. its independence of matter. This sequence of events is indeed basic to all Gnostic systems—however much they vary in detail[40].

The concept of the immanence of matter in God appears to be basically in line with *Hermetic* doctrine. In this the omnipresence of God is emphasized first and foremost.

"There is not anything of all that hath been, and all that is, where God is not." Hence: "The matter, son, what is it without God, that thou shouldst ascribe a proper place to it?" There is no matter that is not made active (*energeitai*—"actuated")—"but if it be actuated, by whom is it actuated" other than by God . . . "for we have said, that Acts or Operations are the parts of God . . . whether thou speak of Matter, or Body, or Essence, know that all these are acts of God. And that the Act of Matter is materiality and of the Bodies corporality and of Essence essentiality; and this is God the whole. And in the whole there is nothing that is not God"[41]. It was God who produced matter (*Hyle*) by separating materiality (*Hylotes*) from essentiality said Jamblichus[42]. Indeed, the formation of the universe is visualized by Hermes

[39] Baur, *ibidem*, p. 23: "Aber auch selbst in diesem Falle, wenn der Begriff der Materie nur auf dieses Minimum reducirt ist, bleibt der Gegensaz zwischen Geist und Materie an sich völlig derselbe . . . so bleibt, wenn auch die Materie nicht als selbständiges Prinzip Gott gegenübersteht, in Gott doch immer der nicht weiter erklärbare Hang, aus sich herauszugehen, und sich in einer Welt zu offenbaren, in welcher die Vollkommenheit des göttlichen Wesens sich nur als eine beschränkte und endliche darstellen kann".

[40] Baur, *loc. cit.*, p. 24: "Dies sind die Hauptmomente der Selbstoffenbarung des göttlichen Wesens und der Weltentwiklung, durch welche sich alle gnostische Systeme bei aller ihrer Variation hindurchbewegen". See also on a monistic view overcoming oriental dualism in the Valentinian Gnosis: W. Bousset, *Hauptprobleme der Gnosis*, Göttingen, 1907, pp. 106 *et seq*. Already in the system of Basilides dualism had been superseded by the monistic perspective of divine emanations.

[41] *The Divine Pymander of Hermes Mercurius Trismegistus*, transl. by that Learned Divine Doctor Everard, London, 1650, p. 156 (XIth Book, 117–125). *Corpus Hermeticum*, ed. A. D. Nock and A.-J. Festugière, Paris, 1960, tract. XII, 21–22, pp. 182–183, and note 71 on p. 191 on *Hylotes*. In 22 the passage given above is translated: "Suppose, mon enfant, que la matière existe séparée de Dieu, quel lieu vas-tu lui assigner pour sa part?"

[42] Jamblichus, *De Mysteriis Liber*, ed. G. Parthey, 1857, VIII, 3, p. 265.5.

as a process that takes place *in* God[43]. "I am that Light, the Minde, thy God, who am before that moyst Nature that appeared out of darkness." When "one of an exceeding great stature and an infinite greatness" manifested Himself to Hermes in a vision he first saw all light, and only "after a little while, there was a darkness made in part, coming down obliquely, fearful and hideous which seemed unto me to be changed into a certain moyst nature, unspeakably troubled, which yielded a smoke as from fire . . ."[44].

On the other hand the Hermetic Corpus extols the glory of God through creation. There is no loss of status connected with it. "And let no man be afraid, because of the variety of things that are made or done, lest he should cast an aspersion of baseness, or infamy upon God; for it is the onely Glory of him to do, or make All things." Nor is there anything evil about the creator—for evil things "are Passions that follow Generation, as Rust doth Copper, or as Excrements do the Body. But neither did the Coppersmith make the Rust, nor the Maker the Filth, nor God the Evilness"[45].

Here then a stand is taken against certain Gnostic doctrines in which the very fact of creation depreciates God's majesty and a distinction is made between the good God-Father and the Creator-God[46]. The optimistic—antignostic—attitude of the *Hermetic Corpus* is not unknown to Paracelsus who extols Creation as the *Magnale* through which we obtain knowledge of God. The Hermetic *Asclepius* tells us that the world exists for man, as man exists for God. Man created as microcosm is called upon to govern the world, following and imitating the pattern of divine government (*Asclepius*, cap. 8–10). Paracelsus' view of the world is "anthropocentric" and may conceivably have been modelled on such Hermetic ideas. Indeed, according to Paracelsus, the creation was good and beneficial in the beginning, but—harbouring the germs of good and evil—it deteriorated owing to the fall of some of the angels. "In the world the beginning of all things was good and pleasing to God, but time has broken the good and it was split into good and evil—from good came evil in the world as well as in heaven . . . thus first the

[43] *Corp. Hermeticum, loc. cit.*, tract. I, *Poimandres*, Introduction: "Formation du monde dans le premier Nous (Père) 4–8".

[44] *Pymander*, transl. Everard, 1650, *loc. cit.*, *Second Book called Poemander*, 1–5, pp. 13–15, and *Corp. Hermet.*, *loc. cit.*, tract. I, *Poimandres*, 1–4, vol. I, pp. 7–8.

[45] *Corpus Hermeticum*, tract. XIV, 7, ed. Nock and Festugière, *loc. cit.*, vol. II, p. 224. Transl. by Everard, *loc. cit.*, 1650, pp. 212–213.

[46] Festugière in *Corp. Hermet.*, vol. II, p. 227, note 18 to tract. XIV, also with ref. to *Asclepios* 15–16, *ibid.*, p. 314, and note 135 on pp. 371–372 on the evil of world and earth.

angels were made miraculously beautiful and good, but some of them sinned and . . . were ejected from the realm of God." (Paracelsus, *Philosophia Sagax*, lib. IV, cap. 1, ed. Sudhoff, vol. XII, p. 417.)

Perhaps it is permissible to compare the Gnostic idea of the negative principle connected with creation with *Kabbalistic* speculation on the supreme Being, the Infinite (*En-Soph*). This is visualized as absolute negation and called *Nothing* (*Ayin*), as it is entirely inaccessible to human understanding and defies definition. More particularly in Kabbalistic tradition it was through an impulse towards creation that God undid the secret inaccessibility of His abstract Being and this impulse is called *Nothing*. It is not the stepping-out of God into activity and creation, but the urge leading to it that is so called and also designated as *I shall be* (*Ehje*). *In* this absolute Nothing creation *from* Nothing unfolds itself, and the Nothing is in some places called aboriginal *Will*[47].

Comparing this with the idea of matter intrinsic to divinity, its designation as Nothing would denote its limitation and descent into the finiteness of matter and the world. Acting as the first cause of *all* that is existent, it would have to be non-existent in itself. Its conversion from incomprehensible spirit into something that is comprehensible, i.e. into matter, would stand for the creation of *something* from *Nothing*.

It is of particular interest that in this Kabbalistic speculation the *Word* emerges with its creative power. The divine Nothing is also seen as the archetypal *light* that forms an *Aura* around the supreme Being in His original state of infinite remoteness and withdrawal. *Qua* first *cause*, this light manifests itself through its *Wisdom* and *Word* as the prototype of the whole creation or macrocosm (*First Adam—Adam Kadmon*)[48]. The infinite Nothing could not manifest itself directly, but needed a mediating instrument—the *sefirot*, i.e. the sum total of creative powers and potentials. One of these is the *Word* for the

[47] G. Scholem, *Die Geheimnisse der Schöpfung. Ein Kapitel aus dem Sohar*, Berlin, 1935, pp. 31–32: "Die erste Sefira, der innerste aller Aspekte, in dem die ewig undurchdringliche Wendung des Schöpfers zur Schöpfung bezeichnet wird, ist der Name *Ehje* 'ich werde sein'. Dies Hervortreten aus dem Ungrund, das noch gar kein 'Hervor'treten ist, sondern nur der Ruck, in dem er die Verschlossenheit seines 'An sich' vernichtet, heisst . . . das *Nichts*. . . . In diesem . . . 'absolut' genannten Nichts, vollzieht sich die wahre 'Schöpfung aus dem Nichts'. . . . An anderen Soharstellen heisst dies Nichts der Urwille". See also: G. Scholem, *Die mystische Gestalt der Gottheit in der Kabbala*, Eranos Jahrbuch, Vol. 29, Zürich, 1961, p. 165.

[48] S. Munk, *Mélanges de Philosophie Juive et Arabe*, Paris, 1859, p. 492, and S. Munk, *Philosophie und philosophische Schriftsteller der Juden mit Anmerkungen* von B. Beer, Leipzig, 1852, p. 53.

"world of the 'sefirot', the total of divine expression—a world aptly called 'internal face'—is conceived as a secret archetypal world of language"[49].

The conceptual elements, then, that are essential to Paracelsian *Prime Matter* can be found in Gnostic as well as Hermetic and Kabbalistic speculation: matter as a part of divinity, forming a hypostasis that subsists *with* God, acts as the Wisdom and *Word* that creates from *Nothing* and becomes ordinary matter (*Flesh*) which calls for liberation and redemption by eventually returning to the supreme Being.

Paracelsian *Prime Matter* in its role as the spiritual pattern of the material world, and the pantheistic version of this idea given by Paracelsus in certain places, compare with the *Prime Matter* of Solomon ibn Gabirol (Avicebron, 1020–1070)—an immediate emanation from the Creator which follows Him in the hierarchy of steps constituting the world both in its real existence and its contemplation by the mind. This *matter* precedes *form*—for it is simple and infinite and it is through form that limitations, diversity, specification and finiteness are imposed upon it. It is well known how this philosophy influenced David of Dinant (d. 1209) and mediaeval Pantheism[50].

Closeness to Gnosticism impresses itself readily in some Paracelsian ideas connected with the concept of *Matter*: first and foremost is that of the creation of the elements in connexion with the Fall and punishment of Lucifer[51].

[49] G. Scholem, *loc. cit.*, 1935, p. 29: "Die Welt der Sefirot . . . wird als eine geheime Urwelt der Sprache aufgefasst . . . Vorstellung vom Wort als Kraft . . .".

[50] See on this point: Pagel, *Paracelsus, loc. cit.*, 1958, pp. 227–236. B. Sart. von Waltershausen, *Paracelsus am Eingang der Deutschen Bildungsgeschichte*, Leipzig, 1936, pp. 128–129, quotes a passage from Valentin Weigel, *Theologia Weigelii*, Newstadt, 1618, cap. 6, fol. 17. In this Weigel claims that David de Dinando, Theophrastus (Paracelsus) and himself agree in saying that God, *materia prima* and heaven are eternal and that God is all this Himself. According to Waltershausen there is but little connexion with mediaeval thinking in either Paracelsus' or Weigel's works and it is characteristic that the latter alludes to a mediaeval pantheist who stands outside the scholastic tradition.

For mediaeval Judaeo-Arabic sources according to which *prime matter* "represents the lowest grade of the spiritual substances, and stands at the gateway, as it were, of the sensible world . . . that prime matter itself is a simple spiritual substance which emanates from the soul and which cannot be perceived by the senses" see A. Altmann and S. M. Stern, *Isaac Israeli. A neo-Platonic Philosopher of the early Tenth Century*, Oxford, 1958, p. 182.

[51] *Prolog, Konzepte und Ausarbeitungen zum Liber Meteororum*, ed. Sudhoff, vol. XIII, pp. 253–254. The *suggested emergence of this view* in the *Jewish religious philosophy of the Middle Ages* is of some interest and may be here noted in passing. Allegedly, according to Gersonides, hell—*sheol*—is the *Hyle-ha-rischon*, the first matter and origin of evil (ad Proverb. XV, 11, and XXVII, 20—quoted from J. C. Wolf, *Manichaeismus ante Manichaeos et in Christianismo redivivus*, Hamburg, 1707, pp. 44–45). Wolf adducing

Among further Paracelsian views that are palpably influenced by Gnosticism, we refer to his recognition of water as a general *matrix* and receptacle for *semina* and to the concept of *cagastrum*—the falsehood inherent in the ever-changing phenomenal world. In ancient tradition this had been aptly symbolized by the dragon which insatiably devours its own tail, standing for darkness and evil[52]. We also refer to the Paracelsian *astral body*, and to his ideas on the passions of the soul and its animal instincts that lead to insanity. Our discussion of this and related doctrines in the light of the Hermetic tradition can be found elsewhere[53] and should be compared with the Paracelsian philosophy of *Prime Matter*—another Platonic-Christian doctrine which forms the subject of the present paper.

[52] See for example Festugière's note 9, p. 12, to *Poimandres* 4 in *Corpus Hermeticum*, ed. A. D. Nock and A.-J. Festugière, 2nd ed., Paris, 1960, vol. I, on Serpent and Darkness with references to Gnostic sources including the *Ouroboros* as represented for example by W. Bousset, *Hauptprobleme der Gnosis*, Göttingen, 1907, pp. 100–101.

[53] The present author in *Ambix*, 1960, vol. VIII, pp. 125–166.

---

51 *continued.*

further literature remarks to this: "Atque hic quidem error de materia mali origine non existimandus est semper Judaeorum inhaesisse animis, sed Philosophorum gentilium debetur lacunis, quas Judaeorum Philosophi sequiores cum S. scripturae canalibus commutarunt". Indeed Jewish philosophy is consonant with the *Placita Platonicorum*, as Maimonides asserted, whom one should follow—rather "quam cum Helmontio in praefat. ad *Alphabetum Natur*. temere negare, Ebraeorúm Philosophiam Platonicis dogmatibus plenam esse".

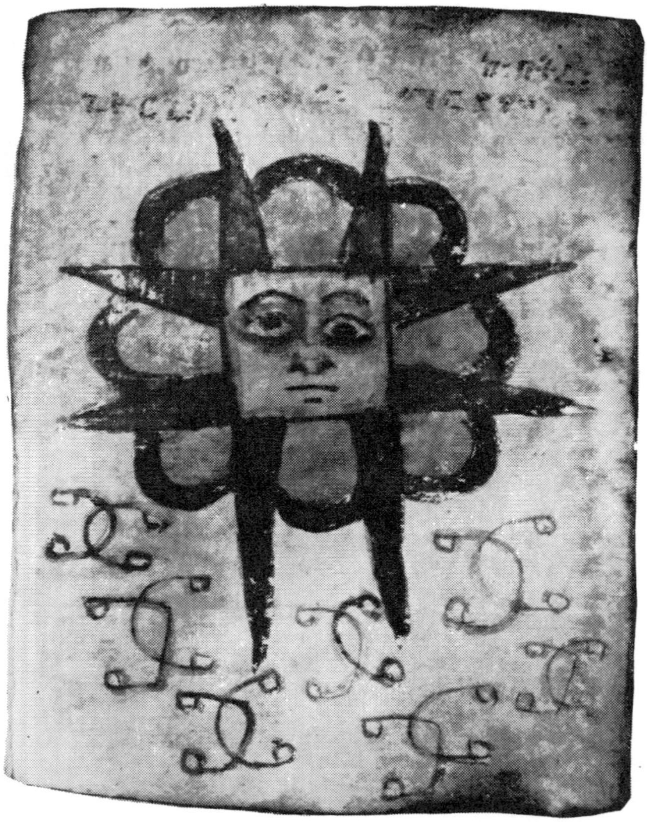

PLATE I. Eight Emanations depicted as emerging from the Divine Face (see *loc. cit.* from Fürst, *Hebräisches Lexicon*, in note 21). From a seventeenth-century Aethiopian amulet in the possession of the London Library, from the Collection of Sir E. A. Wallis Budge. See also Wallis Budge, *Amulets and Superstitions*, OUP, 1930, pp. 186–8. (Photographed from the original by kind permission of the London Library, and reproduced in the original size by the Wellcome Institute). Concerning a possible source, see the solar cross with eight rays from an Assyrian bas-relief as illustrated in J. Menaut: *Pierres Gravées de la Haute Asie*, Paris, 1886, vol. II, p. 71. Reference kindly provided by Mr. H. J. Sheppard, Warwick.

# VIII

## THE EIGHTNESS OF ADAM AND RELATED "GNOSTIC" IDEAS IN THE PARACELSIAN CORPUS

*In collaboration with Marianne Winder*

### Introduction

The accusation of Gnostic heresy was already levelled against Paracelsus (1493–1541) by his first determined critics, notably Thomas Erastus (1523–1583). It was largely based on the theories of Creation as expounded in the *Philosophia ad Athenienses*.[1] A number of doctrines that are common to Gnosticism and the Paracelsian Corpus have already been discussed by the present authors.[2]

These include notably:

(*a*) the pessimistic appraisal of the material world of elements and creatures as something base and excrementitious (*pleroma tes kakias, hell*),

(*b*) the distinction between the highest God of redemption and the lower powers of astral demiurges (*archontes*) who are responsible for creation,

(*c*) *Separatio* in matter uncreated, in contrast to creation *de novo* from nothing, and

(*d*) the role of water as universal matter, the seat of *Behemoth* or devil.

A further example, so far not discussed, is the story of the "Creation of Adam—from Eight Parts". In the present paper we propose to examine its position in the Paracelsian writings and in the light of its historical background.

[1] Pagel, W., *Paracelsus. An Introduction to Philosophical Medicine in the Era of the Renaissance*, Basle, 1958, pp. 91, 315, 204 ff.

[2] Pagel, W., "Paracelsus: Traditionalism and Medieval Sources", in *Medicine, Science and Culture. Historical Essays in Honor of O. Temkin*, Baltimore, 1968, pp. 51–75; Pagel, W. and Winder, M., "Gnostisches bei Paracelsus und Konrad von Megenberg", in *Fachliteratur des Mittelalters. Festschrift für G. Eis.*, Stuttgart, 1968, pp. 359–71; Pagel, W., "Paracelsus and the Gnostic and Neoplatonic Tradition", *Ambix*, 1960, **viii**, 125–66; *idem*, "The Prime Matter of Paracelsus", *Ambix*, 1961, **ix**, 117–35; *idem*, "The Wild Spirit (Gas) of John Baptist Van Helmont and Paracelsus", *Ambix*, 1962, **x**, 1–13; *idem*, *Das Medizinische Weltbild des Paracelsus. Seine Zusammenhänge mit Neuplatonismus und Gnosis*, Wiesbaden, F. Steiner, 1962.

## I. Some Traditional Data Concerning the Eight Pieces of Adam

The story of the eight components of which Adam was created is known to have been often repeated throughout the Middle Ages. It is regarded as part of the Gnostic tradition.[3] In the era preceding Paracelsus, it occurs prominently in the *Book of the Holy Trinity* (*Buch der Heiligen Dreifaltigkeit*)—an alchemical manuscript of the fifteenth century. Here we find a full catalogue of the eight pieces, and this has been compared in detail with a similar catalogue occurring in the *Dialogue between the Emperor Hadrian and the wise child Epithus*.[4]

It is tempting to connect the story with the well known Gnostic idea of the "Group of Eight" (*Ogdoas*). We are told by Irenaeus that Sophia created out of soul substance the Father and King of all things. These are identical with him in that they have a soul-like (right-) and a material (left-sided) aspect. This king creates seven heavens, hence he is also called "Sevenness", whilst Sophia, the mother above him, is called "Eightness". The Mother or "Eightness" is thought to be situated in the middle, namely above the King-demiurge, but below and outside the *Pleroma*, i.e. the realm of divine spiritual fullness of Life.[5]

Elsewhere Ialdabaoth, Sophia's son, together with his offspring, the seven *Archontes*, are said to create the soul of Adam. This is thereby sevenfold and embraces the soul of such constituents as bone, flesh and so on. The remaining

[3] Ganzenmüller, W., "Das Buch der heiligen Dreifaltigkeit. Eine deutsche Alchemie aus dem Anfang des 15. Jahrhunderts", *Archiv für Kulturgeschichte*, 1939, **29**, p. 93. Repr. in his *Beiträge zur Geschichte der Technologie und der Alchemie*, Weinheim, 1956, pp. 231–72, esp. p. 265.

[4] Ganzenmüller, *loc. cit.* (3), 1956, p. 265. See also: Koehler, Richard, "Adams Erschaffung", in *Kleinere Schriften zur erzählenden Dichtung des Mittelalters*, vol. 2, 1900, pp. 1–7; Foerster, M., "Adams Erschaffung und Namengebung", *Arch. Rel. wiss.*, 1907, **11**, p. 477. The authors are indebted to Mr. Desmond Geoghegan for drawing their attention to Jung, C. G., *Mysterium Conjunctionis, An Inquiry into the Separation and Synthesis of Psychic Opposites in Alchemy*. Tr. R. F. C. Hull, London, 1963, p. 387, quoting an English riddle from the fifteenth century: "Whereof was Adam made?" from R. Köhler, as quoted above.

[5] Irenaeus, *Op. Erud.*, ed. Erasmus Roterodamus, Paris, 1563, Lib. I, cap. 34, fol. 58v; ed. G. G. Grynaeus, Basle, 1571, p. 102. See also *ibid.*, Lib. II, cap. 15, p. 145 and Lib. I, cap. 1, p. 19 on the *Ogdoas*. To this see Baur, F. C., *Die Christliche Gnosis*, Tübingen, 1835, pp. 145, 153, 173.

*Additional note*. Celestial and earthly Adam: Reuchlin, *De arte cabbalistica*, Hagenau, 1517, sig. g2 verso, facsimile reprint Frommann, 1964, p. 128.

three hundred and sixty angels create the body of Adam. Hence the latter would consist of eight pieces, namely seven souls and one body. At the same time the complacency and ineptitude of the *Archontes* in this work is emphasized.[6]

In apocryphal Gnostic treatises on Adam,[7] seven emanations or heavens, the sons of Sophia, are mentioned. Ialdabaoth is the first of the seven lower spirits. The other six spirits, being jealous of Ialdabaoth, form the first man according to their own image, a creeping giant monster. Ialdabaoth is then induced by Sophia to breathe his spirit of life into it. He thereby loses the virtue of the light-dew whereas by this act man gains contact with the highest original being, "First Man". It would appear that in this tradition only seven Architects or components of Adam are involved.

In the *Poimander*, Nature is said to be fertilized by "Archetypal Man" (*Anthropos*). Out of the union she produces seven "terrestrial" men. These are by their nature analogous to the seven *dioiketeis* (administrators or *Archontes*). They are androgynous and actuated by heavenly aspirations (*metarsioi*).[8]

In the *Slavonic Henoch-Book* man is said to have been made from seven components—flesh from earth, blood from dew, eyes from sun, bones from stone, reason from the swiftness of the angels and the clouds, tendons and hair from the grass of the earth, and soul from spirit and wind. In addition, it is said that his name was composed of the four directions (East, West, South and North) and that four certain stars were allocated to him and that he was called Adam.[9]

In the *Picatrix*, the well-known mediaeval Arabic book of magic, the body is said to consist of nine substances which form nine concentric circles. However, only eight of these are enumerated, namely: flesh, bone, muscle, nerve,

[6] Jonas, H., *Gnosis und spätantiker Geist*, 3rd ed., 1964, vol. I, p. 396, from *Papyrus Berolinensis* 8502, 47, 16–51, 1. On the arrogance and ineptitude of the *Archontes*: Irenaeus, Lib. I, cap. 33, ed. Grynaeus, *loc. cit.* (5), 1571, p. 99. See also Jonas, *loc. cit.* as above, vol. 1, p. 361. See below, p. 137 and notes (51) and (52).

[7] Preuschen, E., *Die apokryphen gnostischen Adamschriften*, Giessen, 1900, p. 64.

[8] *Corpus Hermeticum I, Poimandres*, Cap. 16–7. Ed. Nock, A. D. and Festugière, A. J., Paris, 1960, p. 12. For the pre-Socratic, Platonic and Greek mythological tradition of androgyny, see Ziegler, Konrat, *Menschen und Weltenwerden. Ein Beitrag zur Geschichte der Microkosmosidee*, Leipzig/Berlin, 1913.

[9] Bonwetsch, N., *Das slavische Henochbuch*, Berlin, 1896, p. 29.

medulla, skin, hair and nail. In other words, one substance is missing. Another Arabic source nominates in addition blood vessels and blood whilst omitting muscle. In this case the result is correctly nine and contrasts with the *Picatrix* tradition.[10]

## II. Paracelsus' Eight Categories of Astrology

### Goethe and C. G. Jung

Not long ago C. G. Jung touched upon our problem.[11] He discussed what he calls archetypal man (*Urmensch*), i.e. the idea of man personified in the workman (*demiurgus*) who makes him. Archetypal man is male and female (*androgynous*).

It should be noted that in the tradition here discussed archetypal man is already a figure at a level below that of the highest divinity (*pleroma*). Archetypal man thus is the Creator-God, in other words, the God of the Pentateuch. Like the latter he creates man in his own image. Adam was created male and female. Hence, we would add, the image according to which he was created should also have been androgynous.[12]

Jung refers to the alchemical treatise entitled *Consilium Conjugii*. In this "Philosophic Man" is said to consist of the "four natures of the Stone". Three of these are earthy or in the earth, whereas "the fourth nature is the water of the stone, i.e. viscous gold which is called 'red gum' (*gumma*) and with

[10] Ritter, H. and Plessner, M., *Picatrix. Das Ziel des Weisen von Pseudomagritti*, London, Warburg Institute, 1962, p. 43. The present authors are indebted to Professor M. Plessner for drawing their attention to this. With reference to the position of *Picatrix* in Hermetic Literature, see Yates, F. A., *Giordano Bruno and the Hermetic Tradition*, London, 1964, esp. pp. 49–57.

[11] Jung, C. G., *Psychologie und Alchemie*, Zürich, 1944, pp. 227–8. (English ed., London, 1953, p. 154.)

[12] To this see *Genesis*, Cap. V, vv. 1–2: "This is the book of the generations of Adam. In the day that God created man, in the likeness of God made he him; Male and female created he them, and blessed them, and called their name (*eth shmam*, as against the Septuagint reading 'called *his* name' — *onoma autou*) Adam, in the day when they were created".

See also: Knorr von Rosenroth, *Kabbala denudata s.Doctrina Hebraeorum*, Sultzbach 1677, vol. I, p. 29 sub verbo *Adam*, paragr. 7: nomen Adam excellentius sit quam nomen *Isch*—Vir . . . nimirum quia in nomine Adam comprehenduntur Malchuth et Tipheret juxta illud Gen. V,2: masculum et feminam creavit eos et vocavit nomen eorum *Adam*. In hac sc. perfectione ut masculi et foeminae notiones concurrant. Nomen *Isch* vero masculum tantum significat.

which the three earthy natures are being tinged".[12a] Divisions into seven and eight parts, though similar in concept, are, according to Jung, much more rarely met with.[13]

It is, however, found in Paracelsus. Jung himself quotes the passage in which Paracelsus develops the idea of *eight* kinds of Astrology.[14] Here Paracelsus first surveys his subject. This deals with the highest—olympic—*Astrum*, i.e. a spiritual power which governs (*a*) lower (animal) reasoning in man, (*b*) sense in animals, and (*c*) the effects wrought by the elements. The *astrum* on High exerts this influence through a corresponding *middle astrum*, i.e. one that lies in the object on which the high astrum acts. He then divides astrology into eight groups. These are as follows:

1. Astrology concerned with the highest—olympic—*astrum* which governs all the others.
2. Astrology dealing with the astral forces that operate in man.

3–6. Four astrologies each connected with one of the (four) elements.

7. Astrology as operative in animal life.
8. An additional astrology which is derived from human imagination. This latter *astrum* is as powerful as the first one.[15]

[12a] *Consilium conjugii de massa Solis et Lunae, Ars Chemica*, Argentor., 1566, pp. 255–6; *Theatrum Chemicum*, Argentor., 1622, vol. V, p. 263. *Gumma* or *gummi* may mean many things in alchemy. The nearest meaning in the present context seems the Dornean: vocatur illud fermentum compositum ex Mercurio et materia prima metallorum et oleo facta inceratione conjunctis (quoted from Castellus, Bartholomaeus, *Lexicon Medicum*, Lipsiae, 1713, p. 374).

[13] In a later work, however, Jung comments: "The double quaternio or ogdoas stands for a totality, for something that is at once heavenly and earthly, spiritual or corporeal . . . it is . . . the microcosm, the mystical Adam and bisexual original man in his prenatal state. . . . In the Scholia to the *Tractatus Aureus Hermetis* there is a quaternion consisting of superius/inferius, exterius/interius. They are united into one thing by means of circular distillation named the Pelican". See *Mysterium conjunctionis*, London, 1963, *loc. cit.* (4), p. 11. See below p. 131 and notes 37 *et seq.*

To this the present authors would add as an example of pertinent quaternions: Knorr von Rosenroth, *Kabbala denudata*, vol. II, *Liber Sohar restitutus*, Francofurti, 1684, p. 383, in *Siphra de Zeniutha s. liber mysterii*, cap. 5, paragr. 36: quattuor sunt domus judicii superiores et quattuor inferiores. Nam scriptum est: non facietis iniquitatem in judicio, in dimensione cubiti, in pondere et in mensura (ubi quattuor haec mystice innuuntur—Lev. 19, v. 35). *Ibid.*, paragr. 29, p. 382: Quattuor reges occurrunt quattuor (i.e. 4 litterae tetragrammati innectuntur quattuor litteris Adonaj: quae) ab illis dependent ut uvae in racemo.

[14] Jung, *loc. cit.* (11), 1944, p. 228.

[15] Paracelsus: *Erklärung der ganzen Astronomei, ein mantischer Entwurf geben zu München* (1536?), in: *Sämtliche Werke*, ed. K. Sudhoff, vol. X, München and Berlin, 1928, p. 645. On the *Eight Virtues of Bliss and Charity* in a Pseudo-Paracelsian treatise see below, p. 135 and note (43).

Heinrich von Mügeln's Eightness of Angels in the contest of the liberal arts

Here, then, Paracelsus stipulates an *eightness* concerning a liberal art. This immediately recalls Heinrich von Mügeln. This fourteenth-century Middle-High-German author describes a contest between twelve liberal arts. The emperor adjudicating the prize says:

die eilften lobt ich immer me:
nu dunkt mich, wie ir tichten ste
swerlich gein dem gelouben min:
sie lert mich, wie acht engel sin:
die letzte engel ane zal
setzet: der ich geleuben sal.

(I would always praise the eleventh, i.e. Metaphisica. Only it seems to me that her invention makes it difficult for me to believe her: she teaches that there are eight angels. The last one, i.e. Theologia, assumes innumerable angels, and I shall believer her).[16]

An additional point of significance in our context is a middle position accorded to *Metaphisica* by Mügeln. He says that she is situated between God and Nature, a description which we shall discuss below with reference to Sophia (p. 128).

Sevenness in Alchemical Literature

Returning to Jung, the latter states more specifically that such eight groups as the foregoing are not normally found in alchemical literature. For the absence of an eighth group he notably refers to the seven figures representing King Sun and the six planetary "metal-homunculi" in the *Pretiosa Margarita Novella* of Janus Lacinius printed in 1546. He continues: "The eighth, however, does not occur here. Paracelsus seems to have invented him in addition". (Der achte kommt hier allerdings nicht vor. Paracelsus scheint ihn dazu erfunden zu haben.)[17]

The Eight Kabiri

Jung wonders whether there may have been a connection between the Paracelsian idea of eight groups and the emergence of an *eighth* member in the group of the *Kabiri*.[18] In literature, they occur, for example, in Goethe's

[16] Heinrich von Mügeln, *Der Meide Kranz*, ed. Willy Jahr, Inaugural Thesis, Leipzig, 1908, p. 113.

[17] Jung, 1944, *loc. cit.* (11), p. 228. See, however, our note (13). Also cf. Jung, *Mysterium conjunctionis, loc. cit.* (4), pp. 399–401: In the *Clementine Homilies* (2nd cent.) Adam is the first of a series of eight incarnations of the "true prophet". The last is Jesus. Comparison is made with the Chinese *P'an Ku* and the Taoist *eight immortals*.

[18] Jung, *loc. cit.*, 1944, p. 222 ff.

*Faust,* Part II, where they are associated with the significance of numbers such as three, four, seven and eight. The terms are reminiscent of the perennial alchemical treatment of the subject.

At the time of Goethe's writing, the question of the *Kabiri* and their number had formed the subject of a learned controversy between Creuzer and Schelling. Schelling had objected that the *Kabiri* were not emanations, but an ascending series of deities to be finally dissolved in the supreme Zeus and depicted as dwarfs. As such they were thought to be magicians who guided the transcendent world into everyday reality. Goethe is said to have made fun of this.[19]

Creuzer, following Herodotus, regarded the *Kabiri* as the sons of Phthas, the father of all great deities. The Egyptians, Creuzer suggests, should have identified them with the seven planets and "worshipped in them and *Phthas* an *Ogdoad* of great potencies". (Gewiss dachte sich der Aegyptier unter den Kabiren die sieben Planeten, und verehrte in ihnen und dem Phthas eine Achtzahl von grossen Potenzen). Creuzer believed in a transmission of the story to the Greeks by the Phoenicians.[20]

The latter saw in the *Kabiri* the seven sons of Sydek (Phthas–Zeus)—the eighth member of the group being called *Esmun.*[21] Creuzer attributed the whole story of the *Kabiri* to an esoteric representation of world harmony as the result of the work of cosmogonic forces. On the authority of Photius, *Phthas* appears as the highest power which creates several "great gods". These, by virtue of their "greatness" can also be called *Hephaestuses.* They are also said to be the children of *Hephaistos* (*legontai de einai Hephaistou*

[19] Cf. Goethe, *Faust, Part II,* ed. Witkowski, G., *Kommentar zu 8071–7,* Band II, Leipzig, Hesse & Becker, 1912, p. 334.

[20] Creuzer, Friedrich, *Symbolik und Mythologie der alten Völker, besonders der Griechen. Dritter Theil,* part three. 3rd ed., Leipzig and Darmstadt, 1841, vol. 3, p. 17.

[21] *Sanchoniatho translated out of Eusebius, Praepar. Evangel.,* lib. I, cap. 10, by R. Cumberland, 1720, pp. 39 and 200. See also Fürst, J., *Hebräisches und chaldäisches Handwörterbuch,* Leipzig, 1876, vol. I, p. 571 under *Kabbir* and *Kabbirim* ("phoenizisch Kabbirim, bei Sanchoniathon p. 22, 38: Kabeiroi, Kaberoi, Name der sieben Söhne des Zdiq (same as Zaddiq) in dem phoenizischen Göttersystem, wozu noch ein Achter mit dem besonderen Namen Eschmon (der Achte) kommt; sie symbolisieren die sieben Planenten. Ebenso hiess der Planet Jupiter nach einer Glosse in Hesychius Melech Kabbir").

See also Fürst, *ibidem,* vol. II, p. 470 under Sch'mon (or Eschmon): ist der Name des phönikischen achten Kabirs, an den acht Strahlen auf seinem Haupt erkennbar (auf Münzen *achter* Sohn des Sadyk), den Himmelskreis versinnbildend, der die sieben Kreisbahnen der Planeten umschliesst (Damascius bei Photius, *Bibl.,* p. 352); Lobeck, C. A., *Aglaophamus sive de Theologiae Mysticae Graecorum Causis,* Königsberg, 1829, vol. II, pp. 1265 and 1277: Esmounos Ogdoos de egeneto epi toutois (scil. the other sons of Sadyk, the Dioskouroi and Kabbiroi) ho Esmounos hon Asklepion hermeneuousin. (With reference to Damascius, in *Vita Isidori,* ccxlii, 573.)

***Additional note.*** **Kabiri inventing *salia* and hence founding *Medicina magica*: Kaau Boerhaave, *Impetum faciens dictum Hippocrati*, Lugd. Batav., 1745, p. 361, with reference to Eusebius — Kabires filii Saduc.**

*paides*), or else they form between them a unit called Hephaistos.[22] It has been inferred (though contested) that they symbolize the tools of the blacksmith.[23]

The connexion of the *Kabiri* with *Hephaistos* is of interest in the Paracelsian context (see below p. 136 and notes 49 *et seq.*).

Perhaps a side-line to the story of the *Kabiri* is indicated in the tradition of the "Eighth King" found in the *Kabbala*. It relates to the "Light of the Name Mah". This emerges from the forehead of (archetypal) "First Man", the *Adam Kadmon*. It is the "Mysterium of the Eighth King" who is mentioned in *Genesis* 36, 39. He is called *Adar*. In his reign there is no mention of death, because he himself did not die as did the seven others who came before him. He rather restored and resuscitated the latter. Scripture apportioned to him a wife deriving from what he took over by his own choice from the other kings—which is expressed by the term *Ben*. And now its place is taken by the name of *Adam* or man because man comprises both sexes. This is why the names *Mah* and *Adam* have the same symbolical value (*per gematriam*).

Death was in this tradition connected with the "Breaking of the Vessels", and the destruction of the "Kings" with the deficiency of male and female harmony in Adam. In the words of Scholem, the vessels had been destined to receive the light emanating from the eyes of *Adam Kadmon*. They were to serve as vessels and instruments in the process of creation. Their breaking indicates a decisive "crisis" of all divine and creature being. It was called by Luria—using Soharistic imagery—the "Dying of the original Kings". For the *Sohar* interprets the list of the Kings of Edom in *Genesis* 36 who reigned and died before Kings reigned in Israel as the pre-existence of Worlds which perished. The fragments of the vessels are interpreted in terms of excretory residues (*Klippoth—cortices, putamina*)—barks and shells—which cannot be assimilated. These take a downward course into the world of creation (*Beriah*) where they persist as demoniac powers.[24]

[22] Creuzer, 1841, pp. 20–1.

[23] Lobeck, *loc. cit.*, 1829, p. 1209 ff.

[24] *Kabbala denudata*, vol. I, p. 510 under *Mah*, paragr. 3.–*mysterium regis octavi*; p. 511–*androgynicity*; p. 542–*vasa confracta, mors, eversio regum*; p. 675–*Klippoth*; p. 580–*productio septem regum*. Scholem, G., *Zur Kabbala und ihrer Symbolik*, Zürich, 1960, pp. 150–51 (cap. III, Kabbala und Mythos). The kabbalistic pattern of unassimilable deposits (klippoth—bringing evil into the world) may well form the ideological background to such Gnostic ideas of Paracelsus as *Tartarus* and *Cagastrum* which notably embrace disease due to indigestible deposits from the food. See Pagel, *Weltbild*, 1962, *loc. cit.* (2), pp. 95–9.

## III. The Adam-story in the Paracelsian Corpus

Nothing as elaborate as the Gnostic stories discussed above (p. 120) can be found in the Paracelsian Corpus. However, it is definitely mentioned that Adam was composed of eight pieces. This occurs in the pseudo-Paracelsian *De Secretis Creationis*.[25] Here the subject is the "subtility" which the four elements have in common with the "eight pieces" or substances of which God has made Adam. This "subtility" appertains to the four elements of heaven and those of earth.

### Middle Nature and the Dark and Bright Fire

In close proximity to the passage from *De Secretis Creationis* just quoted the term "middle nature" is mentioned. This "makes all things under heaven and breaks them again", but remains itself unchanged, just as does the Word of God to which all creation is due. Everything grows through its "Middle Nature". This communicates its heat and humidity to the object, and by this all things are brought together. For "Middle Nature" is a "seed" and *sperma* in all things that grow and is the "fire" and the "sixth essence" in all things; it is "greenness" that makes all things in the earth to become green, the earth being originally black.[26] We shall return to the Paracelsian Middle Nature below (p. 135 and notes 47–8).

Connected with the foregoing there is the contrast between divine light and a fire as contained in the dark flames (*"fewer in einer diesteren flamen"*). Divine light is a spirit made invisible through being covered by a visible body. God is spirit and fire and therefore not apprehensible, an "airy being", a "spiritual body". Before God created heaven and earth, darkness and light had been mixed in the same way as the divine fire is hidden in a body.

We have, then, in *De Secretis* in close proximity to each other the concepts of:

(*a*) the "eight pieces of Adam",

(*b*) "Middle Nature", its role in coming into being, especially in the earth and its products,

(*c*) creating forces (God) compared to an "invisible fire" in "*dark flames*".

[25] Huser, *Chirurgische Bücher und Schrifften des . . . Paracelsi*, Strassburg, Zetzner, 1605, fol., *Appendix*, p. 114.

Die Componierung der Menschenkörper ist die Subtilheit der vier Elementen welche Subtilheit auch sowohl die *acht Stück oder Substanzien in ihr hat von welchen Gott Adam gemacht hatte*, von der Subtilheit der vieren Elementen des Himmels und der Erden.

[26] *De Secretis Creat., loc. cit.* in Appendix to Paracelsus, *Chirurgische Schriften*, 1605, p. 105. To this see Pagel, W., *loc. cit.*, 1962, p. 56, n. 2. *Idem*, *William Harvey's Biological Ideas*, New York–Basel, 1967, p. 277, with reference to Harvey and Van Helmont, and *ibid.*, p. 276, with reference to Dorneus.

VIII

128

These points are at least partly anticipated in the *Book of the Holy Trinity*. In the latter there is first of all the composition of "Adam of eight pieces". This is closely connected with the idea of the "Dark Fire". It says that each piece of Adam consists of two parts, namely of fiery and watery air, the latter being an "eternal black fire". This fire Man has in common with all other things. Each of them, in their turn, also consists of eight pieces.

Finally, there is in the *Book of the Holy Trinity* the intermediary position of the earth which forms a "middle realm" between good and evil. Here the emphasis is laid on the permanent struggle between light and darkness.[27]

Concerning parallels with the Gnostic tradition we have already dealt with the Gnostic *Ogdoas* as a possible pattern of the Adam-story.[28] In addition we would now refer to the Middle Life of *Sophia*,[29] the active creating principle.

It is tempting to connect with this the *Mater in Medio*. This occurs in the *Siphra de Zeniutha* as accessible in the *Kabbala denudata*. Here the Mother is represented by the letter ***Heh***. This stands for "Informative Intelligence" and the "Upper Mother". The letter holds the middle position between ***Jod*** and ***Vav*** in the Tetragrammaton ***(JHVH)***. For on high there is the Father above her, and below she is surrounded by the former's son, the *Microposopus*.[30]

[27] Ganzenmüller, *loc. cit.*, 1956, p. 266 (swarcz sunne fewer), *ibid.* (middle realm).

[28] See above, p. 120 and notes (5) and (6).

[29] Irenaeus, lib. I, cap. 1, ed. Erasmus, *loc. cit.*, in note (5), f. 13v: cum autem universum semen perfectum fuerit, Achamot quidem, matrem ipsorum transire de *medietatis loco* dicunt et intra pleroma introire et recipere sponsum suum salvatorem qui est ex omnibus factus uti syzygia fiat Salvatoris et Sophiae quae est Achamot et hoc esse sponsum et sponsam. Also, Ed. Grynaeus, *loc. cit.* (5), p. 19: Hanc (i.e. Achamoth) autem matrem etiam Octonarium vocant, & Sapientiam, & Terram, & Hierusalem, & Spiritum Sanctum, & Dominum masculino genere. Habere vero ipsam *medietatis locum*, & esse quidem supra opificem, infra vero aut extra complementum usque ad consummationem. *Ibid.*, pp. 24–5, Opificem vero etiam ipsum transire in matris Sapientiae locum, hoc est *in medietatem*, iustorum item animas requiescere etiam ipsas in medietatis loco. Nihil enim animale intra complementum transire. For further references from the *Pistis Sophia*, Bousset, W., *Hauptprobleme der Gnosis*, Göttingen, 1907, pp. 62 and 165.

[30] *Kabbala Denudata*, vol. II, 1684, *Siphra de Zeniutha sive Liber Mysterii*, cap. I, paragraph 41, p. 355:

> Pater residet in principio (i.e. litera Jod quae est symbolum Sapientiae et Patris). *Mater in Medio* (nam litera Heh, quae est nota Intelligentiae informatricis et Matris supernae, inter Jod et Vav medium tenet, prout in supernis a Patre comprehenditur desuper, et a Microposopo, qui est filius ejus, vestitur deorsum, in quo ipsa sese demittit. . . .

Finally we recall the statement of Heinrich von Mügeln's concerning the position of *Metaphisica* between God and Nature in his *Der Meide Kranz*:

Under mir der naturen fluss
ist, über mir der ware got
unwegelich gar sunder spot.[31]

("Under me is the flow of Nature, but above me is the true God, immovable indeed is he".)

The long Gnostic tradition of the "dark fire" is well-known and can be even traced back to the Stoic *pyr noeron* and the *psychikon pyr* of Aristotle.[32]

## IV. The Paracelsian Eight Mothers (Acht Mütter)

Can any further groups of Eight be adduced from the Paracelsian Corpus? This is indeed the case. The author of the Paracelsian treatise on *Gout* introduces the "Eight Mothers".[33]

He first says that there are "four philosophies" and "four astronomies". These are the mirror of all those things which make the physician experienced. Who would say that there is anything true outside these "Eight Mothers"? As little as a child may be born without father and mother, may a physician give birth to his experience (*scienz*) without "the Eight". He must essentially learn the relationship (Proportion) between the limbs of the body. Furthermore there is the fundamental knowledge which comes from the "Eight Mothers" (acht mutern aus welchen der Grund gehet). In addition the physician should also note what natural geometry teaches us and also chiromancy and physiognomy. For these are the books in which we should learn—the book of medicine is nature and as you see yourself in a mirror, in the same way you must see all your experience (*scientias*) in nature. And this is as certain and as little deceptive as if you were to have yourself personally in the mirror.

### The Eight Mothers as the Parts of Limbus and thereby of Man

The Paracelsian treatise discusses the idea of *Limbus*. First of all, we are told, we must know what *Limbus* is. For the latter is the dwelling place of

[31] Heinrich von Mügeln, *Der Meide Kranz*, herausgegeben von Willy Jahr, Inaugural-Dissertation, Leipzig, 1908, p. 110.

[32] Kroll, J., *Die Lehren des Hermes Trismegistos*, Münster, 1914, p. 266; also Lippmann, E. O. von, *Entstehung und Ausbreitung der Alchemie*, Berlin, 1919, p. 197; also Pagel, W., *Das medizinische Weltbild der Paracelsus*, Wiesbaden, 1962, p. 45. For Aristotle on *psychikon pyr* see, *De respiratione*, cap. 21, 478a, 16.

[33] Paracelsus, *Vom Limbo* in *Von den podagrischen Krankheiten und was in anhängig ist*, ed. Sudhoff, vol. I, p. 354 ff.

the "Eight Mothers" which have been mentioned. Man is nothing else but this *Limbus*. There are two *Limbi*, the lesser and the bigger one, and both of them are in Man. *Limbus* as such is the "seed" out of which all creatures grow and are brought forth in the same way as tree grows from seed—with the difference that what the earth is to the tree, the creating word of God is to the *Limbus*. The divine word brings the seeds of all things to their final fruition through what is between seed and end, namely a "middle" (a middle life or the life that is between the seed and its end as a middle—*Mittel*). The bigger *Limbus* is the seed from which *all* creatures have come, the minor *Limbus* is Man, the ultimate creature.

Occasionally this term is merely used synonymously with *Limus*, the earthy clay from which man was made. The essential meaning of *Limbus*, however, embraces far more than this. It is a cosmological concept. *Limbus* stands for prime matter out of which the whole world is being formed. Since in Man the whole outside world (external man) is epitomized, Man is *Limbus* and *Limbus* is Man. Hence the distinction between the Macrocosm as the *Major Limbus* and the Microcosm of man as a *Minor Limbus*.

However, *Limbus* is nothing material. It is rather the realm of spiritual principles (ideas) about to be translated into material objects. *Limbus* thus is, in the true sense of the word, something marginal. It is comparable to the hem of a garment at which creative principles become concrete.

Indeed Adam was created from a *Matrix* that was the whole world. The semen which begot him was the *Limbus* in which the whole world was contained.[34]

If, as in the treatise here discussed, the *Limbus* is identified with the "Eight Mothers", and, as we have seen, Adam is produced from this *Limbus*, a connection with the story of his composition of eight pieces is suggestive.

The "mothers" form a concept that frequently occurs in Paracelsus. As a rule they do not stand for a group of *Eight* (as in the present case), but for a group of *Four*. These are the Elements: Earth, Water, Air and Fire. They are, however, *not* normally used in the sense of the Elements of the Ancients. The Paracelsian "Mothers" are not elemental substances of which natural objects are composed, but they are the "wombs" from which all natural objects receive their origin and the "seal" of specific form and functions. Each object is thus envisaged as the specific fruit of one of the four "mothers".[35]

[34] Pagel, W., *Paracelsus*, 1958, *loc. cit.* (1), p. 228; *Weltbild*, 1962, *loc. cit.* (2), p. 64 with reference to *Opus Paramirum*, liber IV, *De Origine Morborum Matricis*, Sudhoff, vol. IX, p. 192.

[35] Pagel, W., 1958, *loc. cit.* (1), p. 129 ff.

On the face of it we seem to deal here with two traditions reflected in the two groups—that of the "Eight Mothers" in the treatise on *Gout* and that of the "Four Mothers" elsewhere in Paracelsus. In the treatise on *Gout* the "Eightness of the Mothers" is connected with another group of Eight—namely that of the "astronomies" and "philosophies" which the physician must study. The latter group of eight is not isolated however, as it occurs again in the *Erklärung der ganzen Astronomei*.[36]

## The Fertilization of the Four Female Elements by the Four Astral Semina according to Gerard Dorn and Quercetanus (Du Chesne)

In the *Physica Genesis* the Paracelsist Gerard Dorn derives the generation of all objects in nature from an Eightness. This consists of two groups of four: (*a*) the four elements and (*b*) the four astral semina. The former are represented as female, the latter as male. In order to generate objects each of the four astral semina must fertilize each of the four elemental matrices. Their coition takes place in a "middle region" and is made possible by a circulatory process which corresponds to the circulation that takes place in distillation. It is an ever-repeated process of ascending and descending. The force which causes the elements to ascend is the central fire of the earth. Through this the elements are made volatile. They thus ascend to a region which is marked as a centre of activity by the occurrence of celestial phenomena therein. Owing to their volatility, the elements are now enabled to receive the male semina of the astra. They then fall back and conceive each their own foetuses and produce all the generations of things which were ordained by the Highest Creator from the beginning. There are thus *four fathers* and *four mothers* of all objects that are specified in any way.

The generation of specified objects by eight parents should be distinguished from a primary universal process of generation which has only *one* father and *one* mother, namely sun and moon.[37]

The foregoing would appear to be Dorn's main pronouncement on the matter. We have reason to believe that Dorn was also the author of a Commentary to the *Seven Hermetic treatises*. These are probably of early mediaeval-Arabic origin and were first printed in 1566. They were reprinted

[36] See above, note (15). On the *Eight Virtues of Bliss and Charity* occurring in a Pseudo-Paracelsian tract see below, p. 135, and note (43).

[37] Dorneus, G., *Physica Genesis, Dies Tertius, Dixit Quoque Deus, Theatrum Chemicum*, Argentorati, Zetzner, 1613, p. 376. *Physica Trismegisti, ibid.*, p. 408.

with a commentary under the name of Dominicus Gnosicus Belga in 1610.[38] In this commentary the "Marriage of the Elements" is discussed. The author refers to the saying that there is no generation without corruption and that for this reason putrefaction should be studied. Through putrefaction a magnetic attraction of *Arcana* takes place and this is operative in all generation of natural objects. This artifice is like a Jacob's Ladder—for there is a continuous ascent and descent of elements in the great alembic of the world and conversion of one object into another. Hence things of the lower world are united with those of the upper world by the closest bond of marriage achieving perfection of the former through the latter. This marriage was called by Paracelsus, the great doyen of the philosophers, *Gamathea*.[39]

Taking up this concept Quercetanus (Du Chesne, 1544–1609) speaks of that *perpetua circulatio* through which the *semina of the elements* or their matter are copulated with the *semina of the astra*. They thereby produce and perfect their foetuses.[39a]

Perhaps it is in this matrimony—the *hieros gamos*—of the lower elements with the *astra* on High that we should search for the intended deeper–cosmological–meaning of the "Eightness of Adam". The union of elements and astra provides the magisterial pattern for the concept of man as microcosm, as the epitome of the world and all its possible parts and creatures. This at

[38] *First* printed in *Ars Chemica*, Strassburg, 1566, pp. 7–31, under the title *Septem Tractatus seu Capitula Trismegisti Aurei* (in later editions changed to *Tractatus Aureus de Lapidis Physici Secreto in Septem Capitula Divisus*). On its probable origin see Ruska, J., *Tabula Smaragdina*, Heidelberg, 1926, notably pp. 193–203.

An edition of the *reprint*, Lipsiae, 1600, as quoted by Schmieder, K. C., *Geschichte der Alchemie*, Halle, 1832, p. 28, is doubtful. It was reprinted with Commentary both in the *Theatrum Chemicum*, *loc. cit.*, 1613, vol. IV, p. 672, and in Manget, *Bibliotheca Chemica*, 1702, vol. I, pp. 400–45.

On the identity of the author of the commentary with Dorneus see Pagel, W., Paracelsus, "Traditionalism and Mediaeval sources", in *Temkin-Festschrift*, 1968, *loc. cit.* (2), pp. 58–9.

[39] Commentary by Gnosicus Belga to *Hermetis Trismegisti Tract.*, cap. 2, in Manget, 1702, *loc. cit.* (38), vol. I, p. 425.

[39a] Quercetanus, Jos., *Ad veritatem Hermeticae Medicinae*, Paris, 1604, cap. XIV, p. 177. For the significance of the concept in the development of chemistry in the seventeenth century see: Kangro, H., *Joachim Jungius. Experimente und Gedanken zur Begründung der Chemie als Wissenschaft*, Wiesbaden, F. Steiner, 1968, pp. 178 and 189. Kangro refers in this context to J. Thölde, *Haliographia*, Eisleben, 1603, cap. 3 (prime matter of salt is celestial influence and astral impression) and to J. H. Alsted, *Physica Harmonica*, Herborn, 1616, p. 237 (the three principles as receptors of celestial influxes). On the Paracelsian background of all these concepts see Pagel, "The Prime Matter of Paracelsus", *Ambix*, 1961, *loc. cit.* (2). To Jungius and Chemistry (à propos Kangro) see Pagel, W., "Chemistry at the Cross-Roads and the Ideas of Joachim Jungius", *Ambix*, 1969, **xvi**, 100–8.

any rate corresponds to the Paracelsian idea of man and it is not surprising that it finds clearest expression in such Paracelsists as Dorneus and Quercetanus. In the last resort, however, it looks like a paraphrase of an old Gnostic myth—that of the "Eightness of Adam".

## V. Synopsis and Comment

Looking back we have examined the Eightness of Adam. First the report in a fifteenth-century symbolist-alchemical manuscript—*The Book of the Holy Trinity*—and its suggestive Gnostic background. We have then pointed out the close parallels that offer themselves between the account in the manuscript and certain passages in the Paracelsian Corpus—namely the Treatise *De Secretis Creationis*.

From all this it would appear that Eightness as a figure in a symbolic and alchemical context was *not* an invention of Paracelsus or Paracelsian writers.[40]

Eightness in Paracelsus may also be connected with the Eightness of the *Kabiri*. In this, their relationship to *Hephaistos*, their profession as blacksmiths and their role in the creation of the world call for our special attention.[41] We shall return to this presently.

To these two items of Eightness—the "Eightness of Adam" and that of the "Astrologies"—in the Paracelsian Corpus a third item should be added: this is the story of the "Eight Mothers". These again have a role to play in the creation of the cosmos and of man. Their cosmogonic and creative role stems from their connection with the Paracelsian concept of the *Limbus*.[42]

There are several points which should now be discussed in context. The parallel between the passages in *The Book of the Holy Trinity* and the Paracelsian treatise *De Secretis Creationis* not only consists in the Eightness of Adam. Even more striking is the association in both with the concept of "middle nature" and its creative function. The latter is, in its turn, related to the idea of the "dark fire".

All three of these concepts—the eight pieces of Adam, middle nature and dark fire—have their background in Gnostic speculation. Such notably includes the *Ogdoas* as a possible pattern of the Adam story, the *Middle Life* of Sophia, the active creative principle, and the *Dark Fire*. The latter concept can be traced back to Stoic and Aristotelian sources.

[40] As against Jung, C. G., *loc. cit.* (11), 1944, pp. 227–8, with reference to Paracelsus on the "Eightness of the Astrologies".

[41] See above, footnotes (21)–(23). See below, p. 136 and notes (49)–(54).

[42] See above, footnotes (33)–(35).

Gnostic Speculation in the "Authentic" and "Spurious" Paracelsus

Most of the Paracelsian *loci* discussed in the present paper are found in treatises that are not regarded as genuinely Paracelsian. This is not surprising as the same holds good for other Gnostic concepts which we have examined elsewhere. It would appear that the main spokesmen for Pseudo–Paracelsian–Gnostic–speculation derive from the circles of such Paracelists as Gerard Dorn (flor. ab. 1567–?1610), Valentin Weigel (1533–88)[43] and Jacob Böhme (1575–1624).[44]

The pessimistic–Gnostic–view of the world as "excremental" strikes a key-note in Weigel's treatise *Vom Ort der Welt*. Here all bodily things are said to be an "excrement or coagulated smoke from the invisible *astra*". This smoke incorporates three substances, the sulphur, the salt and the mercury; thus a tree is a coagulated smoke consisting of these three substances. Likewise man, *qua* body, is nothing but such a coagulated smoke, an excrement of its inner *sidereal body* or *astrum*. Weigel continues in genuine Paracelsian as well as Gnostic terms that devil and hell are bound up with the elemental world and that no greater pain and punishment could be inflicted on Lucifer than his banishment into this excremental world. Indeed there is no other "hell" than this. In one of the tracts published under the joint names of

[43] Of genuine Weigel treatises we refer in particular to *Vom Ort der Welt* in Valentin Weigel, *Sämtliche Schriften*, ed. W. E. Peuckert and W. Zeller, I, Stuttgart, 1962, cap. 13 on p. 46 sq. for the "excremental" nature of the world and cap. 15 on p. 53 seq. for the elemental world as the seat of Lucifer and Hell. The Paracelsian source for the latter idea has been examined by Pagel in the papers quoted in note (2) and in *Weltbild*, 1962 *loc. cit.* (2), p. 89.

For the "Eight Virtues" see Paracelsus and Weigel, *Philosophia mystica . . . Eilff unterschidene . . . teutsche tractätlein*, Newstadt, 1618, pp. 41–2 in *Theologia Cabalistica de Perfecto Homine*. On this tract and its attribution to Paracelsus, possibly by Huldrich Bachsmeier von Regenbrun who may also be its author see Peuckert, W. E., *Pansophie. Ein Versuch zur Geschichte der weissen und schwarzen Magie*, 2nd ed., Berlin, 1956, pp. 348–52.

From the same collection, *Philos. Mystica*, 1618, we mention: *Kurtze Anleitung zu einem christlichen und gottseligen Leben*, attributed to Weigel. On p. 240 we find *mittel natur* connected with the middle position of the soul between the Divine Spirit and the body of man.

For a source in mediaeval German mysticism Johannes Tauler may be quoted: daran ist die sel edel dz an sy stosset beide zeit und ewigkeit (*Des heiligen lerers Predig fast fruchtbar zu eim recht christlichen Leben*, Basel, Adam Petri, 1521 (3rd ed.), fol. 311 verso). Die sel ist recht ein *mittel* zwischen zeit und ewigkeyt (*ibid.* fol. 18 recto).

[44] On Böhme see, Baur, C. F., *Die Christliche Gnosis*, Tübingen, 1835, pp. 557–611.

Paracelsus and Weigel we find the "Eight Virtues of Bliss and Charity" mentioned in line with the "Four true and main Kabbalistic points" and the "Three Kabbalistic Prima.[43] It is no accident that the treatise of the Paracelsian Corpus in which the Eightness of Adam occurs, namely *De secretis creationis*, and its literary history, are closely connected with the Weigel-circle and notably his pupil Biedermann, as the work of Fritz Lieb has shown.[45]

Inevitably we would ask how far points here discussed are reflected in the "genuine" Paracelsus after all. Three such points offer themselves:
(*a*) the "Mittel-corpus" (middle body). This occurs in the *Opus Paramirum*.[46] Here the outer world is called "Outer Man" (*der eussere Mensch*). Hence, whatever man receives in air, food or medicine, is part of himself. Taking from "Outer Man" he replaces what is deficient in him. In so doing the body of man is called middle body—*Mittel-corpus*.

What is the meaning of *Mittel-corpus*?

First of all, in the passage of the *Opus Paramirum* just quoted the Mittel-corpus of man, receiving material from the outer world, may stand for activity as such. If this were the real meaning, a *locus* in the *Philosophia Sagax* could be adduced.[47] Here Paracelsus speaks of the middle (medium) between prime and ultimate matter. Neither of these is active. Activity and motion (*commotio*), however, are exerted by the middle between them, that is the functioning natural object that has passed the stage of prime matter and not yet reached its end in ultimate matter. It is true that in this passage the astral forces that direct man as well as earth and plant represent the middle. At all events, however, we here again meet with the association of activity with a middle—namely the "middle region" in which the stars dwell. As we have seen (p. 128 and notes 29 *et seq.*) this forms a stock item in Gnostic sources.

A further possible interpretation of man as the *Mittel-Corpus* would refer to the connexion of the Divine Spirit above with the world below through man. In this, Paracelsus sees the nature of man as microcosm—for in him the body, a product of the macrocosm around him, is united with soul (inner man) which is an invisible divine fire. Expressing it in Hermetic terms, Paracelsus speaks of the sulphur or soul as the medium which joins the two contrary things,

[45] Lieb, F., *Valentin Weigels Kommentar zur Schöpfungsgeschichte und das Schrifttum seines Schülers Benedict Biedermann*, Zürich, 1962.

[46] *Opus Paramirum*, lib. I, cap. 3, ed. Sudhoff, vol. IX, p. 53; lib. I, cap. 5–6, *ibid.*, pp. 65–67; lib. II, cap. 3, *ibid.*, p. 97.

[47] *Philosophia sagax*, lib. 1, cap. 11, ed. Sudhoff, vol. XII, p. 257.

namely Divine Spirit and material (macrocosmic) body, and changes them into one being.[48]

(*b*) There are two further *loci* from the genuine Paracelsus which may be regarded as reflecting the Gnostic traditions here discussed.

Paracelsus compares the planets to blacksmiths. It is a product of the planets in us, namely our *astral body* that teaches us "natural widsom". This makes all reasoning and artisan work possible. Moreover, it is in the planets that astral blacksmiths have made their home, and it is from them that all human blacksmiths have learnt. These "planetary blacksmiths" are the masters (*besten schmid*) for in them the art is ingrained and ever-present.[49]

The association of planet and blacksmith stands in one line with the commonplace attribution of metals to planets in alchemical and occult literature in general. In the context of the present paper we are reminded of the *Kabiri*. These were identified with the seven planets and also designated as *Hephaistuses*, i.e. as blacksmiths (p. 126 and note 23). In this connexion Libavius speaks of "Philosophi et Astrologi, qui ex stellis et coeli Vulcanis petunt animas essentiasque rerum"—philosophers and astrologers who try to derive from the stars and the blacksmiths of heaven the souls and essences of things. He was scornful of the idea when he said: Vulcanos aliaque Paracelsica deliramenta.[50]

Finally, Paracelsus speaks of the ineptitude of the Vulcani, "heavenly apprentices and immature master-craftsmen". Their inept "carving and hammering" (*schnizen und schmieden*) accounts for the making of fools—as we

[48] Paracelsus, *De Natura Rerum*, Book I, ed. Sudhoff, vol. XI, p. 319. To this see Pagel, W., *Hist. Essays in Honor of O. Temkin*, 1968, *loc. cit.* (2), p. 61.

Concerning the designation of the soul as "Inner Man" or "Divine Fire" we can again refer to Tauler: der inner mensch und der eusser mensch die habent als verr underscheid als hymel und erd. Gott der hat vil tausent mal meilen darob (*loc. cit.*, 1521 in note (43), fol. 301 verso).

In *Gnostic* parlance "Inner Man" (*eso anthropos*) stands for "Pneumatic Man" (*pneumatikos*)—the highest stage of immediacy to Divinity which man can reach (houtos oun ho sarkinos Adam kata ten phainomenen periplasin Thoyth kaleitai. Ho de eso autou anthropos ho pneumatikos, kai kyroma echeion kai prosegorikon)—Zosimus, III, 49, Peri Organon kai Kaminon, 6, Berthelot, M., *Collection des Anciens Alchimistes Grecs*, Paris, 1887, vol. III, p. 231 (Greek text; transl. vol. II, p. 224).

[49] Paracelsus, *Philosophia Sagax*, Lib. I, cap. 7, ed. Sudhoff, XII, 168.

[50] Libavius, Andreas, *De Universitate et Originibus Rerum Conditarum*. Francofurti, 1610, pp. 8, 73.

are told in the treatise on *The Begetting of Fools*.[51] This is regarded as genuine Paracelsian.

The idea is more clearly expressed in the *Philosophia ad Athenienses*. Doubts have been cast on the authenticity of the latter treatise. However, it is generally recognized to present genuine Paracelsian doctrine. Here the making of mankind in general is attributed to the work not of the perfect masters (*meistern volkommen gut*), but to inferior–perishable–gods (*zergenglichen göttern*).[52]

With this we are again reminded of a Gnostic tradition. According to Barbelo-Gnosticism, Sophia was productive of a work in which ignorance and arrogance were associated with each other in the person of the *Pro-archon*, the maker of this creation.[53]

In a similar tradition, arrogance as well as incompetence in the work of the *Archontes* become instrumental in Sophia's struggle towards regaining the power which she had transmitted to her first son, the first *Archon*, in a state of self-deception.[54]

## In Conclusion

The complex of concepts from the Paracelsian Corpus here discussed has its correlate and predecessor in Gnostic sources. It has kept its identity through the Middle Ages and is recognizable in manuscripts up to the time shortly before Paracelsus—the last port of call being the *Buch der Heiligen Dreifaltigkeit* of the fifteenth century.

Concerning their position in the Corpus the individual concepts fall into two groups:

1. Those which only occur in Paracelsian treatises of *doubtful* authenticity.

[51] Paracelsus, *De Generatione Stultorum*, lib. I, Tractatus I, ed. Sudhoff, vol. XIV, pp. 79–80. Translation by Cranefield, P. F. and Federn, W., "The Begetting of Fools: An Annotated Translation of Paracelsus *De Generatione Stultorum*", *Bull. Hist. Med.*, 1967, **41**, 56–74; 161–74; esp. 63–4.

[52] Paracelsus, *Philosophia ad Athenienses*, lib. II, cap. 1, ed. Sudhoff, vol. XIII, pp. 403–4.

[53] Irenaeus, *Opus Eruditissimum*, ed. Desiderius Erasmus Roterodamus, Parisiis, 1563, lib. I, cap. 33, f. 57r: post deinde simplicitate et benignitate acta generavit opus, in quo erit ignorantia et audacia. Hoc autem opus eius esse proarchonten dicunt fabricatorem conditionis huius: virtutem autem magnam abstulisse eum a matre narrant, et abstulisse ab ea in inferiora, et fecisse firmamentum coeli in quo et habitare dicunt eum. Et cum sit ignorantia, fecisse eas quae sunt sub eo potestates, et angelos, et firmamenta et terrena omnia. To this see Jonas, 1964, *loc. cit.* (6), vol. I, p. 361, note 6.

[54] Jonas, *loc. cit.*, 1964, p. 396.

2. Concepts occurring in *genuine* Paracelsian treatises as well as treatises of *doubtful* authenticity.

Concepts belonging to group (1) include:

(*a*) the Eightness of Adam (*De Secretis Creationis*),

(*b*) the Eight Astronomies and Philosophies (*Erklerung der gantzen Astronomei*),

(*c*) the Eight Mothers (*De Podagricis, Vom Limbo*).

Concepts belonging to group (2) are:

(*a*) the planets as blacksmiths (*Philosophia Sagax*),

(*b*) the ineptitude of the lower creators such as Vulcani and Demiurges (*De Generatione Stultorum*).

(*c*) The middle body (*Opus Paramirum*).

The *loci* here adduced may well not exhaust the story, and to continue the search for further "Eightnesses" in genuine treatises may be rewarding. For the time being our concepts appear to be somewhat diluted in genuine treatises and more prevalent in doubtful treatises, notably those of the Weigel and Dorneus circles.

## Epilogue

A final question: does the "Eightness of Adam" convey a deeper meaning that lends itself to expression in *alchemical* terms? The answer may well be found in the alchemical symbol of *Rebis*. The latter represents *androgyny* and at the same time harmony and perfection as achieved in the completed alchemical Opus. In the same way *Adam* is created *androgynous* and at the same time embodies all the components of the universe. This is symbolically indicated by the figure: *Eight*. Adam is often represented as the product of the four–earthly–elements. That he really consists of *eight* parts, i.e. twice the number of the elements, should imply the highest possible state of completeness and perfection (*pleroumenon*). He embodies not only the four–female–elements, but also the four–male–astral *semina*. It is by way of this androgyny that he ceases to be a mere clot of earth and becomes a true *microcosm*. The figure *Eight* may also stand for initial harmony between male and female, as shown in androgynous–Adam, both archetypal First Man (*Adam Kadmon*) and the first of mankind existing here and now. This male-female harmony is disrupted at a later stage when creation imposes limitation and finiteness on the Deity and the events in Paradise parallel this diminution in status. Androgynous *Rebis* as well as androgynous *Adam* represent the *Stone*—the highest achievement of alchemical creation. In it may be seen the work of the Eight Elemental Gods—four male and four female—who appear in steles of Ptolemaic Egypt, and it may well be the product of very early Graceo-Egyptian religious syncretism.[55]

The subject of the present paper is how Adam was *made* of eight pieces. We would conclude finally with an example which shows how he was *unmade* in eight stages. In Tibetan art the cosmos image known as *Mandala* often displays a marginal wreath which depicts eight burial grounds. These are the places in which body and soul of man disintegrate gradually. In other words, here is Adam divesting himself of the eight parts of which he consists.[56]

*Note added in proof:*
In Dorneus and Du Chesne, the "marriage" of the elements with astral forces, discussed on pp. 131-2, has a genuine Paracelsian source in the *Labyrinthus Medicorum*, cap. XI (ed. Sudhoff, vol. XI, p. 213). However, this does not mention "eightness".

[55] Lepsius, R., *Über die Götter der vier Elemente bei den Ägyptern*, Berlin, 1856 (*Abhandlgn. d. Königl. Akad. d. Wissenschaften*, 1856, pp. 181–234).

[56] Griswold, A. B., Kim, C. and Pott, P., *Burma, Korea, Tibet*, London, 1964, p. 175.

# IX

## THE HIGHER ELEMENTS AND PRIME MATTER IN RENAISSANCE NATURALISM AND IN PARACELSUS

*In collaboration with Marianne Winder*



### I. Introduction. The Upper and Lower Elements and their "Marriage"

In a previous communication[1] the present authors dealt with the conjunction of the upper and lower elements and its role in the Paracelsian *Corpus*. For this a genuine Paracelsian *locus* is extant. It is found in the *Labyrinthus Medicorum*, a late work and part of the so-called *Carinthian trilogy*. Here it says, "Also die elementen frauen von iren mannen entpfahen als von dem obern vulkanischen. . . ."[2] (Thus the element-wives conceive from their men, that is the Vulcans on High.) In this passage the use of the Vulcans is also of interest in view of their Gnostic affiliation and their connection with *Eightness*.[3] In fact, Paracelsians such as notably Dorneus have enlarged on the eightness of partners in this conjunction.[4] These are four male and four female—the four male being the higher or celestial, and the four female components the terrestrial elements. We shall return to Paracelsus and the Paracelsian *Corpus* below.

[1] Walter Pagel and Marianne Winder, "The Eightness of Adam and Related 'Gnostic' Ideas in the Paracelsian Corpus", *Ambix*, **16**, 119–39, 1969.

[2] *Labyrinthus Medicorum*, cap. 11, in Paracelsus, *Sämtliche Werke*, ed. K. Sudhoff, vol. XI, München-Berlin, 1928, 213.

[3] Pagel–Winder (1), "Hephaistuses", 125 and "Vulcans", 136–7.

[4] Pagel–Winder (1), 131.

## Pre-Renaissance Examples of the Conjunction of Celestial (Male) and Terrestrial (Female) Elements

*Elemental Conjunction* is one of the key concepts of Renaissance Natural Philosophy. It will be discussed as such, as well as its emergence in the Paracelsian Corpus. First, however, some ancient sources should be mentioned.

According to Irenaeus,[5] Anaxagoras attributed the generation of animals to *semina* that have fallen from heaven to earth. Irenaeus continues that the Gnostics ascribed these *semina* to the heavenly Mother of the earth. It is this Mother who produces the four earthly elements after the image of an invisible group of four higher elements (*superioris quaternionis, superni quaternarii*). All this calls for collation with the *pneumatikos gamos* in Hellenistic alchemy, notably in Olympiodorus.[6]

In further Gnostic sources, namely the *Gospel of the Egyptians* and the *Gospel according to St. Thomas*, the confluence of the upper and the lower is emphasized. In these it is said that right should be like left, left like right, upper like lower, back like front, and that sex differences should be blotted out: "Only when you make the two one, and in such a way that you make the man and the woman a single One in order that the man is not the man and the woman is not the woman, then you will go into the Kingdom". In alchemical terms this would stand for the perfection of the Work, the *Rebis* which is depicted as hermaphrodite.[7]

[5] *Anaxagoras dogmatisavit facta animalia decidentibus a coelo in terram seminibus* (Irenaeus: *Opus eruditissimum*, Lib. II, cap. 19, ed. Erasmus, Paris, 1563, fol. 94*r*; ed. Grynaeus, Basle, Eusebius Episcopius and Nicolai's brother's heirs, 1571, 156). On semina and Heavenly Mother *ibid.*, Lib. I, cap. 14, ed. Erasmus, fol. 38*v*, ed. Grynaeus, 67. The above Irenaeus passage on Anaxagoras is quoted in Diels-Kranz, *Fragmente der Vorsokratiker*, fragm. 113, 11th edition, Berlin, Weidmann, 1964, vol. II, 31. For Anaxagoras' view see E. Zeller, *Die Philosophie der Griechen*, 4th edition, Leipzig, 1876, vol. I, 907 and n. 1: "Auf dieselbe Art sind ursprünglich auch die Thiere entstanden, indem die schlammige Erde von den im Aether enthaltenen Keimen befruchtet wurde" (Animals developed by earthly mud fertilized by semina contained in the ether.) The implied idea —of form-male and matter-female—can be traced back at least to Aristotle, *Physics*, lib. I, ch. 9; 192a, 20. See J. Ritter, *Historisches Wörterbuch der Philosophie*, vol. 2, Basel-Stuttgart, 1972, col. 982.

[6] M. Berthelot, *Collection des anciens alchemistes grecs*, Paris, 1888, II, *Olympiodore*, 51; *Texte grec*, 102, *Traduction*, 111: "Le but propre de tout l'art, dit Horus, c'est avoir pris secrètement la semence du mâle; tandis que toutes choses sont mâles et femelles. Comme le dit quelque part Marie: Unissez le mâle et la femelle et vous trouverez ce qui est cherché. En effet, sans le procédé de cette reunion, rien ne peut réussir, car la nature charme la nature . . .".

[7] R. M. Grant and D. N. Freedman, *The secret sayings of Jesus*, London, Fontana Books, 1960, 136, Saying 23. On hermaphrodite *Rebis* see W. Pagel, *Das medizinische Weltbild des Paracelsus*, Wiesbaden, 1962, 68.

## Renaissance Sources

### (*a*) Leo Hebraeus

First we refer to Leo Hebraeus (Jehudah Abarbanel, born 1437 in Lisbon, died 1509).[8] The heaven, he says, pours out its most fertile semen into the earth in the same way as male into female. . . . The heavenly body as a whole like a male "embraces" the earth on all sides. The latter, which enjoys rest and stability, is but little moved as a whole, even though agitated and roused by the strong movement of its male partner. Hence not it but its humours, its spirit and natural heat, that is, water, air and fire, are agitated by the virile movement of the celestial body. The earth is like the woman. Through the tempestuousness of intercourse its aforementioned elements are set into motion by the motion of the male. Absence of active movement of her body enables it to receive better and more easily the fertile semen, namely dew and rain. By virtue of the rays of sun, moon, planets and fixed stars all species and all individual bodies composed of elements are begotten and produced in the earth and in the sea. The whole of the heaven through its movement is continuously productive of semen just as the whole of the human body contributes to the formation of semen. Our body consists of six homogeneous tissues (*membra*), namely bones, nerves, veins, membranes, cartilage and flesh that fills the intermediate spaces. In the same way the vast mass of the eighth circle is composed of fixed stars, each with six components. By contrast, the seven planets correspond to the seven heterogeneous organs which in particular co-operate in generating semen. Thus the sun is the heart of heaven, the moon its brain, Jupiter its liver, Saturn its spleen, Mars its bile and kidneys, Venus its testicles and Mercury its penis. In this way things below acquire perfection because of the desire of things above to *love* them and to consummate this love by copulation. This union or conjunction expresses *divine* or *intellectual love*.

It is of some interest, also in connection with Paracelsus,[9] that Leo Hebraeus speaks of the *Chaos* as the spouse of God (*uxor dei*). As the term "matter" is derived from "mother" (*mater*), in Platonic parlance *Chaos* represents the *Spouse* (*Socius*) of the highest God from whom it has sprung in past eternity. From the same *Chaos* the God then produced all the other things in a temporal past.[9a]

[8] S. Munk, *Mélanges de philosophie juive et arabe*, 1857: Notice sur Léon Hébreu, 522–8.

[9] See Pagel, *Weltbild* (7), 64: "Gott ist selbander geworden" from *Liber de Sancta Trinitate* in K. Sudhoff, *Paracelsus Handschriften*, Berlin 1899, 347 seq., No. 88, fol. 264b–76b; *Philosophia sagax*, I, 2, ed. Sudhoff, XII, 49; *Opus paramirum*, IV, ed. Sudhoff, IX, 191–2.

[9a] Leo Hebraeus, *De amore dialogi tres*, Jo. Carolo Saraceno Latinitati donati, Venetiis, 1564, fol. 73v, 74v, 78r, 102v.

(*b*) Adam von Bodenstein

The Paracelsist Adam von Bodenstein[10] says that Man is made through four causes or parents. These are two bodies, *i.e.*, "mothers", namely a material and a celestial body, and two lives or forms, *i.e.*, "fathers", namely a material and a celestial form.[11] All four beget a single son in whom there is "male" life and "female" body. Hence there is need for two categories of medicine, one, ("physic") that preserves and prolongs life, and the other that restores what is lost.

(*c*) Postelius

Guillaume Postel (1505–81) in his work on *Etruria*[12]—to him the oldest inhabited part of Europe—presents a male–female relationship in Heaven itself. This is between the World Soul (*intellectus mundi*) which is utterly male on the one hand, and the stars which are utterly female on the other, the former moving from sunrise to sunset, and the other in the opposite direction.

(*d*) Trithemius

A similar casual allusion is found in a treatise by Johannes Trithemius.[13] Here the author speaks of the four mothers and the four fathers. The former belong to the world of elements and the latter initiate all conjunction. Conjunction represents the *eightness*—two parent quaternaries—through which all things are miraculously unified. In the treatise this unification is linked with

[10] *Medicorum ac philosophorum facile principis Theophrasti Paracelsi eremitae libri V de vita longa . . . una cum commendatoria Valentii de Retiis et Adami a Bodenstein dedicatoria epistola*, Basle, Perna, 1562, c5v: Homo quatuor causis sive parentibus fit: nam duo corpora veluti matres diversae, hoc est naturale et coeleste concurrunt et duae vitae, hoc est, formae quasi patres, naturalis et coelestis una gignunt filium unicum.

[11] See *parentes elementati* below on p. 120 and n. (136).

[12] Guilielmus Postelius, *De Etruriae regionis quae prima in orbe Europae habitatae*, Florentiae, 1551, 112: Prima absolutaque religionis veritas. . . . Hic enim est primus masculeus intellectus mundi . . . pars enim ea tota masculina est et uniformis quae ab ortu in occasum rapitur. Tota est foeminea et mutabilis quae ab occasu in ortum fertur ut sunt stellae fixae et planetae.

[13] Johannes Trithemius, *Von den dreyen Anfängen aller natürlichen Künst der Philosophiae*, in Joh. Schaubert, *Consummata sapientia de lapide minerali Johannis de Padua*, 1681: Es seynd vier Mütter, derer welche in dem Anfang,* dieser aller Knüpfung ist, und das erste in die Zusammenknüpfung, und das lezte einfältig, rein, einig, allein färbend oder tingirend. Die einfältige Erden ist ein rein Element . . . (p. 231) . . . in der Ewigkeit bleibt es Eins, und das dann umbgreiff, macht es den dreyfaltigen Zahl, welchen achtmal umbgreiffend, bringet es alle Ding mit einer wunderbarlichen Natur wiederumb zu Einem (p: 233). To this: K. Arnold, *Johannes Trithemius (1462–1516)*, Würzburg, Schöningh, 1971 (Quellen und Forschungen zum Bistum und Hochstift Würzburg, Band XXIII), 260, under list of letters. The letter of 10 May 1503 to Johannes von Leininger-Westerburg with references to manuscripts and prints prior to Schaubert.

* *Read*: ..., derer welche in der letzten Ordnung und es seynd vier Väter, derer welche ....

the oneness of all contraries—the *Rebis*—which the searcher for the philosopher's stone should finally achieve.

### (*e*) PSEUDO-DREBBEL

In alchemical writings of a later period, even after the first and second generation of Paracelsians, *i.e.*, after Van Helmont (1579–1644), the concept of the conjunction of Heaven and Earth is common. As an example we mention the *Physical Questions* appended to a late German translation of Drebbel's work on the elements.[14] This appendix gives the appearance of being by, or contemporary with, Drebbel (1572–1633). It is easy to show, however, that it was written after 1648, the year in which Van Helmont's works appeared; for the latter, as well as a work by Mynsicht who died in 1632, are cited. The concept is well expressed and may be briefly summarized: heaven is the masculine or agent, earth the feminine; man is light, woman is water. Light and air are *agentia*, water and earth *patientia*. For light works in water, and air in the earth, no other than man and wife. The agent is productive of the *form* of a thing or its *sulphur* or *male semen*. The passive lends *matter* such as the blood of the woman to the embryo.

The author further develops the idea of what he calls *counter-elements*. These are three, namely: darkness corresponding to body, fire to soul, and corruption to the spiritual. Before the Fall corruption was simply the change of created things without any depreciation, consuming fire was light, and darkness the opportunity for quiet and recreation. Now, however, darkness became the habitat of evil spirits, fire the devil's element for doing evil, and hell was born from darkness. Hell has its bodily place on earth, its psychical realm in the firmament, and its spiritual sphere in the devil himself and in his children.

So much then, for sources concerning the conjunction of the upper male and the lower female elements from Renaissance literature and the background to the Paracelsian *Corpus*. By lower elements are understood the classical four—fire, water, earth and air. But what are the four higher elements?

## II. THE HIGHER—CELESTIAL—ELEMENTS, THEIR NATURE AND VIRTUES

### GEORGIUS VENETUS (ZORZI)

Perhaps the best answer to this question was provided by Georgius Venetus (Zorzi). Born at Venice in 1460, he belongs to the generation between Ficinus

[14] Drebbeli, Cornelii *Gründliche Aufflösung von der Natur und Eigenschafft der Elementen mit . . . Anhang . . .*, Frankfurt am Main, 1715, in: Anhang physicalischer Fragen, Questio 61, 98ff. (esp. 101). See John Ferguson, *Bibliotheca chemica*, Glasgow, 1906, repr. London, 1954, vol. I, 223. Regarded as genuine Drebbel, by W.-E. Peuckert, *Pansophie*, 2nd ed., Berlin, E. Schmidt, 1956, 494–5.

and Paracelsus. Early in life he joined the Franciscan order. His works[15] were put on the Roman Index because of Platonic, Talmudic and Kabbalistic doctrines proclaimed in them and sentences from other such authors quoted. His more serious "errors" were also pointed out by Sixtus Senensis (1520–69), Cardinal Bellarmin, Antonius Possevinus (1533–1611) and Marinus Mersennus at the end of his commentaries to the Book of Genesis.[16] Nevertheless Zorzi had dedicated his *Books of Problemata Concerning Passages in the Scriptures* to Pope Paul III,[17] although they, too, had been richly interlarded with Platonic and Talmudic lore.

Zorzi was said to have died in 1510. On the other hand, an encounter with the nun Clara Bugnia in 1514 has been reported;[18] moreover, he dedicated the *Harmonia* to Pope Clement VII (1523–34) and, as mentioned above, the *Problemata* to Pope Paul III (1534–49).[19] Thus it is likely that Zorzi died about 1540. Naturally one of his main sources was Ficinus (1433–99).

We find in Zorzi eight elements, *i.e.*, four lower and four upper elements. What, then, are Zorzi's *upper elements*?

They are the same elements as ours but nobler in structure and with different qualities. He first set out[20] what earlier writers have thought about matter in heaven. Albertus Magnus said there was matter in heaven—matter that is different from that of changeable things. By contrast, Averroes and the other Peripatetics had denied that there was any kind of matter in heaven. Some, he says, to a certain extent rightly called the heavenly matter *quinta essentia*.

Each of the four lower elements belongs to three signs of the zodiac[21] which he seems to locate in the eighth sphere. This correspondence of the elements with parts of the zodiac is a general tenet of ancient and mediaeval astrology:[22] Aries, Leo and Sagittarius are the three fiery signs; Taurus, Virgo

[15] Zorzi's main work was: *De harmonia totius mundi cantica tria*, Venetiis apud Bernardinum Vitalem, 1525, the edition here used throughout; also Parisiis apud Andream Barthelim, 1544 et 1546. His other works are of no interest in the context of the present paper.

[16] Lucas Waddingus, *Scriptores Ordinis Minorum*, Romae, ex typographia Francisci Alberti Tani, 1650, 119 (in British Museum copy misprinted as p. 109).

[17] Henricus Willot, *Athenae Orthodoxorum sodalitii Franciscani*, Leodii, excudebat Arnoldus a Courswaremia, 1598, 127.

[18] *Ibid.*

[19] See note 16 and 99.

[20] *De Harmonia, Cantici III*, Tonus 8, Concentus 5, Canticum III, fol. 89*v* part II.

[21] Signa octavae sphaerae partiuntur per quattuor elementa unicuique assignantes tria signa fol. 90*r*.

[22] Cf. Antiochus of Athens (according to W. and H. G. Gundel, *Astrologoumena*, 1970, 115, n. 40, now thought to have lived in first century B.C.), as quoted by Rhetorios in *Catalogus Codicum Astrologorum Graecorum*, Brussels, 1899, vol. I, 146: 3. Peri tes ton XII zodion kraseos.

and Capricorn the three earthy signs; Gemini, Libra and Aquarius the three airy signs; and Cancer, Scorpio and Pisces the three watery signs.[23]

### HEAVEN FROM FIRE AND WATER

Zorzi continues: "If we are to explain the nature of the upper elements we may follow the Hebrew sages and regard heavenly matter as *fire and water*; not however corruptible and changeable water and fire, but matter of a higher order (*notae*)". This follows from the Hebrew designation of heaven—*hashamayim*, as derived from *mayim* (water) and *esh* (fire). This etymology belongs to the stock of Rabbinical lore up to the era of the *Kabbala Denudata*[24] and even Welling.[25]

It likewise occurs in ancient alchemical sources where a mixture of sulphur or sulphur-arsenic or another sulphuric combination with mercury in the still is compared to a mixture of fire and water. Fire in ancient parlance is sulphur (or sulphur-arsenic) and water represents the female principle of the mixture, identical with the "moist" (*i.e.*, fusible) metal (*selene*, moon).[26]

Fire and water, however, are not the only elements from which heaven is composed but there are also air and earth. Zorzi says:[27] "Astronomers say not without reason that some heavens are fiery, some airy, some earthy and some watery". The reason for this is that fire and water are not sufficient for maintaining stability. In order to sustain the upper waters, there is need in heaven for earthy matter, also for air to make breathing possible.

### HEAVEN IN MAN

In addition, Zorzi says:[28] *Omnes coeli in homine continentur.*[29] For man

[23] Cf. K. Sudhoff, "Daniels von Morley 'Liber de Naturis Inferiorum et Superiorum' ", *Arch. Gesch. Naturwiss.*, 8, 37–8, 1918.

[24] ed. Knorr von Rosenroth, Sulzbach, Lichtenthaler, 1677, vol. I, 720: "*Shamayim*, Coelum, vocatur Tiphereth, quia complectitur *esh mayim*, Ignem et Aquam, et ista conciliat atque perficit: ob quem concursum plurium, etiam plurali numero denominationem habet".

[25] Georg von Welling, *Opus magico-cabbalisticum*, Frankfurt–Leipzig, A. Heinscheidt, 1719, 2: "Hier (Genesis I, 1) setzet Moses die Himmel, die geistlichen feurigen Wasser, zuerst. . . . Der Heilige Geist durch Mosen nennet uns dieses expansum Schamajim, welches ein Nomen compositum ist, und von allen Rabbinen, so da in vera Cabbala geübet und erfahren gewesen, beschrieben worden, dass es zusammengesetzt sey von *Aesch* und *Majim*, Feuer und Wasser".

[26] I. Hammer-Jensen, *Die älteste Alchemie*, København, 1921, 51. Also on p. 46: The fire of the alchemical mixture was to be identified with sulphur (Arsenikon) and sulphur-arsenic because of its "male" nature.

[27] Cantici III, Tonus 8, Concentus 5, Modulus, fol. 89, part II.

[28] Cantici I, Tonus 6, Cap. 17, fol. 111.

[29] There is no need to refer in detail also to *Coelum in homine* as expressed in the

who is the whole world and thus related to heaven in all respects embraces all heavenly powers including the intelligences which rule him. *Heaven in man* is composed of the four incorruptible elements in him.[30]

### DISTRIBUTION OF ELEMENTAL QUATERNARIES IN THE WORLD

Eight elements, four corruptible and four incorruptible—with the addition of the soul—form the first ennead in Zorzi's system of cosmology. He assumes four such sets:[31]

1. in the world below
2. in the firmament
3. above it, *i.e.*, in the realm of the angels
4. in God, *i.e.*, the Archetype.

They are specified as follows:

*Earth*
1. solid in the inferior world
2. in the firmament it forms the heavenly bodies such as sun, moon and stars
3. above this it prepares the Throne of God
4. in the Archetype it is the source of all fecundity.

*Water*
1. washes everything in the inferior world
2. in the firmament it furnishes rain, irrigates and renders things mixable
3. in the realm of the angels it teaches and is productive of gifts
4. in the Maker it washes sins away and regenerates.

*Air*
1. in the lower world enables us to breathe, see, hear and smell
2. in the firmament it makes it possible to see beyond the fixed stars
3. above it it provides the space for the beatific vision of the King and Queen and all the Soldiers of Heaven and the beatific sound of the singing of the Heavenly Hosts. From the realm of the Angels there flows the breath of Life.
4. in the Maker it is the Spirit whereby prophets like Elijah were able to commune with Him.

*Fire*
1. in the lower world heats, cooks and perfects
2. in the firmament it shines and gives the warmth of the sun, and agitates and strengthens like Mars
3. in the realm of the Angels it is expressed as seraphic and fervid love
4. in the Archetype it is the spiritual fire which Moses saw when God revealed Himself in the burning bush.

---

numerous works on Quinta Essentia from Hellenistic alchemy to those of Rupescissa and Ulstadius.

[30] Cantici I, Tonus 5, cap. 10, fol. 91.

[31] Cantici I, Tonus 3, cap. 17, fol. 53.

### PICO AS INSPIRATION FOR ZORZI

Zorzi would seem to have thus elaborated an idea that was preformed in Renaissance philosophy, notably in Pico. Truly, Pico says,[32] what exists in the lower world, also exists in the higher world. The difference lies in the lower quality, condition and purity of the former. With us heat is an elemental quality whereas it is the idea of heat and warming virtue in the minds of the angels. Fire is element with us. The sun is fire in heaven, in the region beyond the world fire is "seraphic intellect". These fires are different in that elementary fire burns, celestial fire enlivens, supercelestial fire loves. There is water with us; but there is also water in heaven, the mover and governor of which is the forecourt of heaven, namely the moon. Finally, there are also waters above heaven—the cherubic minds. The elemental water extinguishes the heat of life, the celestial one feeds it, the supercelestial one ideates it (*intellegit*).[33]

A short and somewhat late account in the Piconian tradition is found in Postelius, who says that matter rejoices in its four elements.[33a] These are situated as well in heaven as in the inferior regions; there they are free from blemish, here they are sordid matter. Therefore, the fire in heaven, air, water and earth which are in the celestial regions nod downwards calling us to that region.

### THE HIGHER ELEMENTS IN AGRIPPA OF NETTESHEIM

It is not surprising that the idea of the higher elements occurs again in Agrippa of Nettesheim. Indeed, the 8th chapter of the first Book of his *Occult Philosophy* is devoted to the way in which the elements are in heaven, in the stars, in demons, in angels, and finally in God Himself. It is, he says, unanimously argued by Platonists that all is in all, both in the archetypal and in the corporeal world, though in different ways according to their nature. Thus elements are not only in the objects of the lower world but also in heaven, stars, demons, angels and the Creator Himself. However, in the former they

[32] *In heptaplum praefatio, Opera omnia*, ed. Basle, 1557, 7.

[33] See also *Heptaplus*, cap. III in *ibid.*, 14, on the three worlds and their correspondences. Pico's analogies outlined above as well as Ficinus' related ideas have recently been importantly considered in connection with Paracelsus by K. Goldammer in "Die paracelsische Kosmologie und Materietheorie in ihrer wissenschaftsgeschichtlichen Stellung und Eigenart", *Medizinhistorisches Journal*, **6**, 5–35 (5 ff), 1971.

[33a] Guilielmus Postelius, *Absconditorum constitutione mundi clavis* (originally 1546), Amsterodami, apud Joannem Janssonium, 1646, the edition used by Abraham of Franckenberg, p. 56: Materia suis quatuor gaudet elementis et in caelo et in inferioribus positis, illic enim sunt defaecata, hic sunt faeculenta materia: ideo Ignis caelestis, Aer, Aqua, Terra quae est in caelestibus, deorsum innuunt nos illuc vocando.

are of dense matter, whereas the latter are of celestial and more excellent matter. For example, the heat of fire does not burn but is simply light and lifegiving to everything through its heat.[34]

In Agrippa an influence of Zorzi has been suspected.[35]

## III. Corollary: The Bright and Dark Fire

Most of the early references to the duplicity of fire have been collected by one of the present authors in connection with Paracelsus and his distinction of essential and material fire.[36]

We mentioned (p. 98) Zorzi's indebtedness to Ficinus. Indeed, the concept of the higher and lower elements is recognizable, in Ficinus, *e.g.*, on the *duplicity of fire*—celestial invisible fire that enlivens, and the visible fire on earth that consumes and destroys.[37]

Zorzi himself speaks of the obscure or compressed (*coarctatus*) fire.[38] This he contrasts with the shining and expanding fire which spells happiness. The context is a discussion of life as bound up with the function of heart and blood vessels. All that is alive lives through immanent heat. As Zoroaster said: Everything is made from fire. Thus fever is due to a fire kindled in man by an abundance of evil deeds that have accumulated in the course of time. This is *dark fire*—it springs from a contracted and indurated heart. The latter thus prevents man from capturing light and wholesome warmth—it is comparable to the sun which, according to the object acted upon, may either liquefy or petrify the latter.

### EARLIER CONCEPTS OF BLACK AND BRIGHT FIRE

#### (*a*) ARISTOTLE

Though elaborated in Renaissance natural philosophy, the distinction between two kinds of fire—white and black—is well documented in ancient sources. Of these Aristotle's vital or psychic fire should be mentioned in the

[34] *De occulta philosophia*, liber I, cap. 8, ed. Lugduni, 1550, vol. I, 20; Lugduni, s.a. (ab. 1600), vol. I, 14.

[35] Wolf-Dieter Müller-Jahncke, *Magie als Wissenschaft im frühen 16, Jahrhundert.* Dissertation, Marburg, 1973, 57ff.

[36] E.g. Hildegard of Bermersheim (Bingen), Hugo of St. Victor, Ficinus, Reuchlin, Agrippa and Khunrath. See W. Pagel, *Paracelsus. An Introduction to Philosophical Medicine*, Basle-New York, 1958, 212–3; *idem*, *Weltbild* (7), 71.

[37] Ficino, *Platonicorum . . . operum philosophicorum . . . libri LIV*, Basle, 1580, 88, to Plotinus, *Ennead II*, 7–8. See also below, p. 103, notes 42 and 43.

[38] Cantici III, Tonus 8, Conc. 1; cap. 17, fol. 78*v*–81*r*, part II.

first place: "All animals with a full-blooded lung require rapid refrigeration because of the small weight of the vital (*psychic*) fire" (*Pyr psychikon*).[39]

In the Renaissance it was said of Aristotle that he distinguished between a life-giving fire in the cavity of the moon and a burning fire with excessive heat, the former serving Nature for the generation of animals, the latter is perfecting Nature's work.[40]

This would refer to the well-known rôle attributed by Aristotle to "astral heat" in generation:

> In all cases the semen contains within itself that which causes it to be fertile—what is known as "hot" substance (*to kaloumenon thermon*), which is not fire (*pyr oude*) nor any similar substance, but the pneuma which is enclosed within the semen or foam-like stuff, and the natural substance which is in the pneuma; and this substance is analogous to the element which belongs to the stars (*en to pneumati physis, analogon ousa to ton astron stoicheio*). That is why fire does not generate any animal . . . whereas the heat of the sun does effect generation, and so does the heat of animals.[41]

The Aristotelian *locus* is also related to the Ficinian commentary to Plotinus' discussion of heavenly fire:[42] "But heavenly fire is the only pure fire, and it neither suffers nor causes violence: shining wonderfully but glowing so blissfully that it surpasses even the beauty of its aspect when it is touched in any way. But the generally visible and burning fire is not pure fire but rather a fiery element".[43]

[39] *De respir.*, cap. 21, 478a, 15: "deitai tes katapsykseos dia to mikran einai ten rhopen tou psychikou pyros". *The Works of Aristotle*, trl. and ed. W. D. Ross, Oxford, 1908, translates, "there is little scope for deviation from the normal amount of their vital fire". In addition to the psychic fire, the Aristotelian *pyrigona*—creatures living in fire—should be mentioned because of the Paracelsian salamander tradition; cf. Paracelsus on essential and material fire in *Liber de renovatione et restauratione*, ed. Sudhoff, vol. III, 209; *Liber Azoth*, Sudhoff, XIV, 577: "the salamander is said to live in the essential fire". Aristotle, *Historia Animalium* V, 19 552b, 10, also Aelian, *Natura Animalium* II, 2; Apuleius, *De Deo Socratis*, 8; *Kore Kosmou*, Stobaeus I, 996. To these ancient sources see Philo, *Philosophische Werke*, ed. trl. L. Cohn and I. Heinemann, vol. IV, Breslau, 1923, 59, note 3 (*De Gigantibus*) by H. Leisegang.

[40] Nicolaus Leonicenus, *Opuscula*, Basle, 1532, f. 86*r*.

[41] Aristotle, *De Generatione Animalium*, 736b, 35ff., trl. Peck, London, Loeb Library, W. Heinemann, 1953, 170–1.

[42] Marsilius Ficinus, *Platonicorum . . . Operum Philosophicorum . . . Libri LIV*, Basle, Perna, 1580, to Plotinus, Ennead II, 1, 7–8, p. 88.

[43] "Est autem caelestis ignis, solus purusque ignis, neque vim patiens, neque inferens: mirifice lucens, sed super aspectum suavissime calens si quo modo tangatur. Manifestus autem ignis atque comburens non ignis est purus, sed ignitum potius elementum". (Ficinus, *Platonicorum . . .*, Basle, Perna, 1580, 88).

### (b) GNOSIS AND HERMES

A dark fire, *skoteinon phos*, is the term given to all cosmic light in Gnosticism.[44] A distinction is made, too, between visible and invisible fire.[45] In passing it may be noted that in the *Hermetic Corpus* the dragon, otherwise known as fire-spitting being, is identified with *skotos* (darkness) and thereby with matter and primeval matter, *i.e.*, water.[46]

Finally, the "turbid fire" (*tholodes pyr*) of Iamblichus may be mentioned. He connected it with impure matter by which the purity of the soul is impaired. This is the result of a mixture with "dissimilar" and "contrary" material under demoniac influence.[47]

### (c) RABBINICAL AND KABBALISTIC SOURCES

Of the latter the most unequivocal is Reuchlin's reference to Ramban Gerundensis (Nachmanides). Here it says: Kabbalists assert that God wrote His law into a fiery globe through dark fire superimposed on light fire, whence it is clear to us through the Kabbala that Scriptures were in dark fire on the "back" of bright fire.[48]

According to Scholem, the Kabbalistic source goes back to Isaac the Blind (*c.* 1165–1235). He distinguished (*a*) an original law (*Ur-Torah*) from (*b*) written law and (*c*) oral law. The first comprises ideal or potential signs destined to be actualized. The second stands for law with the colours of (invisible) white fire and the third for the colours emerging from black (visible) fire. Of the latter—black fire—it is said that it burns against the background of the white fire just as ink "burns" on the white surface of a sheet of vellum. In the "white fire" no forms of letters are visible, and where they are we are already dealing with black fire. Hence the written *Tora* cannot assume visible form other than through the force of the oral law. In other words, the written law cannot be understood without the oral law. Only when the black flames come apart in moments of intuition and contemplation is the white

[44] Hans Jonas, *Gnosis und spätantiker Geist*, Göttingen, 1954, vol. I, 149.

[45] Hippolytus, *Refutatio Omnium Haeresium*. ed. L. Duncker et F. G. Schneidewin, Göttingen, 1859, lib. VI, cap. 9, 236–9.

[46] *Corpus Hermeticum*, ed. Nock and Festugière, vol. I, 15, fn. 11, referring to Bousset, *Hauptprobleme der Gnosis*, Göttingen, 1907, 100.

[47] Iamblichus, *De Mysteriis*, lib. II, cap. 4, ed. Parthey, Berlin, 1857, 77; W. Pagel, *William Harvey's Biological Ideas*, Basle, S. Karger, 1967, 294, n. 40.

[48] *De arte cabalistica*, 1517, LXIII, reprint 1964, 238: "Qua re apparet nobis per Cabbalam, quae fuerit scriptura in igne fusco super dorsum ignis candidi". Also ed. Pistorius, *Artis cabalisticae scriptores*, Basle, Henricpetri, 1587, 705. See Pagel, *Paracelsus* (36), 212.

light or sphere of divine compassion accessible to prophets, with the exception of Moses to whom it was accessible all the time.[49]

The basic idea had been well substantiated in earlier Talmudic and Rabbinical literature. The main *locus* is in Raschi's Commentary to the last chapter of Deuteronomy[50] interpreting the phrase *esh dath*, "fiery doctrine". Here Raschi says that the Scriptures were before His face in dark fire on top of white fire.

Further *loci* are found in *Shekalim* (*Talmud Jerushalmi*)[51] where Rabbi Pinchas in the name of Rabbi Simon b. Levi says that the Torah which the Holy One has given to Moses was rooted in white fire and written in dark fire, and also in Tanchumah to *Genesis*: How was the Torah written? On top of white fire with black fire as it is said in the Song of Songs, ch. 5, v. 11: His head is as the most fine gold, his locks are curly and black as a raven. The substance of the tables of the law themselves was white fire, and the letters written on them were dark fire.[52]

In *Sota* (*Jerusalem Talmud*) the blank "skin" (vellum) of the Torah which God has given is said to have consisted of white fire, whereas the letters engraved on it were from black fire, the Torah itself being fire, mixed with fire, carved out of fire, given by fire, from the right hand.[53]

### (*d*) A SEVENTEENTH CENTURY TEXT

In the seventeenth century we still find a double fire in Henricus Alstedius' *Theologia Naturalis*,[54] to wit, a fundamental ("elementary") and a focal fire. The former is a pure heat which is not nourished, not visible, gives life and nurture to others, is vital, health-giving, preserves everything, nourishes, gives increase, sustains, and acts through *sensus*. The focal fire is mixed with water, earth, and concrete qualities. It is visible and is not maintained without fuel. It is instrumental, consuming, and disturbs and dissipates everything where it has invaded.

### SUMMARY TO THE NATURE OF THE HIGHER ELEMENTS

In *conclusion*, it would appear that the *higher elements* are basically the

[49] Gershom Scholem, *Zur Kabbala und ihrer Symbolik*, Zürich, Rhein-Verlag, 1960, 71 and note 38 on 268. *Idem*, *Ursprung und Anfänge der Kabbala*, Berlin, 1962, 254.

[50] Raschi, to *Soth ha-b'rakha*, *Deuteronomy*, 33, 2.

[51] Shekalim 80, 5.

[52] *Tora th'mimah al d'barim* 33, 2.

[53] Sota fol. 22b. We are indebted for these Talmudic *loci* to Rabbi Raymond Apple lately of the Hampstead Synagogue communicated to us by Dr. F. T. Glasson, D.D.

[54] *Theologia naturalis exhibens augustissimam naturae scholam, in qua creaturae Dei communi sermone ad omnes pariter docendos utuntur adversus Atheos, Epicureos et Sophistas huius temporis*, s.l., apud Antonium Hummium, 1615, 317.

same as the lower elements, with the difference that each of the former is more spiritual in substance and more active in function than each of the lower ones.

## IV. The Higher Elements in the Prime Matter of Paracelsus—Created or Uncreated

How far are the higher elements related to Paracelsus' views of *Prime Matter* and its *creation*?

### (*a*) position of the elements

Paracelsus' attitude towards the elements is ambiguous. On the one hand he recognized the four traditional elements, as for example (though by no means exclusively) in his chemical work, the *Archidoxis*. He also interpreted them originally in terms of the *Four Mothers* (see below). The latter stand for elemental sources, each of which impresses its specific seal on its specific products such as water on metals and minerals, and earth on plants.[55]

On the other hand, instead of the four traditional elements, Paracelsus visualizes as the fundamental components and directing principles of matter the three "primaries": salt, sulphur and mercury. These emerge when matter steps out from a non-corporeal state into a still invisible primeval water.[56]

The point which interests us in the context of the present paper is the use by Paracelsus of "sophic" preformation of principles and elements in his concept of *Prime Matter*. This and their linking with sex differentiation[57] is reminiscent of the higher elements and their relationship with the lower elements which we have discussed from Renaissance sources.

### (*b*) prime matter (iliastrum) and creation

To understand the position of elements (higher and lower) in Paracelsus their relationship with Prime Matter must be discussed as well as the origin of Prime Matter itself—for it is in this that the elements develop. First, was it created or eternally existing? Secondly, how does Paracelsian Prime matter compare with matter in the sense generally accepted today?

The creation of man and the objects of his ambient world from nothing is consistently emphasized and asserted in the Paracelsian *Corpus*, in the authentic as well as the suspect treatises. It is difficult, however, to be certain about the position of the world as a whole—the world that is in its embryonic stage before any separate objects existed. This is known under various names such as *Chaos*, *Iliastrum* and *Prime Matter*. All these convey uni-

[55] W. Pagel, *Paracelsus* (36), 208.

[56] W. Pagel, "The prime matter of Paracelsus", *Ambix*, **9**, 121, 1961.

[57] See W. Pagel, *Weltbild* (7), 77.

versality and absence of form and separateness. They certainly do not indicate matter in the generally accepted sense, but rather something that is neither spirit nor ordinary matter. All these terms stand for a frontier separating no-thing from thing—the field in which the challenge lies for the Creator, the "seam" (*limbus*) at which materialization and separation of individual species and objects from no-thing take place. It can be substantiated that Paracelsus believed in the creation of objects not as such, but in the form of *semina* and that these were created all at the same time to be developed by demiurges (*vulcani*) in the due course of world history and to reach their predestined end then and there—basically the Augustinian idea of *germinal forms*.[58]

God, then, created heaven and earth and all that they contain. But did he also create *de novo* and as such *Chaos, Iliastrum*, and that *Prime Matter* which is synonymous with Chaos and Iliaster? We have reason to believe that Paracelsus regarded it as a medium *in* or *out of which* He created rather than that itself had been created first. At all events, there is more than one locus, which is suggestive of prime matter un-created, but it may well be that Paracelsus was not consistent in this.

The *locus classicus* comes from the *Opus Paramirum*, perhaps the most characteristic and mature of all his treatises. "The prime matter of the world was Fiat" (dieweil aber materia prima mundi fiat ist gewesen).[59] The text is well and consistently transmitted. As it stands, the passage "sits" perfectly in its context, and any emendation, such as "from" the fiat, or "out of it" does not necessarily seem to be called for. That a true identity of Prime Matter with the Divine Word (*Fiat*) is really meant, also emerges from the context. For it continues: "Who will try to explain this Fiat?" In other words, the Fiat qua divine is inscrutable to man. This inscrutability removes Prime Matter from the realm of Nature which is accessible to human

[58] *Ibid.*, 121, with reference to Hans Meyer, *Geschichte der Lehre von den Keimkräften von der Stoa bis zum Anfang der Patristik*, Bonn, 1914, 128ff.

[59] *Opus paramirum*, I, cap. 2, ed. Sudhoff, IX, 48. There are no text-variants in Sudhoff's critical apparatus to the *locus* in vol. IX, 667. W.-E. Peuckert's *Studienausgabe*, vol. II, 9 (Basel and Stuttgart, 1965) has the text identical with F. Strunz, *Th. Paracelsus, Volumen paramirum und Opus paramirum*, Jena, 1904, 92, and Sudhoff, *loc. cit.* (IX, 48). The Latin translation, *Liber paramirum . . . Theophrasti Paracelsi*, ed. Basileae, P. Perna, 1570, according to Sudhoff, *Bibliographia Paracelsica*, Berlin, 1894, No. 122, p. 205, by Forberger, has (19): "ad huiusmodi formarum proprietates tradendas et explicandas pertinebat et primam mundi materiam declarare. Ceterum istam constet fuisse Fiat, quis audebit illud Fiat explicare?" Fridericus Bitiskius, *Paracelsus, Opera omnia medico-chemico-philosophica*, Genevae, 1658, vol. I, 34 gives: "opus habemus cognitione materiae primae. Cur vero prima materia mundi fuerit Fiat, quis hoc Fiat explicare conabitur?" Huser, Folio ed. 1603, I, 27: "dieweil aber Prima Materia Mundi Fiat ist gewesen".

research. In this way it is placed on the same level as the *Arcana* (virtues), for of them Paracelsus said that they were divine and not "natural".[60] Moreover, it is by content *not isolated* in the *Corpus* of the *genuine* works.[61] In the earlier work *On minerals* prime matter of the world (here called "ultimate" matter), "the first", the "beginning" was "with God" (nun ist das erst gewesen bei got, der anfang, das ist ultima materia).[62] It is this first ("ultimate") beginning that is then "made by God" into a second product (here called "prime matter") which contains the *semina*. It is not said, however, that the first, the beginning ("ultimate matter") was "made" by God, but that it was merely *with Him*.

The Paracelsian topos *bei got* (with Him) indeed implies "non-created". For Paracelsus says that God created herbs and fruit, but He did not create the virtue which is in the herb or fruit. The latter are things "natural" and therefore created, whereas the virtues are divine and therefore uncreated.

> The natural objects, they are His, the herb He has created, but its inherent virtue He has not created; for each virtue is uncreated, that is, God is without beginning and not created, and thus all virtues and forces were in God before heaven and earth and before all things had been created, at the time when God was a Spirit and hovered over the water. . . . Nobody should say that the virtue of things, their power, be natural, but it is supernatural and without beginning. . . . Herbs are created just as trees and stars; for they were not with God in the beginning of the Godhead, that is before heaven and earth were created.[63]

[60] *De vera influentia rerum*, tract. I, ed. Sudhoff, vol. XIV, 215. "Die ding die sind sein, das kraut hat er beschaffen, aber die tugent darinnen nit. Dan ein jetliche tugent ist unbeschaffen; das ist, got ist on anfang und nicht beschaffen. So sind alle tugenden und kreft in got gewesen, vor himel und erden, und ehe alle ding beschaffen sind worden, da got ein geist war und schwebet uber die wasser . . ., so mag niemant sagen das die tugent der dingen, ir kraft etc. natürlich seie, sonder ubernatürlich, on end und anfang. . . . Die kreuter sind beschaffen, wie auch die beum und das gestirn; dan sie warn nit bei got im anfang der gotheit, das ist, ehe himel und erden geschaffen ward". It may be pertinent to mention Johannes Tauleri, *Des heiligen lerers Predig, fast fruchtbar zu eim recht christlichen Leben*, Adam Petri, Basel, 1521, fol. 311*r sub fine* (Predigt uff Martini oder Nicolai): "Gott is us wendig aller natur unn ist selbs nit natur".

[61] Therefore we would hesitate to agree with Goldammer, *Medizingeschichte in unserer Zeit, Festgabe für Heischkel-Artelt*, Stuttgart, 1971, in note 106 on 144: "Vielleicht ist vor 'fiat' ein 'durch' oder 'aus' zu ergänzen". The same applies to the attribution of the passages where the Fiat is said to be Prime Matter to "deutero-Paracelsian" sources *ibid.* on 133.

[62] *Das buch De mineralibus*, ed. Sudhoff, vol. III, 34.

[63] *De Vera Influentia Rerum, Philosophia Magna*, X, Tractatus I, ed. Sudhoff, vol. XIV, 215. "Die ding die sind sein, das kraut hat er beschaffen, aber die tugent darinnen nit. Dan ein jetliche tugent ist unbeschaffen; das ist, got ist on anfang und nicht beschaffen. So sind alle tungenden und kreft in got gewesen, vor himel und erden, und ehe alle ding

In both passages, then, the *Prime Matter* from which the world derives is presented as part of God rather than subordinated to Him as a created object. Both passages, too, are reminiscent of the Prologue to the Gospel of St. John, in which the world is presented as founded on the *Word* that was *with God*. Moreover, *qua logos* and being *with God*, the "first", the "beginning" of the world is marked out as something spiritual and as non-matter in the usual sense of "matter".[64] It is an immaterial spirit that existed by itself in the beginning and later on "became flesh" in Gospel-terms, or in Paracelsian terms: "The word *fiat* was made material, apprehensible and a body in which there lies and is hidden all that is predestined" (Yliastrum ist die erste materia . . . wie das verbum Fiat materialisch, greiflich und ein leib ist worden, darinnen nun alle praedestinata stecken und verborgen ligen).[65]

Again, that it was the word *fiat* that became material, namely in the form of salt, sulphur, mercury, is not said at one isolated place—so, for example, we read: also dass das word fiat geworden ein dreyfach corpus, das ist getheilt in dreyerlei corpora.[66] Moreover, Prime Matter *qua tripartite* is juxtaposed to God who is likewise—*wie got also materia prima*. As the latter has only one name, *i.e.*, Prime Matter, in spite of the different functions of its three parts, so has God in spite of the disparate "offices" of God the Father, the Son and the Holy Spirit.[67]

---

beschaffen sind worden, da got ein geist war und schwebet uber die wasser. . . . So mag niemant sagen, das die tugent der dingen, ir kraft etc. natürlich seie, sonder ubernatürlich on end und anfang. . . . Die beum und das gestirn warn nit bei got".

[64] *bei got*, further passages: dise erden . . . darumb so ist das selbig alein im ersten anfang bei got (*Liber de inventione artium*, ed. Sudh., XIV, 251). Bei wem sollen wir denn anderst die ding suchen als alein bei got? (*Lib. de invent. art.*, *Prolog*, ed. Sudh. XIV, 249). Alle ding sind gewesen unsichtbar, bei Gott . . . gefasst in ein limbum, das ist ein sichtig corpus das selbig corpus ist die grosse welt worden (*De podagricis, I, De limbo*, ed. Sudh. I, 316. Huser, Fol. ed. 1603, vol. I, 565). Among the Paracelsians, Valentin Weigel seems to have been particularly impressed by the Paracelsian attribution of prime matter to being *bei Gott*. "Diese grosse sichtbare Welt . . . hat eine materia, und ist doch ohne materia gemacht worden . . . denn Gott hat keine leibliche materiam gehabt . . . sie ist wohl materialisch, sichtig, aber von keiner materia herkommen, sondern ausz dem unsichtigen . . . diese gantze welt und alles was man sihet, was *bey Gott* und in seinem Wort unsichtig, Unleiblich, und wie es *bey Gott* war, also war es auch in der Schöpffung, den engeln gegeben, da Gott sprach, fiat lux . . ." (Valentin Weigel, *Vom ort der welt*, Kap. 13, in *Sämtliche Schriften*, ed. W.-E. Peuckert and W. Zeller, Stuttgart, 1962, 46, our italics.)

[65] *Liber Azoth*, cap. I, ed. Sudh. XIV, 549.

[66] Fiat ist worden ein dreyfach corpus (*Buch meteororum*, cap. 2, *De prima materia coeli et stellarum*: Huser, Fol. ed. 1603, vol. II, 72, ed. Sudh. XIII, 134).

[67] *Buch meteororum*, cap. II, ed. Sudh. XIII, 136.

(*c*) ILIASTRUM—PRIME MATTER PRIOR TO ALL CREATION

Perhaps the most concise passage in which *Prime Matter* and *Iliastrum* are identified and given priority to all creation is found in the small glossary at the end of Paracelsus' tract on the virtues of the mineral waters of Pfäfers: Iliaster ist die erste Materia vor aller schöpfung ("Iliaster is prime matter prior to all creation").[68]

The priority of a medium *from* which creation took place rather than that this medium was created first is expressed in several passages. For example: "how many species God has created from the single iliaster" (wie vielerlei species got us dem einigen iliaster geschaffen hat),[69] or, "Prime Matter of the world was a uniform *Chaos*; out of this same *Chaos* God has made the greater world, separated and divided into four different elements" (prima materia mundi was ein einiger Chaos, aus demselbigen Chaos hat got gemacht maiorem mundum, gescheiden and abgesöndert in vier unterscheitliche element).[70]

(*d*) CREATION—"INFORMATION" OF PRIME MATTER (SOPHIC WATER)

In all this the biblical tradition that the spirit of God hovered over the waters leads to the stipulation that *water* stands for *prime matter* from which God created. As Rabbinical tradition has it, water was indeed the first, and there is no indication in *Genesis* that, and when, it was created.[71] This water was, of course, not ordinary water, but a "sophic" prefiguration and idea, an *aquaster* with the connotation of a passive, *female* medium (matrix) in which some active, *male* force operates by introducing form into something formless and homogeneous—"informing" it. "Creation" is "information". Indeed, this is the wording of the Latin translation of Paracelsus' Pfäfers tract by Forberger.[72]

Paracelsus speaks about the invisible *matrix* whose *first matter* cannot be seen by anybody. The world is born out of this *matrix* and so are man and all creatures. Before heaven and earth were created the spirit of God hovered on the water. The water was *matrix*, for in it heaven and earth were created and in no other *matrix*. The spirit of God was carried (*getragen*) in it, the spirit that is, of God which is in man and which is lacking in all other creatures. Now, as the world was nothing but a water, and the spirit of the Lord was on the water, this water became the world; this is now the *matrix* of the world, and in it subsequently are all creatures (was sol man sagen von der matrice das

[68] *Vonn dem Bad Pfeffers Tugenden*, ed. Sudh. IX, 658.

[69] *Ibid.*, ed. Sudh. IX, 644.

[70] *De natura rerum, VIII, De separationibus rerum naturalium* (Huser I, 903; ed. Sudh. XI, 360). According to Sudhoff, this treatise is not genuine.

[71] For the Rabbinical tradition see Raschi's *Commentary to Genesis*, 1.2.

[72] Forberger, *Liber Paramirum*, 1570, *loc. cit.* (59), 364: "Iliaster est prima materia ante rerum informationem". See above, note 68.

sie unsichtbar ist und niemand sicht ir erst materiam . . .? dis wasser war matrix; dan in dem wasser ward beschaffen himel und erden und in keiner andern matrix nicht. In deren ward der geist gottes tragen . . . nun also die welt nichts war sondern ein wasser und der geist des herrn war auf dem wasser, so ward das wasser zu der welt . . . und in im weiter alle geschöpf.)[73] In a similar vein salt, sulphur and mercury—the first bodily manifestation, the "flesh" of the *logos* or *Prime Matter*—are said to be of a watery nature (also das der sulphur und mercurius und salz, so in dem stern seind, ein wasser natur seind und sonst nichts in inen haben als all ein die wasser natur, dorauf sie dan geordnet seind).[74]

### (*e*) GOD AS SEPARATOR OF THE ELEMENTS

God operates like the chymist—separating rather than creating *de novo*. This is the well known position of the *Philosophia ad Athenienses*,[75] a lively treasure of heretic doctrines whose authenticity is in doubt. However, in the same *Von des Bades Pfäfers Tugenden* in which we found the *Iliaster* as pre-creation Prime Matter and whose authenticity is beyond doubt God is presented to us through the light of nature as separator of each thing that was to stand by itself (also beweist uns das liecht der natur das got von einander geschieden hat ein ietlichs das besonders stan solt.)[76] Similarly, also in a genuine tract: The *Yliaster* was divided . . . and has given the four elements.[77] Moreover, in the genuine treatise *De meteoris*, God is said to have created all things in the prime matter that they should be, but Himself separated again each thing out into what it was destined to be . . . extracted, separated, formed ultimate matters out of prime matter, that is, created each individual. . . . Who, to begin with, had created and put in all things together at once and afterwards, within six days, pulled out what had lain in it.[78]

[73] *Opus Paramirum IV*, Huser I, 72; Sudhoff IX, 190–1.

[74] *Philosophia de generationibus et fructibus quatuor elementorum*, Book II, Tractatus 3, cap. 1, Sudhoff XIII, 33.

[75] *Philosophia ad Athenienses*, I, text 7, Sudhoff XIII, 392.

[76] *Von des Bades Pfäfers Tugenden*, Sudhoff IX, 643.

[77] "am ersten ist der Yliaster geteilet worden, der dan nichts ist, und hat geben die vier elementen". *Philosophia de generationibus et fructibus quatuor elementorum*, Book I, cap. 1, Sudhoff, XIII, 9.

[78] "Got in der ersten prima materia alle ding geschaffen hat zu sein, aber selbs gescheiden wider heraus, ein jetlichs in das, das es hat sollen sein . . . extrahirt, separirt, geformirt hat aus der prima materia ultimas materias, das ist, ein jetlichs geschöpft . . . der am ersten alle ding in eins geschaffen und gelegt hat, darnach in sechs tagen heraus gezogen, was im selbigen gewesen ist". Paracelsus, *De meteoris*, cap. 3, *De stellarum prima materia et essentiis*, ed. Sudhoff, vol. XIII, 149.

Finally and unmistakeably, Paracelsus speaks of God—the highest fabricator—as separating and withdrawing from primary unformed iliastric mass.[79]

## (*f*) PRIME MATTER AS CREATED IN SPURIOUS ("DEUTERO-PARACELSIAN") TREATISES

None of the passages cited tell us that *Prime Matter, Chaos, Yliaster* or Water (*Aquaster*) from or out of which creation took place was first created by God. One passage in which this is expressly stated comes from a treatise which is unanimously regarded as non-authentic: in *De pestilitate* we read that through the Fiat first water was created and thereafter all other creatures (dan durch das Wort FIAT ist am ersten das wasser beschaffen worden und hernach aus dem wasser alle andere creaturen.)[80]

It is of some interest that a second passage which looks as if it pointed to the creation of original "matter" also occurs in a non-authentic work. Here the author speaks of a "tincture"[81] that was made before "Prime Matter", *made* that is by Him who has created all things. He calls this "tincture" *ante Prima Materia*—precursor of Prime Matter—and it is in the latter that the tincture operates by "tinging" and "transmuting", *i.e.*, like an alchemist, like a *vulcanus*. God, the highest *vulcanus*, is productive of the most perfect and miraculous composition. The key word is making *semina* and committing all things to them. It is in the course of this creative mechanism that such "rods and whips" emerge which transform a morbid change ("body") into a syphilitic one (welche ante prima materia in der prima materia sein tingirn und transmutirn verbringt. Nun ist die selbig ante prima materia ein tinctur, die da gemacht wird von dem, der alle ding beschaffen hat, welches machen als ein geisel oder ruten zu sein . . . was nun der obrist vulcanus macht, das ist ein volkomene composition . . . nach der kürz also alle ding seind in

[79] "Also ist dises erst corpus yliastri ein kloz gewesen, in dem alle kreuter, alle wasser, al gemmae, al mineral, al stein, al chaos gelegen seind, die allerin der höchst fabricator hinweg geschiden hat und gebildet also subtil, das das, so hinweg genomen ist worden, ein anders gewesen ist. Als am ersten hat er hinweg genomen den luft, und aus dem ubrigen seind noch drei geworden, das feur, wasser und erden; aus disen hat er hinweg genomen das feur, noch seind zwei bliben; also bis zum end. (Philosophia de generationibus et fructibus elementorum". Sudhoff, XIII, 13.)

[80] *De Pestilitate—Cabala*: Sudhoff XIV, 601; Huser I, 328.

[81] On the various meanings of the term see Bartholomaeus Castelli, *Lexicon medicum*, ed. J. P. Bruno, Leipzig, 1713, 722. The meaning here intended is that of a secret *arcanum* that has the power of transmuting substances into something similar to itself—*assimilating* it. In Paracelsian usage it involves colour change and curative effects. The tincture is prepared through extraction and concentration. Of mediaeval alchemical sources see for example Avicenna, *Ad Hasen regem epistola de re recta* in *Theatrum Chemicum*, vol. IV, Argentorati, Zetzner, 1613, 973, *De tincturis*.

die samen gemacht und gesezt . . . aus dem folgt nun generatio corporis morbi gallici, in dem nun wird der sam geseet, iezt wachsen die franzosen.)[82] However, the *Tincture Ante Prima Materia* of this passage is hardly relevant in our context. It is *not* the Prime Matter of the world and its implied creation which seems to be at issue here, but any seminal force that acts on and in an undifferentiated body whereby a new being is created, in the present case a special *ens morbi*. More specifically, a part morbid or disposed to disease is "made syphilitic"—for syphilis, in Paracelsus' concept, is not an independent disease of its own, but a secondary change albeit with its own characteristics. "Prime Matter" in this instance would, then, really be the bodily organ or substance worked upon by a divinely created seminal force which is spiritual and thus above and "before" it. With this Paracelsus believes to have superseded traditional humoral and materialistic terms of pathogenesis.

(*g*) IN CONCLUSION

Not one but several passages from *authentic* Paracelsian treatises present Prime Matter not as matter in the sense accepted today, but as a spiritual medium in and from which the world was created. In some places it is identified with the divine Fiat—the Word (*logos*). As such it was uncreated and *with God*.[83] It is also represented as a "sophic", *i.e.*, ideal prefiguration of water with the connotation of something homogeneous, or, formless into which forms are introduced through creation. *Creation* means *Information*[84] and this takes place in Prime Matter (*Iliaster*) that was before all creation. This is accomplished by the active divine power hovering on or operating in "Prime Matter" or else transmuting it as such into the three first principles: salt, sulphur and mercury. The latter in their turn were not yet "matter" in the modern sense but rather spiritual directives causing corporeal matter to assume certain states such as the solid, the combustive or the smoky state. Creation of the elements from the formless mass (*yliaster*) is represented as operating by *separation* and gradual *withdrawal* of one element after the other. This statement is not restricted to the *Philosophia ad Athenienses*—generally regarded as spurious ("deutero-Paracelsian") but is found in the genuine Paracelsian *On the generation and fruits of the elements*—the latter treatise probably forming the source of the unauthentic one.

[82] *Paracelsus' sogenanntes III. Buch der Wundarznei, Liber III, cap. 7*, Sudhoff X, 463–4.

[83] "Nun ist das erst gewesen bei got der anfang, das ist ultima materia, die selbige ultimam materiam hat er gemacht in primam materiam". *De mineralibus, cap. 1*, Sudhoff III, 34. See above, p. 108, and notes 62 and 64.

[84] Ante rerum informationem—Forberger's Latin translation of the sentence quoted in the text to note 68. *Liber Paramirum, accessit . . . de thermis, De thermarum Farvariae . . . virtutibus*, Basel, 1570, 364. See above, n. 72.

In the concepts here reported Paracelsus may appear to voice pantheistic views which are also suggested elsewhere in his genuine work.[85] However, Paracelsian philosophy has many "mansions"—theist, panentheist,[86] mystical and other views can be found therein. It is true that heretic–Gnostic doctrines are much more outspoken and prominent in non-authentic treatises in which the name of Paracelsus may well have been used to make them popular.[87] In a somewhat diluted form, however, they can be found in the genuine Paracelsus as well.

The idea, finally, of higher and lower elements and its place in Paracelsus will be clarified in our discussion of the *Mothers* as *Eightnesses* below (p. 120).

## V. Eightnesses

### INTRODUCTION

In our previous communication[88] we started with Eightnesses and finished with the conjunction of the higher and lower elements. In the present paper we started with the conjunction of the higher and lower elements, and propose to conclude with further material on *eightnesses*, ancient, mediaeval and Renaissance. In the light of what we have said about the conjunction of the higher and lower elements, it would seem reasonable to suggest that it is this very conjunction of two elemental quaternaries on which the whole concept of eightnesses is based—despite the remoteness of its ramifications.

### A CHRISTIAN KABBALISTIC SOURCE OF THE EIGHTNESS OF ADAM—ZORZI

Previously we investigated *the Eightness of Adam*. In the present paper our main source has been Georgius Venetus (Zorzi). Again it is Zorzi who provides evidence for Adam's eightness, and this in a most appropriate Kabbalistic context. He says that Adam consists of two quaternaries because of the main two letters in his name—d (*daleth*) and m (*mem*)—each stands for a quaternary, the former for "four" and the latter for "forty". The third letter in Adam—a (*aleph*)—stands for his "perfusion with divinity". In other words, Adam comprised two quaternaries, *i.e.*, an eightness: "Adam duas esse litteras quadrarias daleth vero quattuor et mem quae quadraginta

[85] E.g. Das da ist materialisch und leiblich geworden got und sein werk . . . der centrum . . . geblüe. (*De Generationibus et Fructibus Elementorum*, lib. 1, Sudhoff XIII, 12).

[86] "Prima Materia, das ist aller anfang ist im vater" (*Buch von den tartarischen Krankheiten*, cap. 7; Sudhoff XI, 51).

[87] To this Goldammer in his excellent essay, "Bemerkungen zur Struktur des Kosmos und der Materie bei Paracelsus", in *Medizingeschichte in unserer Zeit.* Festgabe für E. Heischkel und W. Artelt, Stuttgart, 1971. Cf. note (61), 133.

[88] W. Pagel and M. Winder (1).

importat. Ex quibus innuunt hominem ex duabus quadraturis compositum et aliquali divinitate perfusum denotatur ipsum a (aleph)".[89]

## THE EIGHTFOLD ADAM IN THE SLAVONIC HENOCH BOOK AND RELATED EIGHTNESSES

References to the Slavonic Henoch Book in our previous essay were based on the edition by N. Bonwetsch. Attention should be drawn, however, to the much fuller text and commentary by R. H. Charles.[90]

The following passages may be listed from Charles:

(1) The pseudo-Hippocratic *Peri Hebdomadon*[91] enumerates the following correspondencies: 1. stony earth—bones; 2. soft earth—flesh; 3. soft moisture in the earth—marrow, brain, sperm; 4. river water—blood; 5. bog water—bladder, gut; 6. sea—entrails moisture; 7. air—breath; 8. moon—diaphragm.

(2) Aetius in *Stoicorum Veterum Fragmenta*:[92] "The Stoics say that (the soul) consists of eight parts, *i.e.* the five sense faculties, voice, generative and leading faculty from which, like the feet of a polypod, all parts are extended throughout the organs where they are at home".

(3) St. Augustine:[93] "This is the seventh day, our Sabbath whose end is not the evening but the Lord's day like an eighth day belonging to eternity".

(4) Of mediaeval sources, according to Honorius Augustodunensis, our body resembles the musical *octave*. As in the latter seven tones can be distinguished, the human body is likened to four elements and the human soul to three powers.[94]

(5) In an Anglo-Saxon ritual called *Octo pondera de quibus factus est Adam*, man is said to be made out of eight substances:[95]
Pondus limi, inde factus est caro;
Pondus ignis, inde rubeus est sanguis et calidus;
Pondus salis, inde sunt salsae lacrimae;
Pondus roris, inde factus est sudor;
Pondus floris, inde est varietas oculorum;

[89] Zorzi (15), fol. 63 verso to Cant. III, tonus 6, cap. 12 (pagination beginning after fol. 338).

[90] R. H. Charles, *Apocrypha and Pseudepigraphica of the Old Testament*, Oxford, 1913, vol. 1, XIX and *The Book of the Secrets of Enoch*, ed. Morfill and Charles, 1896, 40. W. H. Roscher: *Die hippokratische Schrift von der Siebenzahl in ihrer vierfachen Ueberlieferung*, Studien zur Kultur u. Geschichte des Altertums, VI, 3/4, Paderborn, 1913, 10ff.; E. Littré, *Oeuvres complètes d'Hippocrate*, Paris, vol. 8, 1853, ch. 6, 637–8 and vol. 9, ch. 6, pp. 436–7.

[91] For an appraisal of this pseudo-Hippocratic work and its probable Iranian sources, see Albrecht Götze, "Persische Weisheit in griechischem Gewande. Ein Beitrag zur Geschichte der Mikrokosmos-Idee". *Z. Indol. Iranistik*, **2**, 60–98, 167–77, 1923.

[92] Ed. Arnim, vol. 2, p. 226, no. 827. Cf. also Plutarch, *Placita*, Book, IV, cap. 4, 21.

[93] *De Civitate Dei*, *22*, 30.5.

[94] De imagine mundi libri tres, I, 82 (in Migne, *Patrologia Latina*, vol. 172, 140.)

[95] *Rituale Ecclesiae Dunelmensis*, ed. J. Stevenson, Publications of the Surtees Society, vol. 10, London, J. B. Nichols, 1840, 192.

Pondus nubis, inde est instabilitas mentium:
Pondus ventis, inde est anhela frigida;
Pondus gratiae, inde est sensus hominis.

### IRANIAN SOURCES

Oriental sources were emphasized by Reitzenstein and Schaeder.[96] They refer to the eightfold nature (*ogdoadike physis*) and the eight parts of which archetypal man is composed. In this connection, Goetze's notes on the Iranian origin of the pseudo-Hippocratic *Peri Hebdomadon* must be mentioned.[97]

### PLATO'S EPINOMIS

Here we are told that five genera of elements exist in living beings. These with the addition of three classes of demons represent an *eightness*—the demons standing between fiery astral divinities—the upper pole in the realm of the living—and the earthly beings alive. The demons are formed from ether and air and mediate between men and gods, and form an *ogdoas* of eight powers akin to each other. There are also semi-divine dwellers in water.[98]

In all this we recognize the genuine Platonic idea of two quaternaries. These underlie the gradual harmonic unfolding of the existence of the physical world—divisible and changing—from existence—indivisible and eternally unchanging.[99]

### A POSSIBLE NEW TESTAMENT ALLUSION

A New Testament passage from the *Book of Revelation* may also be mentioned. Here to a group of seven kings an eighth member is added, the

[96] R. Reitzenstein and W. H. Schaeder, *Studien zum antiken Synkretismus aus Iran and Griechenland*, 1926, 6, 18, 32, 119, 130, 225–6.

[97] A. Goetze (91), 71.

[98] Plato, *Epinomis*, Greek text with English translation, W. R. M. Lamb, Loeb Classical Library. Plato, vol. 8, London, Heinemann, 1927. 981c (for five elements), 984e (for *daimones*), 986e (for eightness). The *Epinomis*, according to Karl Praechter, *Die Philosophie des Altertums* in Ueberweg's *Geschichte der Philosophie*, vol. I, Berlin, 1926, 325–6, has been suspected to be spurious and really not by Plato, but by Philipp the Opuntian of the fourth century, B.C., but this is very doubtful. See also Eduard Zeller, *Die Philosophie der Griechen*, vol. II, 1, 3rd ed., 1875, 891ff.—author of the *Epinomis*: "ein wirklicher Plantoniker".

[99] *Timaios* 35. To this F. M. Cornford, *Plato's Cosmology*, London, 1937, 68. For a topical application of the Platonic principle in Renaissance architecture through the influence of Zorzi see: Rudolf Wittkower, *Architectural Principles in the Age of Humanism*, London, Warburg Institute, 1949; 2nd ed., London, A. Tiranti, 1952, 90–1, concerning a document relating to S. Francesco della Vigna at Venice. On 15 August, 1534, the Doge Andrea Gritti laid the foundation stone of the new church. . . . He had commissioned Francesco Giorgi (Zorzi) of the monastery attached to that church to write a memorandum

"beast".[100] "And there are seven kings: five are fallen, and one is, and the other is not yet come. . . . And the beast that was and is not, even he is the eighth, and is of the seven". We referred in our previous paper to the Kabbalistic tradition of the eight kings of Edom.[101] Edom in Rabbinical parlance also means "Rome", and the passage from *Revelation* about the seven kings with the beast (of Rome) as the eighth may perhaps be connectible.[102]

THE EIGHT-CORNERED STAR OF HELLENISTIC AND ARABIC ALCHEMY

A compound of alum (*stypteria strongyle*) is symbolized by an eight-cornered star as reproduced by Berthelot from manuscript sources.[103]

THE EIGHT-VICES THEORY (ACHTLASTERTHEORIE)

Marie Luise Gothein has pointed out[104] that in Gnostic–Byzantine tradition the number of the deadly sins was eight and not seven as in the later Western tradition, the eighth being *vana gloria* (vanity). This theory must have also existed in India, for the *Vārāha Purāna* observes that there are eight Mātṛkas

---

about Sansovino's—the architect's—model. The memorandum on the proportions of S. Francesco is a practical application of his book on the harmony of the universe. Zorzi bases his deductions on the *Timaeus* where cosmic order and harmony are represented by the squares and cubes of the double and triple proportion starting from unity, which led him to the two geometrical progressions, 1, 2, 4, 8 and 1, 3, 9 27. Traditionally represented in the shape of Lambda

1<br>
2 3<br>
4 9<br>
8 27

the harmony of the world is expressed in the seven numbers which embrace the secret rhythm in macrocosm and microcosm alike.

[100] *Revelation*, 17, 11.

[101] W. Pagel and M. Winder (1), 126.

[102] For a basic and general biblical commentary see T. F. Glasson, *The Revelation of John. The Cambridge Bible Commentary on the New English Bible*, Cambridge, 1965, 97. See also: Albrecht Götze (91) and R. H. Charles, *A critical and exegetical commentary on the Revelation of St. John*, Edinburgh, 1920, vol. II, 70-1 (the "beast" being probably Nero, as generally accepted and not Domitian).

[103] M. Berthelot, *Introduction a la chimie des anciens et du Moyen Age*, Paris, 1889, 108, line 6 and 112, line 21; *idem, La chimie au Moyen Age*, Paris, vol. 2, 1893, paragraph 64, p. 134: "serapha qui éprouve l'argent—d'une signe chez les chimistes". Sculptures of eight-cornered stars occur for example in ancient ossuaries in Jewish art of the Talmudic period. See B. M. Lerner, "Note to Berakhoth 17b", in A. Ehrman, *Talmud, translated into English with Commentary*, Tel Aviv, 1972, 410.

[104] Maris Luise Gothein, "Die Todsünden", *Arch f. Gesch. Religionswiss.*, **10**, 416–84 (439), 1907.

(goddesses) who personify the eight morally bad qualities: desire, greed, pride, anger, illusion, envy, malice and the spreading of slander.[105]

CELSUS

In Celsus' *True Word*[106] the soul passes through eight gates. Each of seven gates represents one of the seven *metals* and their corresponding *stars*. They are accessible by means of a ladder. The eighth gate, however, is above this ladder. A variation on the same theme is the Arabic *Dream of Ostanes* in which Egyptian, Indian and Persian influences are mentioned. In it a version is presented of seven gates from whose guardians the aspirant has to demand the keys in order to reach perfection and omniscience after having passed through the last gate.[107]

A further point is the Kabiri mentioned by Celsus in connection with the idea of the seven gates. Their number was eight as we discussed in our previous paper.[108] The kinship of the Kabiri with corresponding metals and planets was at all times regarded as essential. The seven metals corresponding to seven planets have also been visualized as transmitters of astral impulses towards committing sin in mediaeval morality plays as Gothein has pointed out.[109]

MIDRASH RABBAH

In the Midrash Rabbah, a Rabbinical Bible Commentary dated about 650 A.D. we find a paraphrase to *wayyizer* (He created):

> There were two formations (one partaking of the nature) of the celestial beings (the other) of earthly creatures. . . . He created him with four attributes of the higher beings (*i.e.*, the angels) and four of the lower creatures (*i.e.*, beasts): he eats and drinks, like animals; procreates, like animals; excretes, like animals; and dies, like animals: he stands upright, like the ministering angels, and speaks, understands and sees, like the ministering angels. . . . The Lord reasoned: "If I create him of the celestial elements he will live (forever) and not die; while if I create him of the terrestrial elements, he will die and not live (in a future life). Therefore I will create him of the upper and the lower

[105] P. Pott, *Yoga and Yantra*, The Hague, M. Nijhoff, 1966, 84.

[106] *Celsus' wahres wort. Aelteste Streitschrift antiker Weltanschauung gegen das Christentum vom Jahr 178 n. Chr.* Wiederhergestellt, aus dem Griechischen übersetzt von Theodor Keim. Zürich, Orell, Füssli, 1873, 85.

[107] M. Berthelot: *La chimie du Moyen Age*, Tome III, *La chimie arabe*, 1893, 119–23; Bidez-Cumont, Paris, 1938: *Les mages hellénisés*, II, 347–52.

[108] W. Pagel and M. Winder (1), 125–6.

[109] M. L. Gothein, Die Todsünden (104), 480.

elements; if he sins he will die, and if he dies he will live (in the future life)".[110]

### HILDEGARD VON BERMERSHEIM

Hildegard von Bermersheim or Bingen (1098–1179) says:

> Just as the soul vivifies and consolidates the body, the sun, moon and other planets warm and strengthen the firmament with their fire. For the firmament is like the head of man, / sun, moon and stars like the eyes, / the air like the sense of hearing, / the winds like smell, / the dew like taste, / the sides of the world like arms and like touch; / and other creatures which are in the world are like the belly, the earth, however, like the heart.

In other words, Hildegard compares the parts of the macrocosm with the five senses plus the seats of the rational, vegetative and sensitive soul respectively amounting to eight components.[111]

### THE EIGHT ASTROLOGIES OF DANIEL OF MORLEY

In our previous communication we did not connect the *Eight Astronomies of Paracelsus* with anything more concrete than the general tradition of the liberal arts. However, a closer association seems to be suggestive, namely with the *Liber de Naturis Inferiorum et Superiorum* of Daniel de Morley (*fl.* 1175–1217).[112] In this "eight astrologies" are distinguished. According to Thorndike this goes back to a Gundissalinus quotation from Alfarabi.[113]

[110] *Midrash Rabbah*, trl. H. Freedman and Maurice Simon, London, Soncino-Press, 1939, 112: To Genesis XIV, 3.

[111] Sicut anima corpus vivificat et consolidat sic etiam sol, luna et caeteri / sic / planetae firmamentum cum igne suo fovent et confirmant.
Nam firmamentum est velut *caput* hominis,
sol, luna et stellae ut *oculi*,
aer ut *auditus*,
venti velut *odoratus*,
ros ut *gustus*,
latera mundi ut bracchia et ut *tactus*;
et aliae creaturae, quae sunt in mundo, sunt ut *venter*,
terra autem ut *cor*.
(Hildegard von Bermersheim or Bingen, *Causae et Curae*, ed. Paulus Kaiser, Leipzig, Teubner, 1903, Book I, 10, lines 30–7.)

[112] edited by K. Sudhoff in *Archiv f. d. Gesch. d. Naturwissenschaften u. d. Technik*, **8**, 1–40 (34), 1918.

[113] L. Thorndike, *History of Magic and Experimental Science*, New York, 1923, vol. II, 171–87 (177). Discussion also in Haskins, *Studies in the History of Mediaeval Science*, 2nd ed., 1927, 127.

By content the categories of Paracelsus can be suggested to mirror those of Morely as follows:

| Morley | Paracelsus |
|---|---|
| Judgment (of effects of planets) | Olympic-governing-astrum |
| Medicine | Astral forces in man |
| Nigromancy (earth)<br>Agriculture (water)<br>Illusions and magic (air)<br>Alchemy (fire) | Four astrologies, each connected with one of the four elements |
| Images | Astrology as operative in animal life |
| Mirrors | Astrology derived from Imagination. As strong as Olympic astrum |

(The elemental correspondencies are suggested by the present authors).

JOHN DEE

In his *Monas Hieroglyphica*[114] John Dee (1527–1608) describes the symbol of a cross in the centre of the occult sign of *mercury* to which that of *Aries* is attached. A ternary is formed by the central cross—two crossed lines with the point connecting them being taken as the third component. This point presumably symbolizes the Holy Ghost as connecting God the Father with the Son. On the other hand, he says, the cross is a *quaternary* by virtue of its four right angles. But it also presents an *octonary* "in the most secret manner of which I doubt whether our predecessors, the magi, ever beheld it, and which you will especially note". The *octonary* emerges when the two horizontal arms are divided into two equal parts. The vertical arm is divided into one longer (inferior) part comprising three units and a shorter (superior) part comprising one unit of length.

## VI. The Eight Mothers of Paracelsus and the Ilech and the Parentes Elementati

So far we have dealth with:

(1) the conjunction of the higher and lower elements in ancient and Renaissance sources;

(2) the question: what are the higher elements? (Zorzi and the double fire);

[114] John Dee's text and C. H. Josten's translation in *Ambix*, **12**, 1964, Theorema VI, pp. 156–7: Ternarium quidem: ex duabus Rectis, & Communi utrisque, quasi Copulativo Puncto. Quaternarium vero: ex 4 Rectis, includentibus 4 Angulos rectos. Singulis, bis, (ad hoc) repetitis; (Sicque, ibidem, secretissime, etiam Octonarius, sese offert: quem, dubito an nostri Praedecessores, Magi, unquam conspexerint: Notabis maxime.)

(3) the *Prime Matter* of Paracelsus created or non-created?
(4) Eightnesses as based on the conjunction of higher and lower elements.

Our discussion should have led us to a better understanding of *Eightnesses*—a concept so often turning up unexpectedly from Hellenistic and Gnostic times throughout the Middle Ages and after. It would seem to be based in all its remote ramifications on one fundamental idea; four higher and four lower elements and their conjunction. What the "higher elements" were we have submitted in the present paper.

There is still one more *topos* which now appears accessible in the light of the conjunction of the higher and lower elements. It is the *Eight Mothers*—a *topos* of great importance because (*a*) it is Paracelsian, and (*b*) because of the difficulties experienced by previous interpreters.[115]

THE EIGHT MOTHERS AS TWO QUATERNIOS

We venture to suggest that these *Eight Mothers* are simply another version of the many *Eightnesses* which we have discussed. Like these, they indicate the two sets of *quaternios*, namely the higher and the lower elements, and their conjunction. Each of the traditional four elements would, then, form a *mother*, *i.e.*, a field that consists of two parts—one higher celestial and one lower earthly. Each of these four twin elements is productive of groups of natural objects, each with its specific hallmark of origin.

THE QUADRIPARTITE AND DOUBLE QUADRIPARTITE WORLD OF PARACELSUS

However, it would seem that, apart from the *eight mothers*, Paracelsus does not anywhere give expression to eightness in his natural philosophy. On the contrary, in one place he emphasizes that "God set up the world in a quaternary and let it be completed therewith although he could have made eight" (Got die welt in ein gevierts gesezt, und lassen genug sein damit, der wol hett mögen acht machen.)[116]

And yet, when we look for it we can hardly avoid meeting the two quaternaries in various genuine Paracelsian places. For example, the world com-

[115] Goldammer, *Artelt-Festschrift* (61), 134, n. 62: "Zur Achtzahl, die wiederum religionsgeschichtlich eine uralte, weit über die Gnosis hinaus- und zurückreichende Bedeutung hat (vor allem in Aegypten) und bei Paracelsus—allerdings mehr beim untergeschobenen als beim echten—eine gewisse Rolle spielt, vergleiche Walter Pagel und Marianne Winder: The eightness of Adam and related 'Gnostic' ideas in the Paracelsian Corpus. In *Ambix*, 1969, *16*, 119–39. Aufklärung darüber, was nun eigentlich die acht Mütter an unserer dunklen Stelle sind, vermögen die Autoren auch nicht zu verschaffen (vgl. p. 129 ss.)".

[116] *Philosophia de generationibus et fructibus elementorum*, I, cap. 8; Sudhoff XIII, 15.

prises a lower and an upper heaven. The former consists of the two lower elements, earth and water, and the latter of the two upper elements, namely fire which should be called *astrum* and air which also stands for *chaos*. In order that the earth can bring forth fruit there is need for four more agents, namely sun, moon, star and air. These together would give us the two quaternaries, *i.e.*, the eightness we are looking for. At the same time we would be justified in regarding the former elemental quaternary as female and the latter as male.[117]

At all events, Paracelsus evidently recognized invisible upper and spiritual elements as distinct from lower corporeal elements in a way comparable to that of Zorzi.[118] Moreover, Paracelsus stipulates the *spiritual* nature and essence of elements in contrast to their corporeal manifestations.[119]

A hidden and somewhat abortive eightness in Paracelsus' elemental theory may be found in the *Opus Paramirum* where a distinction is made between *Two Anatomies* (*zwo anatomien*). One is that of the greater world, and the other that of the lesser world of man. The latter is divided into a male and a female anatomy. Still in the same place, Paracelsus makes man *concordant* to the greater world with its four elements, in other words, man, too, should consist of such a quaternary. He says that the generations of the outer world repeat themselves in man—the lesser world being like the four mothers belonging to the greater world.[120]

### CONJUNCTION OF QUATERNARIES IN PARACELSUS

Moreover, Paracelsus introduces the *conjunction* of two quaternaries. This conjunction is entered into by one upper and one lower quaternary. The matter occurs where he says that a *conjunction* takes place (*a*) in man (as a microcosm) between the various "fruits" of each elemental *matrix* in him and (*b*) in the corresponding elemental "fruits" in heaven. For example, microcosmic Saturn meets Saturn, the fruit of the celestial element fire, microcosmic melissa the fruit of celestial earth, microcosmic metal the fruit of celestial water, and microcosmic dew the fruit of celestial air.[121]

This passage not only reveals a hidden eightness but also the concept of higher—celestial—elements. These, as *matrices*, are productive of each of the specific *higher* elemental "fruit" which corresponds to a specific lower elemental

[117] *Opus Paramirum* IV *De matrice*; Sudhoff IX, 177, 184.

[118] *Philosophia de generationibus et fructibus elementorum*, I, cap. 4, Sudhoff, XIII, 12.

[119] *Liber meteororum*, cap. 2, Sudhoff XIII, 138.

[120] *Opus paramirum* II, cap. 2; Sudhoff IX, 95.

[121] To this see the important essay by K. Goldammer, "Paracelsus, Kosmologie und Materietheorie in ihrer wissenschaftsgeschichtlichen Stellung und Eigenart", *Medizinhistorisches Journal*, **6**, 5–35 (26–7), 1971.

"fruit" in man. In other words, we encounter here an analogue to the higher and lower elements of the Renaissance authors discussed above.

### SPIRITUALIZATION OF THE "HIGHER" ELEMENTS AND THE POSITION OF FIRE

Paracelsus' distinction between higher—spiritual and invisible—elements such as air and fire, and lower—corporeal visible—elements such as earth and water reflects a spiritualization of the former.[122]

Closely related to this is Paracelsus' denial of the elemental nature of fire. This is merely destructive—hence not elemental. In reality, what is meant by fire is a higher celestial agent, an *elementum coeli*, the firmament.[123] However, it is true that Paracelsus does not seem to have been consistent in this matter; for *loci* can be adduced in which fire—the *elementum ignis*—occurs as elemental *matrix* on the same level as the other elements. Thus it is said that crystals, beryls, ice and thunderbolt "descend from the element fire" (*ex elemento ignis descendunt*).[124] This is in some way connected with Paracelsus' version of *graded medicine* as expounded in the treatise *De gradibus*. Galen associated each of four grades of qualities (heat, cold and so on) with a number of individual substances; by contrast, Paracelsus associated each of four grades with one element: for example, pepper displays the fourth degree of heat in Galen whilst all "fruit" belonging to the element fire represents a fourth degree in Paracelsus.

Fire as an element on the same level as the elements air, water and earth is found where Paracelsus presents the act of creation as one of *separating* and *removing*. As we mentioned (p. 111 and n. 79), this basically chemical version of creation is found in genuine treatises, perhaps most succinctly in that *On the generation and fruits of the elements* and not only in the *Philosophia ad Athenienses* which is regarded as spurious. This is a point of great interest in the light of Paracelsus' ideas on the *prima materia*.[125] Here he says:

> Thus this first Iliastric body was a mass (*kloz*) in which all herbs, all water, all gems, all minerals, all stones, all chaos lay. These the highest fabricator alone has separated off and fashioned so subtly that that which he had taken away became something different. First he has separated off the air, and from the rest three more came into being,

[122] *Philosophia de generationibus et fructibus elementorum*, lib. I, cap. 4, Sudhoff XIII, 11–12.

[123] *Liber meteororum*, cap. 1, Sudhoff XIII, 133.

[124] Collectanea to *De gradibus et compositionibus medicamentorum simplicium*, cap. 4, Sudhoff IV 94.

[125] See above, pp. 106–14.

namely fire, water and earth. From these he took away fire so that two remained, and so to the end.[126]

ILECH AND PARENTES ELEMENTATI

Our story of elemental conjunction in the upper and lower world requires a look at still another Paracelsian topos: *Ilech.* This has more than one meaning. Traditionally and largely it is interpreted as an instance of *conjunction*—the union, that is, of earthly beings, including man, with supercelestial forces.[127] This is visualized as prolonging life, and the classical locus is found in Paracelsus' treatise *On Long Life.* Here the union is said to operate through outside objects. The latter are called "mansions of supercelestial things". They transfer virtues, such as heavenly dew—*tereniabin, i.e.*, a sweetness transmitted by the air, and *nostoch, i.e.*, an astral missile. Any elemental "fruit" that comes to man from outside can be effective when it communicates a virtue of a "foreign microcosm" and is thereby enabled to govern the physical body. The forces resulting from such a union (*syncoelestis conjunctio, colligatio*) are enormous (*ingentes, eximia virtute*). They explain the admirable forces which can be displayed by a plant such as *melissa* (balm) when it has achieved *conjunction* with the outside cosmos. It thus prolongs life just as *urtica* (nettle) burns and *flammula* is exceedingly bright coloured. Such effects are *magnalia*—divine mysteries. The carriers of such supernatural forces are called *bamahemi*.[128]

When incorporated in elemental matter (*elementatus*) nothing that happens

[126] *Philosophia de generationibus et fructibus elementorum*, cap. 6, Sudhoff XIII, 13, as quoted above, p. 112, note 79 in the original German.

[127] *Supranaturale et primum ex astris coniunctio supercoelestis et siderum firmamenti cum astris rerum inferiorum unio.* Martin Ruland, *Lexicon Alchemicum*, Francofurti, 1612, 262.

[128] Paracelsus, *De vita longa*, lib. IV, cap. 8, ed. Sudhoff, vol. III, 284. According to Gerard Dorn, the Paracelsian meaning of *bamaheu* is *Curriculi supernaturalium.* See G. Dorneus, *Dictionarium Theophrasti Paracelsi continens obscuriorum vocabulorum, quibus in suis scriptis passim utitur, definitiones.* Francofurti, 1584, 23; Bartholomaeus Castellus, *Lexicon Medicum*, ed. J. P. Bruno, Lipsiae, 1713, 99 sub *Bamahemi.* The present authors suggest that *Bamahemi* recalls the Hebrew *Bamah, i.e.*, a high place, most frequently used for the site of an altar and idolatry. See Julius Fürst, *Hebräisches und Chaldäisches Hand-Wörterbuch*, 1853, vol. I, 195–7. According to Buxtorf, it is Ara idolis consecrata vel cui idola imponuntur, corruptum a Graece *Bōmos* (*Lexicon Chaldaicum Talmudicum et Rabbinicum*, ed. B. Fischer, Leipzig, 1875, 166). For the *Talmudic sources* see Zwi Weinberg in A. Ehrman, *Talmud El-Am*, translation and commentary, Jerusalem–Tel Aviv, 1965, to: *Berakoth*, fol. 14a, 318, referring to Akkadian *Bam-tu*(*m*), *ban-tu*, the back ridge of a mountain. In the Bible used for altars in the high places of cities, also whole shrines and temples of pagan worship, in some periods of Jewish history permitted, in others banned. In Talmudic parlance *bama* stands for the idolatrous act of scarificing on an unauthorised altar.

through the "exaltations" of both worlds "can be taken from it",[129] *i.e.*, from "plainly Ilech". Through Ilech, spiritual man (*Aniadus*) is regenerated in us, and our life is prolonged through the latter's union with the macrocosm—*celestial man*. Such supernatural and marvellous powers (*exaltations*) can be also transferred to inert elements (*matrices*) through *Ilech*. Similarly *Ilech* is said to achieve the union of an astral force with the members of the body, thus becoming an indwelling moving power. A member is thus moved according to its *Ilech*. This includes such movement as cerebral paroxysm with unconsciousness and "turbulentia ventorum" affecting any internal organ.[130]

More remotely *Ilech* is used as the source for active force of any kind such as a mineral force (*spara*, *i.e.*, a hunting spear) which is said to stem from the *Ilech* of prime matter.[131] It lies in the internal-elemental constitution of an object. Thus the internal constitution—principle—of a river or of wine is said to be from the *Ilech* and not from its surface[132]—and a stone with certain properties is called Ilech.[133] The provenience of Ilech from air in sweet dew and its action on brain, heart and spleen are emphasized.[134]

The whole concept is, of course, reminiscent of the practice common in natural magic, ancient, mediaeval and Renaissance, of transferring powers and virtues to objects of nature and art.[135]

## THE PARACELSIAN PARENTES ELEMENTATI PATER ELEMENTATUS AND MATER ELEMENTATA

The union of a higher male and a lower female partner is evidently intended when Paracelsus introduces the *Pater Elementatus* and the *Mater Elementata*. These occur at an isolated place and as isolated termini in a chapter heading.[136] The concept is not developed in any detail. However, its occurrence in a

[129] *De vita longa*, liber IV, cap. 8. Sudhoff III, 284.

[130] Kolleg-niederschrift zu Liber III, *Paragraphorum de caducis*, cap. 2, Sudhoff V, 291.

[131] Sudhoff V, 158, *Annotationes in libros duos Theophrasti De tartaro in librum I, tr. 4, in cap. I*, here also called *Idestrum*—a conjunction which may be *humoralis*, *naturalis* or *mineralis* (*e.g.*, vis crystalli), Kollegienheft to Liber I, *De gradibus*, cap. 2, Sudhoff IV, 92.

[132] Kollegienheft to *De Morbis ex Tartaro Oriundis*, I, tr. 5, cap. 2, Sudhoff V, 42.

[133] "Lapis est ad scindendum facilis" (as differing from amethyst). Sudhoff IV, 128: "Ilech lapis est". (*De gradibus V, In caput secundum*).

[134] *De Gradibus et Compositionibus Receptorum et Naturalium*, lib. IV, cap. 6, Sudhoff IV, 38.

[135] For ancient sources: P. Festugière, *La révélation d'Hermes Trismegiste*, I, Paris, 1950, 196 and 222; E. R. Dodds, *The Greeks and the irrational*, Berkeley and Los Angeles, 1951, 246; Dietlinde Goltz: *Studien zur Geschichte der Mineralnamen in Pharmazie, Chemie und Medizin von den Anfängen bis Parcelsus* (Sudhoff's Archiv, supplement XIV), Wiesbaden, 1972, 26–8.

[136] Paracelsus, *Liber Meteororum*, ed. Sudhoff XIII, 128.

genuine Paracelsian treatise can claim our attention. Moreover, it may be correlated with the thesis of Adam von Bodenstein, the early Paracelsist, that "man is made through four parents", two mothers and two fathers, each with a material and a celestial component. (See above p. 96 and note 10.)

## Summary and Conclusions

(1) The main subject examined is the "marital" conjunction of "higher"–male, celestial–elements with "lower"–female, earthly-elements, as propounded by Renaissance philosophers, and its emergence in the genuine Paracelsus.

(2) To understand the nature and significance of the "higher" elements a full analysis of the concept as found in Georgius Venetus (Zorzi) has been provided, also with reference to such predecessors as Ficino and Pico. Additionally, new material has been adduced concerning the distinction between a "higher"—non-destructive, but generating, bright—celestial-fire and its opposite—the dark, consuming-fire, a distinction extant in the authentic Paracelsus (*essential* versus *material* fire). The idea has been followed up from Aristotle through Stoicism, Gnostic and Kabbalistic/Rabbinical sources to Zorzi himself and Alstedius. The ambivalent position of fire in Paracelsus's elemental doctrines has also been examined.

(3) The "higher" and the "lower" quaternaries of elements provide another instance of *Eightness*—a symbol widely used and with extensive, remote and unexpected ramifications in Gnostic, mediaeval and Paracelsian philosophy. The examples given in a previous communication have now been supplemented, and the concept of Eightness of Elements has been shown to elucidate a genuine Paracelsian idea which has so far baffled Paracelsian scholars: that of the *Eight mothers*.

(4) Conjunction of the four "higher" and four "lower" elements appears to underlie two further genuine Paracelsian topoi: *Ilech* and the *Parentes elementati* (*pater elementatus et mater elementata*).

(5) The "higher" elements are finally reflected in Paracelsus' idea of *Prime matter* as a divine spiritual "boundary"-stage *before* all creation and "information". This position has now been further documented through not one but a variety of loci from the *genuine* Paracelsus.

(6) While it is true that some of the "unorthodox" doctrines receive more emphasis in spurious "deutero-Paracelsian" tracts, those here analysed are genuine Paracelsian, though sometimes not so outspoken and somewhat diluted. Occasionally it is just in unequivocally spurious treatises that religious-orthodox opinions are vented—in contrast to treatises of recognized authenticity. The examples from authentic treatises include divine creative activity as an act of separation and addition rather than creation *de novo*.

*Acknowledgment*

W.P. wishes to recall with gratitude the many discussions which he was privileged to have with the Rev. T. F. Glasson, D.D., and with Professor Gershom Scholem and the inspiration and literary help he derived from them for the present paper.

# X

## Das Rätsel der „Acht Mütter" im Paracelsischen Corpus

*Paracelsus* weist in seinem naturalistischen Weltbilde den vier Elementen ihre traditionelle Stelle an. Dies gilt besonders von seinem chemischen Werk und umfaßt auch das Feuer, obschon er an anderer Stelle dessen Charakter als Element leugnet und es durch ein „elementum coeli", das Firmament, ersetzt[1]. Die traditionelle Elementenlehre wird aber bei *Paracelsus* überschattet durch seine Auffassung der klassischen Elemente nicht als Komponenten individueller Naturobjekte, sondern als spezifische Keimböden mit spezifischen Produkten oder „Früchten". In diesem Sinne ist jedes der vier „Elemente" eine „Mutter", die gebiert: „Aus den vier mütern werden alle ding geboren der ganzen welt"[2]. Damit setzt sich *Paracelsus* in Gegensatz zur herrschenden Tradition – ein Gegensatz, der nicht nur der elementaren Zusammensetzung der Objekte, sondern vor allem den elementaren „Complexionen" gilt. Es ist „unnüz geret, das das element ein complex an im habe, heiß oder trocken, kalt oder feucht . . . dan sie seind alle vier in im: die erden ist kalt und trocken, kalt und feucht, heiß und trocken, heiß und feucht . . . das ir nit nach den complexionen die element sezen, sonder nach irer form, das ist wie die vier müter an inen haben"[3]. Es sind also nicht vier Elemente in einem Ding und daher auch nicht die Mischungen von „Complexionen" oder Qualitäten, die zu jedem dieser Elemente gehören und vorwiegen oder mangeln. Vielmehr besteht in „ietlichem ding" nur „ein complexion und nicht mer und mag auch kein ander element in im haben, dan sovil es von seiner muter hat"[4]. Das Objekt ist mithin eine „Frucht" mit spezifischen Eigenschaften seiner spezifischen „Mutter", nämlich des einen Elements, zu dem es kraft der Eigenschaften gehört, mit denen es gesiegelt ist. So sind z. B. „alle

[1] Feuer, Firmament, elementum coeli: *Paracelsus:* Liber meteoror. cap. I (Hrsg. *K. Sudhoff*; Bd. XIII, S. 133; im folgenden Sudh. mit Band und Seitenzahl).

[2] Elemente, vier mütern: De generatione et fructibus elementorum I, 3 (de elemento aeris; Sudh. XIII, 10).

[3] Complexion: l. c. XIII, 11.

[4] Liber meteor. I, 2 (Sudh. XIII, 135). Vielleicht besteht hier ein Zusammenhang mit der paracelsischen Wendung in der Lehre von den „Graden der Stoffe". Diese bezeichnen bei *Paracelsus* nicht mehr die Qualität individueller Substanzen, sondern die Eigenschaft der „Mutter", aus der eine Gruppe verwandter Stoffe stammen. So wären z. B. alle Abkömmlinge des Feuers „im vierten Grad" usw.

frücht des elements aquae . . . salia, mineralia, gemmae et lapides"; Pflanzen, Tiere und Mensch sind „Früchte" der „Mutter Erde"[5].

*Plato* spricht im Timaeus von dem, was „ist" und nicht „entsteht" und dem, was „entsteht" und nicht „ist". Das erstere sind die immer bestehenden und sich gleich bleibenden „Modelle" (εἴδη) und das letztere die immer wechselnden, aus einem etwas anderes, „dies oder das" werdenden, sie nachahmenden Bilder (εἴδολα); das sind die sicht- und tastbaren Körper. Außer diesen „zwei" muß aber noch ein „drittes" unterschieden werden, nämlich ein fortdauerndes in sich gleich bleibendes Aufnahmegefäß für die sich verändernden, entstehenden und vergehenden Objekte. Dieses Rezeptakel (ὑποδοχή) ist gestaltlos, aber ein bewegliches „Magma", das unter dem Druck von seiten der Abbilder, die ein- und austreten, Gestalt anzunehmen *scheint.* Es ist sozusagen eine „Pflegerin" (τιθήνη) für die Abbilder, eine Pflegemutter oder, da sie dauernd alle Dinge aufnimmt, einer „Mutter" schlechthin vergleichbar (προσεικάσαι πρέπει τὸ μὲν δεχόμενον μητρί)[6]. In diesem Vergleich nehmen die ewigen Vorbilder die Stellung von „Vätern", der gestaltlose „empfangende" Raum („Materie")[7] die der „Mutter" und die

[5] Früchte des Wassers: De gen. et fruct. element. IV, 1, 4 (Sudh. XIII, 88).

[6] Timaeus 50 D – 51 B. Dazu *F. M. Cornford:* Plato's Cosmology. The Timaeus of Plato transl. with running comment. London 1937. S. 187. – Das Rezeptakel (50 A), dazu *Cornford* l. c. 181–185. – Rezeptakel als Raum: 51 E – 52 D, dazu *Cornford* l. c. 191–201. – *A. E. Taylor:* Plato Timaeus and Critias transl. London 1929. S. 47–51. – *K. J. Windischmann:* Platons Timäos. Eine ächte Urkunde wahrer Physik. Hadamar 1804. S. 77–83. Zur Modifikation der platonischen Lehre s. Aristoteles, Physik I, 9, 192 a 20 und 192 a 13: ἀλλὰ τοῦτ ἔστιν ἡ ὕλη, ὥσπερ ἂν εἰ θῆλυ ἄρρενος καὶ αἰσχρόν καλοῦ . . . ἡ μὲν γὰρ ὑπομένουσα συναιτία τῇ μορφῇ τῶν γινομένων ἐστίν, ὥσπερ μήτηρ. In *C. Prantl:* Aristoteles Acht Bücher Physik. Leipzig 1854. S. 50 f.: „dies ist das Wesen des Stoffes etwa wie wenn das Weibliche Stoff des Männlichen und das Häßliche Stoff des Schönen wäre" . . . S. 49: „jenes Substantielle, welches bestehen bleibt, ist allerdings Mitursache für die Gestaltung des Entstehenden gleichsam wie eine *Mutter*".

[7] Raum-Materie: *Clemens Baeumker:* Das Problem der Materie in der griechischen Philosophie. Münster 1890. S. 113: „so ergibt sich für Plato die Notwendigkeit eines zweiten Prinzips neben den Ideen für die Erklärung der Weltbildung. Es ist dasjenige Element der Wirklichkeit, welches er im Timaeus als das allgemeine Receptaculum, als Mutter und Pflegerin alles Werdenden bezeichnet und welches wir nach dem Vorgang des Aristoteles mit einem aristotelischen, für Plato freilich nicht völlig zutreffenden Ausdrucke die platonische Materie zu nennen gewöhnt sind. Daß der Name *hyle* dem Plato fremd, hebt Chalcidius in Tim. c. 308 mit Recht hervor. Der Ausdruck findet seine volle Erklärung als technischer Terminus in der Tat erst mit dem aristotelischen Begriff der Materie als des Gestaltbaren, Potentiellen"; vgl. *Zeller* (3. Aufl.) II a 605, 1.

X

256

flüchtigen Dinge die der geborenen Produkte an. Daraus folgt, und dies wird ausdrücklich hervorgehoben, daß die „Mutter“ (Raum-Materie) keineswegs Erde oder Luft, Feuer, Wasser oder irgendeine ihrer Verbindungen oder Bestandteile genannt werden darf. Denn sie ist bloße Pflegerin oder Ziehmutter, die dem Erzeugnis des Vaters Nahrung und Raum gewährt.

Der Timaeus kann mithin nicht als Quelle für die paracelsische Auffassung der Elemente als „Mütter“ gelten, oder doch nur in sehr entferntem und übertragenen Sinne. Viel näher liegt hier die Tradition der jüdisch-arabischen Gnosis und Mystik, wie sie im Buche der Schöpfung (Sepher Jezirah) und in den Schriften der *Lauteren Brüder* Niederschlag gefunden hat. Das Jezira-Buch, auf neupythagoreischer Zahlensymbolik und hebräischer Buchstabenmystik gegründet, stammt wahrscheinlich noch aus vorchristlicher Zeit und ist im Mittelalter vielfach besprochen und kommentiert worden. Dadurch war es den christlichen Kabbalisten vor und in der Lebenszeit von *Paracelsus* bekannt, obschon es im Druck erst 1552 in der lateinischen Übersetzung und Paraphrase von *Guil. Postelius* und dann hebräisch 1562 in Mantua erschienen ist[8]. Hier sind deutlich die drei „Elemente“ Luft, Wasser, Feuer als „Drei Mütter“ (*Sch'losch Immoth*) eingeführt. Sie sind mit ihren Entsprechungen in „Welt, Mensch und Jahr“ übersichtlich im Buche „Kusari“ des *Jehuda ha-Levi* (1130) zusammengestellt[9]:

| Drei Mütter: | Aleph | Mem | Schin |
|---|---|---|---|
| In der Welt: | Luft | Wasser | Feuer |
| Im Menschen: | Brust | Leib | Kopf |
| Im Jahr: | Feuchte | Kälte | Hitze |

[8] Sefer Jezirah, Liber de creatione. In: *Joh. Pistorius Nidanus:* Artis cabbalisticae Tomus I. Basel (Henr. Petri) 1587. S. 870, cap. 3. – Liber Jezirah translatus et notis illustratus a Jo. Stephano Rittangelio. Amsterdam 1642. Cap. III, sect. 2–4. S. 201 f. – *Lazarus Goldschmidt:* Sepher Jesirah – Das Buch der Schöpfung. Frankfurt 1894. III, S. 56. – Zur Lit.: *A. Franck – Ad. Gelinek (Jellinek):* Die Kabbala oder die Religionsphilosophie der Hebräer. 1844. S. 112 f. – *Christ. D. Günsburg:* The Kabbalah. London 1865. S. 151. – *E. O. von Lippmann:* Entstehung und Ausbreitung der Alchemie. Bd. II. Berlin 1931. S. 150. – Grundlegend und kritisch: *G. Scholem:* Ursprung und Anfänge der Kabbala. Berlin 1962. S. 23–25; der zahlen-mystische Teil des Lib. Jezirah als neu-pythagoreisch (*Nikomachus von Gerasa,* um 140 n. Chr. im Ost-Jordanland), die Buchstaben-Mystik innerjüdisch-talmudisch aufgefaßt. Sprachlich spricht nichts gegen das 2.–3. Jahrhundert als Verfassungszeit. In der hier erheb-

Die drei „Mütter" sind zunächst durch drei der 22 Buchstaben bezeichnet[10]. Von diesen entspricht der erste der Luft (*Avjr*) und der Welt, dem Makrokosmos, der zweite dem Wasser (*Majim*), der Seele und dem Menschen als Inbegriff der Schöpfung, d. h. als Mikrokosmos und der dritte dem Feuer (*Esch*) und den Jahreszeiten. „Welt, Mensch und Jahr" bilden weitere Kategorien von Entsprechungen. Die Erde ist unter den Elementen nicht genannt, da sie als emanatives Verdichtungsprodukt des Wassers (*tholdoth erez majim*) aufgefaßt wird, ähnlich dem Himmel, der vom Feuer, und dem Wind, der von der Luft emaniert. Nach *Jehuda ha-Levi* ist die Erde nicht erwähnt, da sie den Stoff hergibt, aus dem *alle* Erzeugnisse gemacht sind, während man wohl von feurigen, luftigen und wässerigen Körpern spricht. Das Wasser ist als Urstoff passend gewählt – ein dichterer Körper als das Wasser wäre unbildsam in allen seinen Teilen gewesen. Die Natur bearbeitet den Stoff nur und bildet ihn nach ihrem Gefallen, solange er in Wassergestalt ist.

Weiterhin finden wir die vier Elemente als „die *Mütter* alles Seins, aus denen Minerale, Pflanze und Tier entstanden" in den Schriften der *Lauteren Brüder* aus dem 10. Jahrhundert[11]. Es heißt dort auch: „die vier Elemente, die so genannten Mütter, sind Wasser, Feuer, Luft, Erde"[12] und „die Körper unter der Mondsphäre bestehen aus sieben Arten. Vier davon sind die Allmütter (Elemente) und drei die erzeugten Teilwesen, Tier, Pflanze und Mineral"[13]. Ferner wäre aus dem islamischen Kulturkreis *al-Qazwini* zu erwähnen (1203–1283)[14]. In

lichen Stelle wird meist *Immoth* als „Mütter" gelesen. Aber Saadja- und Geniza-Manuskripte lesen nicht *Immoth*, sondern *Ummoth* „Fundament" (*Scholem* l. c.).

[9] *Jehudah ha-Levi:* Das Buch Kusari, nach dem hebräischen Text des Jehuda ibn Tibbon her, übers. u. komment. von *David Cassel.* Leipzig 1853. Tract. IV, 25; S. 348 f.

[10] Elemente – Stoicheia – Buchstaben des Alphabets: *Hermann Diels:* Elementum. Eine Vorarbeit zum griechischen und lateinischen Thesaurus. Leipzig 1899. S. 81 f.

[11] *Fried. Dieterici:* Die Philosophie der Araber im IX. und X. Jahrhundert n. Chr. aus der Theologie des Aristoteles, den Abhandlungen Alfarabis und den Schriften der Lauteren Brüder. I. Einleitung und Makrokosmos. Leipzig 1876. S. 133.

[12] l. c. II (1879), 200.

[13] l. c. V (1876), 55. – S. auch *E. O. von Lippmann:* Entstehung und Ausbreitung der Alchemie. I. Berlin 1919. S. 372: „Arkan", Elemente, „Allmütter", „Mütter alles Seins" bei den Lauteren Brüdern.

[14] *Zakarija ben Muhammed ben Mahmud el-Kazwini's* Kosmographie nach der Wüstenfeldchen Ausgabe aus dem Arab. übers. von *M. Ethé.* Leipzig 1868. Teil II über die Erscheinungen der sublunaren Welt (S. 182). S. auch Lippmann a.a.O. (Anm. 13) S. 412.

seiner (vielleicht nicht authentischen) Kosmographie wird der elementarische Urstoff (*el-ansar*) den sogenannten *maudu'at* zugrunde gelegt. Damit sind die erst gesetzten Elementkörper unter der Mondsphäre, die „Mütter", *ummahat,* gemeint. Aus diesen gehen die „Erzeugnisse" – *muwalladat* – Mineralien, Pflanzen und Tiere, hervor. Die Elemente schlechthin werden auch *arkan* genannt und ihrer gibt es vier, Feuer, Luft, Wasser, Erde. Die Urmaterie als „Mutter" ist der „Strom", der aus Eden ausgeht, in einem Fragment über das Paradies des *Salomo ibn Gabirol* (1021–1058), das durch *Abraham ibn Esra* überliefert ist[15]. Die „Mutter"-Urmaterie spaltet sich in die „vier Häupter" oder Elemente alles Daseienden (*hanahar ch'em l'chol ha-gwijoth w'arbah roschim hem ha-schorschim*).

In der *Alchemie* wird dem *Gefäß,* mit dem gearbeitet wird, eine besondere symbolische Bedeutung zuerkannt. Es ist das *ovum Philosophorum,* in das „unser Stein" zu legen ist, damit er durch „Feuer und Kunst" Vollendung erreicht. So sagt König *Haly:* das Gefäß ist die Wurzel und gleichsam die *Matrix,* wie sie in den Tieren empfängt und den Conceptus ernährt[16].

Es liegt nahe anzunehmen, daß *Paracelsus* an diese „Mütter"-Tradition angeknüpft hat, wie er auch sonst arabische und hebräische Termini verwendet hat. Beispiele sind: *Tereniabin* für den Himmelstau und *Bamahemi* als Träger übernatürlicher Kräfte[17]. *Reuchlins* Buch „De arte cabalistica" war seit 1517 im Druck zugänglich. *Paracelsus* verwendet vielfach den Ausdruck „Kabbala" und „kabbalistisch" für seine tiefere Weisheit, die die oberflächlichen traditionellen Lehren ersetzen müsse. Ob er das Werk von *Reuchlin* oder ähnliches in der Hand gehabt oder davon gehört hat, wissen wir nicht. Es ist aber nicht unwahrscheinlich. Auf jeden Fall hätte er bei *Reuchlin* die Lehre des Buches

[15] *David Kaufmann:* Studien über Salomon ibn Gabirol. Budapest 1899. S. 69.

[16] Ludus puerorum in: De alchimia opuscula complura veterum Philosophorum. Frankfurt 1550. fol. 138r. – Artis auriferae. II. Basel 1610. S. 115. Dazu *M. A. Atwood:* Suggestive enquiry into the Hermetic Mystery with a dissertation on the more celebrated Alchemical Philosophers. 3rd ed. Belfast 1920. S. 146. – Im Text des „Ludus" heißt es: „vas est tamquam matrix in animalibus, quia in eo generant et concipiunt generationem pariter et nutriuntur" (de vase sive ovo philosophorum in quo lapis noster ponendus est, ut igne et arte perficiatur).

[17] Zu „Tereniabin" und seiner alchemistischen Tradition vgl. *E. O. von Lippmann:* Geschichte des Zuckers. Leipzig 1890. S. 83–85 (2. Aufl. Berlin 1929. S. 145). – Zu „Bamahemi" vgl. *W. Pagel* u. *M. Winder*: The Higher Elements and Prime Matter in Renaissance Naturalism and in Paracelsus. Ambix 21 (1974), 93–127 (S. 124 und Anm. 128).

„Jezira" von den drei Elementen als „Müttern" finden können, sowie weitere Anführungen aus ihm. Es heißt dort, daß die Kombinationen und Permutationen der zwei und zwanzig *Elemente* (das heißt hier zunächst Buchstaben des hebräischen Alphabets) in keiner Weise als „bäurisch" und „ungelehrt" anzusehen sind. Denn es handelt sich um Dinge des göttlichen Geistes. So „steht geschrieben im Buche Jetzira, mit jenem Geiste hat Gott die zwei und zwanzig Buchstaben ausgehauen, *drei Mütter,* sieben doppelte und zwölf einfache". Dies gehört zu den Mysterien der heiligen Schriften, dem Geistigen, das Gegenstand der Kontemplation und des frommen, glücklich machenden und nicht zu verspottenden Glaubens ist. Im Glauben an die Buchstaben gelangen wir leicht zum Nachdenken über Höheres und vertrauen darauf, daß Geheimnisse in den Buchstaben gefunden werden können, wie die Anrede Gottes an Mose in der Dunkelheit [18].

Woher auch immer die Anregung, *Paracelsus* hat der „Mutter-Theorie" eine Wendung gegeben und sie in eigener Weise durchgeführt und systematisiert. Dabei bleibt er allerdings bei der alten aristotelischen Tradition, nach der z. B. die Minerale und Metalle vom Wasser abgeleitet werden [19].

*Paracelsus* spricht gewöhnlich von den Elementen und „Müttern" in der Vierzahl der Tradition. Er sagt sogar: „got die welt in ein gevierts gesezt, und lassen genug sein damit, der wol hett mögen acht machen" [20]. Man möchte glauben, daß hierin ein Hinweis auf die sehr alte und mindestens gnostische Tradition der *„Achtheiten"* gegeben ist. Diese kommen wirklich im Paracelsischen Corpus zum Ausdruck [21], und die angeführte Stelle scheint zu zeigen, daß sich *Paracelsus* selbst der Bedeutung der Achtheiten, ihrer Symbolik und Tradition bewußt war. Der „achtteilige" Adam und die „acht Astronomien" gehören nicht authentischen, „deutero-paracelsischen" Traktaten an. Die *„acht Mütter"* dagegen finden sich in der als früh angesehenen Abhandlung „Von den podagrischen Krankheiten" [22]. Es ist in einer Spekulation über das,

[18] *Joh. Reuchlin:* De arte cabalistica. Lib. III. Hagenau 1517. fol. LXXII v. Als Appendix zu *Joh. Picus de Mirandola:* Opera. Basel 1557. S. 878 f. (Nachdruck Stuttgart – Bad Cannstadt. S. 256).

[19] Siehe oben Anm. 5.

[20] got-welt-gevierts: Phil. de gener. et fruct. element. I, 8 (Sudh. XIII, 15).

[21] Achtheiten: vgl. *W. Pagel* u. *M. Winder:* The Eightness of Adam and related Gnostic ideas in the Paracelsian Corpus. Ambix 16 (1969), 119–139. – Ferner „The Higher Elements ..." in Ambix 21 (1974), 114–123 (vgl. Anm. 17).

[22] „Von den podagrischen Krankheiten", lib. I vom Limbo (Sudh. I, 355).

was der Arzt als *Elementar*-wissen erwerben und besitzen muß, wo der Begriff auftaucht. Dies sind die „vier Philosophien" und die „vier Astronomien". Die letzteren umfassen die himmlischen, die ersteren die irdischen Dinge. Zusammen ergeben sie die „Acht Mütter". *Paracelsus* gibt ihnen mithin das gleiche Prädikat, das er sonst den traditionellen vier Elementen gibt, nämlich das der *Mutter.* Astronomie und Philosophie sind daher die *Elemente* des ärztlichen Wissens, die eine Korrespondenz von Himmlischem und Irdischem umfassen. Diese „Acht Mütter" sind in dem sog. „Limbus" oder „Samen" aller Kreaturen enthalten. Es ist der „Samen", der „sein erden hat gehabt in dem wort gottes"[23]. In ihm sind Himmlisches und Irdisches noch nicht getrennt. Anderweit identifiziert *Paracelsus* das Wort *Fiat* mit der *Prima materia,* die „vor aller Schöpfung war"[24]. Der „Limbus", in dem sich die „Acht Mütter" finden, steht also für die unkörperliche Vorform der Schöpfung, eine unsichtbare ideale „Erste Materie", ein Prolog im Himmel, dem ihre „Fleischwerdung" zunächst in Gestalt der „Tria Prima" (Mercur, Schwefel und Salz) und sodann der Elemente folgt[25].

Besitzen wir ein Modell oder eine Quelle, auf die sich die „Acht Mütter" zurückführen lassen? Da sie nach ihrer Definition acht „Elemente" sind, vier himmlische („Astronomie") und vier irdische („Philosophie"), so liegt es nahe, ein solches Modell in der Lehre von den Entsprechungen der „oberen" und der „unteren" Elemente zu finden. Diese Lehre war in der Naturphilosophie der Renaissance weit verbreitet. Sie hat einen mittelalterlichen Vorgänger in *Daniel de Morleys* „Acht Astrologien", ein Lehrstück, das auf *Alfarabi* zurückgeht und von *Gundissalinus* verbreitet wurde[25a]. Ihr Hauptvertreter in der Renaissance, *Georgius Venetus* („Zorzi", 1460 bis ca. 1540), hat *Ficinus* (1433–1499) und *Pico della Mirandola* (1463–1494) als Vorläufer, und *Agrippa von Nettesheim* (1487–1535) ist unmittelbar von ihm abhängig[26]. Sein Hauptwerk war die „Harmonia totius mundi", erschienen

[23] l. c.

[24] „Von dem Bad Pfeffers Tugenden" (Glossar i. f.; Sudh. IX, 658), folgend Opus Paramirum I, 2 (Sudh. IX, 48).

[25] *W. Pagel:* The Prime Matter of Paracelsus. Ambix 9 (1961), 117–135 (S. 121). – *W. Pagel* u. *M. Winder:* Higher Elements ... (vgl. Anm. 17), S. 106–111.

[25a] *Daniel de Morley:* Liber de naturis inferiorum et superiorum. Hrsg. v. *K. Sudhoff.* Arch. für Geschichte der Naturwiss. u. Technik 8 (1918), 1–40 (S. 34). Dazu *Lynn Thorndike:* History of Magic and Experimental Science. Vol. II. New York 1923. S. 181–187 und *C. H. Haskins:* Studies in the History of Mediaeval Science. Cambridge, Mass. 1927 (2nd ed.). S. 127.

[26] Vgl. *Pagel* u. *Winder:* Higher Elements . . . (Anm. 17), S. 97–102. Zu *Pico* und *Ficino* vgl. *K. Goldammer:* Die paracelsische Kosmologie und Materietheorie

1525 in Venedig. In diesem werden *acht Elemente* unterschieden, vier zerstörbare und vier unzerstörbare. Sie verteilen sich auf vier Reiche: die Welt hinieden, das Firmament, die Sphäre der Engel über dem Firmament und die des Archetyps (i. e. Gottes). Jedes der vier Elemente, Erde, Wasser, Luft und Feuer findet sich in allen vier Reichen, aber in Formen, Funktionen und Zuständen von Grobheit oder Feinheit, die der Würde und Bedeutung des betreffenden Reiches angepaßt sind. Es ergibt sich folgende Anordnung von je vier Quaternionen[27]:

| | Untere Welt | Firmament | Engelreich | Gott |
|---|---|---|---|---|
| Erde | Festigkeit der Körper | Himmelskörper | Gottes Thron | Fruchtbarkeit |
| Wasser | Wäscht | Regen, Mischbarkeit | Nähren und Schenken | Wegwaschung der Sünden Regeneration |
| Luft | Atmung, Sinne | Sicht jenseits der Fixsterne | Selige Sicht d. himml. Heerscharen, Hauch des Lebens | Geist d. Propheten, Kommunikation mit Gott |
| Feuer | Hitze, Kochen, Vollenden | Sonnenschein, Wärme | Seraphische – „glühende“ – Liebe | Geistiges Feuer im „brennenden Busch“ |

in ihrer wissenschaftsgeschichtlichen Stellung und Eigenart. Med. hist. J. 6 (1971) – grundlegend für den Vergleich der Materie- und Elementenlehre von *Ficinus, Pico* (Onkel und Neffe) und *Agrippa* mit der von *Paracelsus.* Siehe auch *K. Goldammer:* Bemerkungen zur Struktur des Kosmos und der Materie bei Paracelsus. In: Medizingeschichte in unserer Zeit (Heischkel-Artelt-Festgabe). Stuttgart 1971. S. 121–144 (S. 128 f. Erwähnung der „Acht Mütter als Bestandteil des Limbus“). – Zur Abhängigkeit des *Agrippa* von *Zorzi* vgl. *Wolf-Dieter Müller-Jahncke:* Magie als Wissenschaft im 16. Jahrhundert. Die Beziehungen zwischen Magie, Medizin und Pharmazie im Werk des Agrippa von Nettesheim. Diss. Marburg 1973, umfassend und von akutem Interesse. S. auch *Pagel u. Winder:* Die Konjunktion der himmlischen und irdischen Elemente in der Renaissance-Philosophie und im echten Paracelsus. Festschr. f. *K. Goldammer.* Internat. Paracelsus-Ges. Salzburg 1975/76 (in Vorbereitung).

[27] *Georgius Venetus (Zorzi):* De harmonia totius mundi. Venedig 1525. Cant. I, tonus 3, cap. 17 (fol. 53).

Die Elemente als solche sind mithin gleich, aber unterschieden durch Konstanz, Spiritualität, Feinheit und Reinheit. Der Mensch vereinigt in sich beide Quaternionen, die himmlischen und die irdischen. Daher wird, nach alter gnostischer Tradition, Adam aus acht Stücken bestehend und erschaffen vorgestellt[28]. Dies wird auch von *Zorzi* – in einer kabbalistischen Wendung[29] – und im paracelsischen Corpus zum Ausdruck gebracht. In diesem Sinne wird dann der in der alten und mittelalterlichen Alchemie geläufige Begriff des „Himmels im Menschen" gedeutet (*caelum in homine*), wie auch der Himmel selbst als ein Gemisch von Wasser und Feuer angesehen worden war. Es war *Johannes von Rupescissa,* einem häretischen Franziskaner des XIV. Jahrhunderts, auf der Suche nach den „Quintessenzen" in Pflanzen und Tieren, gelungen, ein solches „Feuerwasser" in Gestalt von Branntwein zu destillieren, die „Seele" oder den „Geist" von Wein, das „Wasser des Lebens" der hellenistischen Alchemisten-Philosophen und Spiritualisten. Es ist verschieden von den „einfachen" Elementen, denn, obwohl „heiß", wirkt es kühlend und entzündungswidrig. Indem es Fäulnis und Verderben verhindert, bewahrt es den elementaren Aufbau des Körpers vor Zersetzung und Zerfall in die ursprünglichen Elemente, die ihn zusammensetzen. Auf diese Weise bringt es den erhaltenden „Himmel in den Menschen", wie auch der Himmel erschaffen wurde zur Bewahrung und Erhaltung der Welt[30].

Auch *Paracelsus* spricht von den „oberen Elementen". Es heißt in der „Philosophia sagax": „also sol auch der mensch wissen, das der elementisch leib dermaßen an sich zeucht die siderisch kreft aus kraft der coniunction, so beide corpora miteinander haben, wie sie dann einander verfügt seind, also das der mensch der eußern elementen sol genießen, der underen und der oberen und das in eines magneten art zusamen komen in centro des menschen, da das licht der natur ligt"[31]. Hier ist die Konjunktion der „oberen" und „unteren" Elemente betont, an anderer Stelle ihr bloßer Parallelismus: „dan wie die vier matrices außerthalb wonen, in solche ist der leib auch gesezt. darumb sich hie scheiden die philosophei und astronomei"[32]. Hier begegnen uns wieder die beiden Quaternionen, die wir oben bei den „Acht Müttern"

[28] *Pagel* u. *Winder:* Eightness of Adam . . . (vgl. Anm. 21), S. 114 f.

[29] *Georgius Venetus* (vgl. Anm. 27), cant. III, tonus 6, cap. 12, part II (fol. 63 v).

[30] *W. Pagel:* Paracelsus. Basel – New York 1958. S. 263–265.

[31] Philosophia sagax I, 3 (Sudh. XII, 67).

[32] Blatern, leme, beulen, löchern u. zitrachten der franzosen IV, 1 (Sudh. VI, 368).

als vier „Astronomien“ und vier „Philosophien“ und als Vertreter der vier himmlischen und vier irdischen „Elemente“ – Mütter – kennengelernt haben. Weiterhin: „ir wissent aus andern beschribnen büchern, das die große Creatur der Parens ist Microcosmi. Daraus folget nun, vier teil sind in der großen Creatur, also seind auch vier teil in microcosmo“ [33]. Endlich ist die Rede von „quattuor elementa duplata“ [34], wo über die Extraktion der pflanzlichen Quintessenzen für die Beförderung langen Lebens verhandelt wird. In jeder Pflanze sind die vier Elemente verdoppelt. Dies gilt nicht für die Quintessenz, die ein ungeteiltes Ganzes als Teil der Pflanze ausmacht.

Die Vorstellung oberer und unterer Elemente liegt auch der Unterscheidung von Erde und Wasser auf der einen und Feuer („Astrum“) und Luft („Chaos“) auf der anderen Seite zugrunde. Die beiden letzteren werden als „zwei Himmel“ bezeichnet und der Erde und dem Wasser gegenübergestellt. Damit die Erden-matrix Früchte hervorbringen kann, werden vier weitere Faktoren benötigt: Sonne, Mond, Stern und Luft. Wie in der Erde nichts gedeihen kann, „es sei dan das solche *element* beihendig sind“, so kann auch die Gebärmutter des Menschen nichts hervorbringen ohne diese „Elemente“ [35]. Wenn alle die genannten Faktoren Anspruch auf den Titel „Element“ haben, würde hier wiederum eine Achtheit von „Elementen“ oder „Müttern“ gegeben sein.

Wir erwähnten die „Conjunction“ – diese spielt eine große Rolle für *Paracelsus* auf allen Stufen des Geistes- und Körperlebens. So liegt für ihn das Wesen der Erkenntnis in der Konjunktion des Erkennenden mit seinem Objekt. Es ist die Vereinigung ihrer Astralleiber, wodurch mit Hilfe der „Imagination“ seitens des Erkennenden die „verborgene Natur“ des Objekts hervorzukommen gezwungen wird. Denn nicht der Beobachter „weiß“, sondern das Objekt „weiß“, nämlich was es zu tun hat, um sein eigenes Wesen zu gestalten und zur Vollendung zu bringen. Das muß der nach dem Wissen Strebende dem Objekt „ablernen“ [36]. Das gilt besonders für die den Arzneidrogen innewohnende „scientia“. Auf diese Weise gelangt „mein geist“ in seinen Gegenstand.

[33] Zwei Bücher von der pestilentz u. iren zufällen. Cap. 2 (Sudh. VIII, 377).

[34] Quattuor elementa duplata in „De vita longa“ III, 5 (Sudh. III, 275).

[35] Opus paramirum IV: De matrice (Sudh. IX, 184).

[36] Scientia abzulernen: „so du nun der scamonea ir scientiam ablernst, also das in dir ist wie in der scamonea, so hast du experientiam cum scientia“ (Labyrinthus medicorum, cap. 6; Sudh. XI, 191).

„Nun sind geist im himel, geist in kreutern, geist im lufft, also im wasser. dieselbigen geist und mein geist, die komen zusammen"[37]. Ebenso gibt es die Konjunktion des Menschen mit dem Makrokosmos oder übernatürlichen Kräften, die ihn vertreten (*Ilech*), wodurch langes Leben oder sogar Unsterblichkeit erlangt werden kann[38]. Für unser Thema ist die Konjunktion der oberen und unteren Elemente in dem lapidaren Satz ausgesprochen: „also die elementen frauen von iren mannen entpfahen als von dem obern vulkanischen"[39]. Es ist die alte Idee des *hieros gamos* zwischen Himmel und Erde, der Befruchtung der letzteren durch himmlischen Tau und Regen, der Erzeugung von Lebewesen durch Samen, die vom Himmel herabfallen – Vorstellungen, die sich auf die alt-griechische Mysterien- und Tragödientradition, auf Vorsokratiker und schließlich auf die Gnosis zurück verfolgen lassen[40]. Hier ist es die himmlische „Mutter" der Erde, die nach dem Muster der oberen „Quaternion" von samenhaften, unsichtbaren Elementen die vier irdischen Elemente hervorbringt. In rabbinischer Lehre wird der Regen als „Gatte der Erde" bezeichnet[41]. Die „vulkanischen" oberen nennt *Paracelsus* auch „Archei" oder an einer isolierten Stelle „patres elementati". Diesen entsprechen die „matres elementatae"[42]. Wie bei *Plato* und *Aristoteles* ist die Rolle des Weiblichen lediglich, Platz und Nahrung für das Erzeugnis des Vaters zu stellen[43]. Durch Bezeichnung der „Schmiede" und des „Vulkanischen" als „Archei" wird eine Assoziation hergestellt mit den „Archonten" der Gnosis – jenen bösartigen „Verwaltern" (διοικητείς), astralen Demiurgen, die den Seelen auf ihrem Herabstieg das „gegenspielerische" schlechte Pneuma der Leidenschaften anhängen und ihrem Aufstieg Hindernisse in den Weg legen[44].

[37] Geist komen zusammen: De lunaticis, tr. III (Sudh. XIV, 58).

[38] De vita longa IV, 8 (Sudh. III, 284).

[39] Labyrinth. medicor. cap. 11 (Sudh. XI, 213).

[40] *Pagel* u. *Winder:* Higher Elements . . . (vgl. Anm. 17), S. 94–97.

[41] mijtra baalah d'ara – pluvia est maritus terrae – nach *Raf Jehuda* in *Joh. Buxtorf:* Lexicon Chaldaicum, Talmud. et Rabbinicum. Ed. *B. Fischer.* Leipzig 1875. S. 1085 unter „R'wijah, Regen, quod facit ut coeat terra cum ea (sc. pluvia) ad producendum concepta semina mense Octobri".

[42] Liber meteoror. (Sudh. XIII, 128).

[43] *F. M. Cornford* zu „Plato Timaeus" (1937), 187 (vgl. Anm. 6).

[44] Lit. in *W. Pagel:* Das medizinische Weltbild des Paracelsus. Seine Zusammenhänge mit Neuplatonismus und Gnosis (Kosmosophie I). Wiesbaden 1962. S. 35 f., 40–42, 74. Zu Archonten und Dämonen als Vermittlern allen Wissens – inest enim illis cognitio rerum – *Isidor:* Etymolog. VIII, 11, 15; *Barthol. Anglicus:* De proprietatibus rerum II, 18 (Straßburg 1491, sig. a 8 v.). – *Isidorus* gibt nach Instit. divin.

Vor *Paracelsus* lassen sich nicht wenige Quellen beibringen für die „Umarmung“ der Erde durch den männlichen, Samen-bereitenden Himmelskörper und das „Chaos“, die „materia communis“, die „mater et verbo et re ipsa“ ist und als „Gottes Gemahlin“ (*uxor dei*) apostrophiert wird, wie z. B. bei *Leo Hebraeus*[45]. *Trithemius* spricht von vier „Müttern“, und vier „Vätern“, die ersteren, welche „in der letzten Ordnung“ und die letzteren, welche „in dem Anfang . . . aller Knüpfung“ sind. Das Resultat der „Verknüpfung“ ist ein reines, einiges Etwas, ein „Element“. So ist die „einfältige Erden ein rein Element“[46].

Fassen wir zusammen, so hat sich uns der Begriff der *Acht Mütter* als sehr beziehungsreich erwiesen und aufgeschlossen als ein Ableger des Glaubens an die Entsprechung der „oberen“ – himmlischen – und „unteren“ – irdischen – Elemente. Daß dem so ist, ergibt sich aus dem Zusammenhange, in dem sie im paracelsischen Buch „De podagricis“ eingeführt werden. Hier zerfallen sie in die vier „Astronomien“ und die vier „Philosophien“ – die ersteren mit himmlischen, die letzteren mit irdischen Naturdingen befaßt. Beiden wird das Prädikat „Mutter“ zugeteilt, das bei *Paracelsus* für „Element“ steht. Diese zweimal vier „Elemente“ müssen in dem Wissen und Können des Arztes zusammen kommen. Sie sind sozusagen für ihn „elementar“. Im Bilde der *Acht Mütter* sehen wir mithin die Korrespondenz der oberen und unteren Elemente – in der Naturphilosophie der Renaissance, besonders bei *Zorzi*, breit angelegt und auch sonst bei *Paracelsus* zu belegen. Beziehungen lassen sich anknüpfen zur Mutter-Element-Spekulation des Jezirah-Buches und der *Lauteren Brüder* und mehr spezifisch zu den

II, 14 d. *Lactantius* die Etymologie: „daemonas a Graecis dictos aiunt, quasi daemonas, id est peritos ac rerum scios“ (Wortstamm: *dao* „lehren, lernen“). Dazu *Paracelsus:* De inventione artium, tr. I (Sudh. XIV, 251): „so wissen die geister die ding all“. – Zur älteren Geschichte der Dämonen vgl. *Ingeborg Hammer-Jensen:* Die älteste Alchymie. Kopenhagen 1921. S. 119 über die „Egregoroi“, hebr. „Irin“ – „Wächter“, im Henoch-Buch, die Menschen über Astrologie und Metallurgie belehrend, und die gefallenen Engel mit Bezug auf. Gen. VI, 1, wo die „Egregoroi“ nach den schönen Töchtern der Menschen Lust empfunden und die Riesen erzeugt haben sollen.

[45] *Leo Hebraeus:* De amore dialogi III. Jo. Car. Saraceno Latinitati donati. Venedig 1564. fol. 102 v.

[46] *Joh. Trithemius:* Von den dreyen Anfängen aller natürlichen Künst der Philosophiae. In: *Jo. Schaubert:* Consummata sapientia de lapide minerali Joh. de Padua. Frankfurt 1681. S. 231–233. Ein Brief vom 10. Mai 1503 an *Jo. von Leiningen-Westerburg* nach *K. Arnold:* Johannes Trithemius 1462–1516 (Quellen und Forschungen z. Bistum u. Hochstift Würzburg XXIII). Würzburg 1971. S. 260 (Liste der Briefe).

„Acht Astronomien“ von *Daniel von Morley* (bzw. *Alfarabi*) und der weithin verbreiteten gnostischen Tradition der „Achtheiten“ im Natur- und Geistesleben.

*Summary*

The „Eight Mothers“ – a concept of the *Paracelsian Corpus* emerges from the belief in the correspondence of the upper-celestial- and the nether terrestrial-elements. This belief is common to Renaissance naturalist philosophers and stated in detail by Georgius Venetus ("Zorzi"). Its connexion with the "Eight Mothers" is evident from the context in which they are introduced in the Paracelsian "De podagricis". Here they fall into two *quaternios*, namely the "Four Astronomies" and the "Four Philosophies" – the former concerned with matters celestial and the latter with matters on earth. Both are designated as *Mother* which in Paracelsus stands for *Element*. These twice-four "Elements" must be joined in the knowledge and art of the physician – they are "elementary" for him. The correspondence of the four upper and four lower elements is also evident elsewhere in Paracelsus. "Mother"-element speculations that seem to be basic are extant in the Sefer Jezirah, the works of the Lautere Brüder and more specifically in the "Eight Astronomies" of Daniel de Morley (and his sources Alfarabi and Avicenna) and the influential *Gnostic* tradition of *Eightnesses* in the life of Nature and Spirit.

# XI

## The Paracelsian Elias Artista and the Alchemical Tradition

Of Goldammer's most admirable Paracelsus-interpretations which have inspired me for more than thirty years one point stands out as essential: the messianic idea concerning a future realm of equity and justice for the pious and the poor.[1] It was to remedy the pressure of religious prosecution, the uncertainties, anxieties and the penury of the time in a world on which the shadow of destruction in the *Platonic Year* was already cast.[2] Yet it was not blind forces that were here at work. There is a meaning, a divine purpose in history as reflected in a new concept of Time.

Time is no longer seen as "empty" successive movement, is not a continuum of uniform and homogeneous moments. Time is rather "filled" by a series of purposeful "nows". Each of these indicates the point in time in which a certain object reaches the fulness of perfection, its "monarchy". What matters regarding time is therefore not past and future, but the present, the "now".[3] This is how God works in history and man is bound to appreciate history as the expression of His will. It is from this that the pessimistic vein is somewhat ambivalently corrected and our own world the prospect of some perfection is not refused. It is strangely juxtaposed to the *New Jerusalem* and the *Golden World* beyond.[4] The matter laid before the reader in the following pages belongs to the optimistic aspect envisaging some messianic era in our own world in which Paracelsus divines the realisation of transmutation, the alchemical dream of elevating base metal to the perfection of gold.

### *Elias Artista and Paracelsus*

Elijah, the prophet, also called *Helias,* and Elishah, called *Heliseus,* supplied sobriquets for the attribution of anonymous alchemical treatises in the Middle Ages. To Paracelsus Helias represents various features of an ideal through which enlightenment and happiness will descend upon future generations and lift the veil of obscurity which still blinds him and his age. Helias is the perfect adept to come. The example he gives is a phenomenon

[1] Kurt Goldammer, Paracelsische Eschatologie, II, Nova Acta Paracelsica 1952, VI, 68 – 102 (p. 90 seq).

[2] Goldammer, ibidem, I, vol. V, 1948, p. 61.

[3] „Zeit als sinnerfüllte Augenblicke der Geschichte", Goldammer, Paracelsus. Natur und Offenbarung. Hannover 1953, p. 92. To the object-specific "nows" as composing "biological time" in Paracelsus see W. Pagel, Das medizinische Weltbild des Paracelsus (Kosmosophie, I, ed. K. Goldammer), Wiesbaden 1962, p. 101 – 105 and idem, Paracelsus als Naturmystiker, in: Epochen d. Naturmystik (A. Faivre, R. C. Zimmermann, eds.). Berlin 1979, p. 59.

[4] Goldammer, Natur und Offenbarung, l. c., p. 92; idem, Paracelsus. Sozialethische und Sozialpolitische Schriften. Tübingen 1952, p. 323.

that had long been known and even occurred in a natural-philosophical treatise of Nicolaus Cusanus (1401–1464). The latter mentions a "story" to the effect that a certain spring-water in Hungary owing to its vitriol-content can transmute iron into copper. It supported the evidence for water being a complex substance which can harden or even petrify things brought into touch with it. Indeed plants should derive most of their substance from water.[5] Transmutation of iron added to a copper-vitriol solution into copper was accepted up to the middle of the seventeenth century, as for example by Libavius and Sennert although it had been refuted by Guibert (1603, 1614) and Angelus Sala (1617) and subsequently on a more solid experimental basis by Van Helmont (1624) and Joachim Jungius (1630).[6] Paracelsus naturally still subscribed to the transformation of iron into copper. This, he said, is achieved by Nature who has her "particular freedom as received by God". It can be also accomplished by us using vitriol and he will indicate how. Hence there should be many more such transmutations possible that are still unknown such as notably the conversion of iron into gold. "Many arts are withheld from us because we have not ingratiated ourselves to God so that he would make them manifest to us. To make iron into copper is not as much as to make it into gold. Hence what is less God has allowed to emerge. What is more is still hidden up to the time of the arts of Helias when he will come. For the arts have Heliam in the same way as other fields have their's."[7]

Helias here serves the optimistic view of a messianic future in which the adept philosopher will perform feats that are not yet given to human endeavour. His prowess is bound up with transmutation. Elsewhere, in a metaphysical context, transmutation of iron into copper is quoted as an achievement of "celestial magic" on the same level as conversion of man into wolf, sapphire into diamond and other such changes. It is connected with the power of becoming invisible as shown in the transfiguration of Christ and hence "celestial".[8]

The story was modified in a treatise regarded as unauthentic. Here the alchemist is credited with power that supersedes Nature – he puts one thing to another and thus produces from a variety of ingredients a single substance what "does more than Nature could do by herself". And this in the face of such "transfigurations of natural things", as seen at Gastein where lead is converted into copper, in Carinthia where silver is made from

[5] Nicolaus Cusanus, De staticis experimentis (Idiotae de sapientia, lib. IV), Opera, Paris 1514, fol. 96 v and r. Tr. H. Menzel-Rogner, Leipzig 1944, p. 30–31.

[6] Hans Kangro, Joachim Jungius' Experimente und Gedanken zur Begründung der Chemie als Wissenschaft. Wiesbaden 1968. To this: W. Pagel, Chemistry at the Cross Roads, the Ideas of Joachim Jungius (1587–1657), in: Ambix, 1969, XVI, 100–108.

[7] Paracelsus, Von den natürlichen Dingen, I, von terpentin ... vitriol, cap. 8, ed. Sudhoff, II, p. 163.

[8] Philos. sagax, II, 4, ed. Sudhoff, p. 333.

mercury, in Hungary where gold is gained from silver. The alchemist who receives from God the gift of producing such effects also knows through God how to conceal such *arcana* "up to the coming time of Helia artista when what is occult will be manifest".[9]

*Heliseus* (Elishah) was possessed of magic power by virtue of godliness. He was thus productive of long distance-effects. He is the holy one whose body God will not allow to be mocked. When his baldness was held to derision he, the "celestial magician", exercised his supernatural "black magic" *(nigromantia coelestis)* – he "created" the bears which devoured the children who had scoffed at his bald head.[10] The bears "were made" (wurden) super-naturally (uber die natur) by virtue of his devout belief in God; this made him a *magus* whose curse wrought unheard of physical effects.[11] It was a "necromantic" vision in which Helias and Moyses appeared before Christ.[12] It had been Helias whose prayer had "closed heaven" in the same way as Ezechias arrested the sun-dial by entreaty and Josua stopped the course of the Sun.[13] It is in a related context that the *Heliezati* are bracketed together with the *Enochdiani* and the *Aquaster*[14] – individuals and forces endowed with long life and even immortality through their union with the macrocosm, the *Iliaster.*[15] Similarly Heliseus and Elias close the ranks of those who like Sampson, David, Salomon, Enoch, Adam and Moises understood much of the "heavenly treasure" *(himmlische thesaurinella),* namely the scope of the "aquastric and pyromantic" art. It is the art of the "aquastric magus". He can prevail upon the world of spirits (the *trarames, durdales, turba magna)* to teach him the marrow of theology. This one would assume should provide the magical means of producing real objects and effects from shadowy and ideal fore-forms from their germinal soil, the *aquaster* – itself the fore-form of the real hotbed of real objects, namely water.[16]

---

[9] Tinctura physicorum, cap. 4, ed. Sudhoff, XIV, p. 396.

[10] With ref. to II Kings, 2, 23–24. Philos. sagax, II, 3, ed. Sudhoff, XII, p. 328; nigromantia coelestis, ibidem, cap. 4, p. 335. Magia "taught" by Apocalypsis Johannis, Moises, Aaron, Elias, Enoch, Bildad, David, Salomon, Daniel, Baruch, Jeremiah, Hesekiel and all other prophets each of whom was a magus and a "born" cabalist and diviner, De pestilitate, ed. Sudhoff, XIV, p. 637.

[11] Philos. sagax, II, 6, ed. Sudhoff, XII, p. 370.

[12] Ibid. II, 4, p. 381.

[13] Prognosticatio ad XXIV. annum . . . anno 1536, ed. Sudhoff, X, p. 624.

[14] De vita longa, IV, 3, ed. Sudhoff, III, p. 281. – Enoch and Elias and others whose spirit and celestial body were taken by God into heaven: Philosophiae tract. V (vom schlaf und wachen der Geister), ed. Sudhoff, XIII, p. 358. Enoch and Elias who properly knew their mind live eternally and never die, Lib. de imaginibus, cap. XII, ed. Sudhoff, XIII, p. 383. Enoch and Elias as also David, Moises and Aaron were led out of hell, namely the elemental world, the matrix mundi majoris, Lib. Azoth, practica lineae vitae, ed. Sudhoff, XIV, p. 581.

[15] De vita longa, loc. cit., note 14.

[16] Lib. Azoth, cap. 2, XIV, p. 552. On aquaster: C. G. Jung, Paracelsica. Zürich u. Leipzig 1942, p. 91 94, spinning out the aspects of psychical principles with bodily connections.

Paracelsus, then, reserved for Helias and Heliseus a whole spectrum of functions. These ascend from the lowest, namely his role as the chemical light of future generations. By him miracles of the chemical art will be achieved which were so far only obtainable to Nature. Helias, the artist, will then transform objects such as notably metals, for example iron, into gold. He will act with natural means, as a *natural magus*. Beyond this Helias represents super-natural forces. They follow from his devout belief as well as his union with cosmic forces and spirits. It is these which teach him how to produce real objects and phenomena from the shadows of ideas, their fore-forms or "prologues in heaven"; it is from an all-comprising treasure-house of such fore-forms, the fore-form of fore-forms that they derive. This is the *aquaster* – an ideal fore-form of water, the "prime matter" which provides the building-material for all objects in the world. *Helias artista,* the chemist of the future achieving effects so far out of reach, thus joins the ranks of the prophets of old. These had been capable of super-natural feats and by dint of belief and union with cosmic forces had attained to long life and indeed immortality.

*Mediaeval Sources*

Paracelsus' *Helias artista* with his messianic associations and the vision of a super-chemistry coming true in a distant future ties up with a strong mediaeval tradition. This is bound up with the activities of the Franciscan order, in the first place of Brother Elias of Cortona, companion and successor to St. Francis. When deposed from his generalship in 1239 he faced among other things the accusation of having occupied himself with alchemy. Alchemical tracts were consequently assigned to his name, however improbable their authenticity. Roger Bacon, a Franciscan, left alchemical treatises. Arnald of Villanova is known for his intimate connections with Franciscan divines and exponents of chiliastic and Joachimite ideas including French Beguines. He too became a great name in Alchemy. Franciscan alchemy and chemistry may be said to have reached its climax with John de Rupescissa towards the middle of the fourteenth century.

In the present context the work we have to consider is the *Speculum Alchymiae Heliae Monachi Franciscani.* It was printed for the first time in full in *Opuscula quaedam Chemica,* Francofurti 1614. Its substance had been printed before in 1603 as *Arnaldi de Villanova Speculum alchimiae liber nunc primum in lucem editus,* also at Francfort, and reprinted in the *Theatrum Chemicum,* vol. IV, Francofurti 1613, also assigned to Arnald of Villanova. The latter two versions differ from the 1614 text in several important respects. On the whole they are shorter and less rich in quotations which are chiefly from Arabic writers such as notably Geber, Morienus and Hermes. They have, however, one more chapter at the end, an "octava dispositio", and a summary *(recapitulatio)* to wind up the treatise.

From Thorndike's account of the manuscripts the 1614 edition would appear to be closer to the mediaeval tradition, although Thorndike apparently considered only the 1603 and 1613 text for comparison. This emerges for example in what he says about the Hermes quotations. Several of these are found in the 1614, but missing in the earlier version.[17] Nor is there any *recapitulatio* in the manuscripts. Assigning the text to Helia, the Franciscan monk, the 1614 version would follow some of the continental manuscripts, whereas others as well as British manuscripts attribute it to Nicolaus de Comitibus "of the Trevisan march", possibly the astrological writer of the middle of the fifteenth century.[18] Dedication to Pope Benedict XIth would exclude Elias of Cortona, the companion of St. Francis, as the Pope was only 13 when Elias died and the text is by contents obviously much older anyway.[19] Assignation to Arnald as in both of the earlier printings is just as arbitrary. The present author came across a passage in the 1614 edition which amounts to a quotation from Arnald. Here it says: the *Rosarius* "de Villa nova" states that sublimation is dignifying in that a *maximum* is achieved from a *minimum*, or something spiritual from corporeal and the spirit is nobler than body. This passage is omitted from the earlier printed versions attributed to Arnald.[20] It would exclude Arnald as author at least of the 1614 version. The mysterious Dausus (Dausten, Dastin) is mentioned by name in 1603, but merely as "quidam" in the same place in 1614.[21] This may suggest a late date, possibly in the middle of the XIVth century for the composition or editing of the tract.

At all events the *Speculum* is solid evidence for the broad mediaeval roots of *Elias artista*. It could be added to from a number of further items extant in the manuscript catalogues[22] with a great variety of alchemical themes including the use of *Helias* as author of a treatise normally ascribed to Rhazes.[23]

---

[17] Hermes quotation common to both versions: aurum nostrum ... Pater est Sol et argentum nostrum ... mater Luna, 1614, p. 79; 1603, p. 45, both in septima dispositione. Hermes dicens, sublima subtile a spisso, 1614, p. 62; missing at this place on p. 20, 1603. Dixit Hermes: vis ejus integra est, si versa fuerit in terram, 1614, p. 82; missing 1603. Lynn Thorndike, A History of Magic and Experimental Science, vol. III, New York 1924, p. 169 says that a Hermes quotation in the manuscripts is missing in the printed editions (in the sixth disposition).

[18] Thorndike, Hist. of Magic, III, p. 83 and 163.

[19] Thorndike, loc. cit., p. 163 seq.

[20] In an analogous passage in the 7th disposition, 1614, p. 76, the "Rosarius de villa nova" ibidem, p. 72, becomes: "quidam consilio Rosarii ductus dicit", also with respect to the overriding dignity of sublimation: quisquis scit perfecte sublimationem, scit totum magisterium facere. "Sublimatus, honoratus" are the attributes of a powder ascending from earthy deposit in Arnaldus, Rosarium, in Opera chymica, Francofurti 1603, p. 50. Similarly: iste homo sublimatus est id est in dignitate positus. Flos florum, 1603, p. 111.

[21] "Dausus philosophus", 1603, p. 35; 1614, p. 71: quidam (on calx).

[22] Lynn Thorndike and Pearl Kibre, Catalogue of Incipits of Mediaeval Scientific Writings in Latin. London 1963, p. 1817 (10 items).

[23] Liber utilitatis naturae secretorum compositus per fratrem heliam ordinis fratrum minorum. Thorndike and Kibre, loc. cit. in note 22, p. 822. In: L. C.

*After Paracelsus*

The Paracelsian tradition of *Elias artista* with all its magical and messianic overtones became common currency in XVIIth century chemical philosophy.[24] It provided the watchword in one of the ordinary alchemical treatises of the time: the *Cheiragogia Heliana de auro philosophico* of Raphael Eglinus Iconius (1559–1622) – "anagrammatizomenos" to "Nicolaus Niger Hapelius". His distinguished career as Professor of New Testament and archdeacon at Zürich came to an abrupt end when he had squandered his fortune by his addiction to alchemical experimentation. He removed to Marburg again to take up a theological professorship, after 1601.[25] His preoccupation with prophets and prophecies is evidenced by his *Conjectura halieutica characterum piscium* in which he taught how to forecast events from certain marks found in fishes.[26] What is of greater interest and more significant is his contact with Giordano Bruno at Zürich – the last refuge on Bruno's wanderings from Helmstedt and Francfort before his fateful return to Italy. It was Bruno's *Summary of metaphysical terms to grasp the study of logic and philosophy* which Eglinus published from dictated notes at Zürich in 1595, after Bruno's disappearence into the dungeons of the Inquisition. What is even more: Eglin had the courage to bring out a second edition nine years after Bruno's martyrdom at the stake (Marburg, 1609). Eglin (together with another alchemist, Joh. Henr. Heinzel – "Einzellius") thus forms at least a personal link between Bruno and Hermeticism.[27]

Eglinus (– Hapelius) is deeply imbued with the truth and reality of alchemical transmutation. He militates against two Jesuit scholars who denied sulphur and mercury as the original and principal components of mineral and metal. He crowns his argument with the demonstration *in vitro* of what he believed to be the conversion of mercury into a variety of metals and their reversion into mercury.[28] This does not embrace silver and gold,

Witten II and R. Pachella, Alchemy and the Occult. III, Mellon Collection, Yale U. L., Manuscripts. New Haven, 1977, MS. 7, p. 49. Ibidem, MS. 29, p. 188, Elias Cortonensis, Lumen luminum, resembling a work, sometimes ascribed to Rases, Thorndike and Kibre, p. 1237, by contents possibly related to MS. 7.

[24] For relevant titles see H. Kopp, Die Alchemie in älterer u. neuerer Zeit. Heidelberg 1886, I, p. 250–252. Adam Bruxius, author of Helias tertius, 1616, is reminiscent of Gaspar Bruschius, in whose Hodoeporicum Bavaricum of 1553 a Vaticinium of "Thesbaeus Helias" is quoted. Thorndike, Hist. of Magic, V, p. 373.

[25] For biography and bibliography: J. Ferguson, Bibliotheca Chemica, 1906, I, p. 232–233 and 364–365.

[26] Ferguson, ibid., p. 233.

[27] D. W. Singer, Giordano Bruno. New York 1950, p. 153. W. Pagel, Review of Yates, F. A., Giordano Bruno and the Hermetic Tradition. London 1964, in: Ambix 1964, **XII**, 72–76.

[28] Disquisitio Heliana de metallorum transformatione adversus Hagelii et Pererii Jesuitarum opiniones, Lipsiae 1606, also Marburg 1608 and 1612 – the latter the edition used (in this the Disquisitio appears as part II of Cheiragogia Heliana de auro philosophico necdum cognito), p. 168: ostendimus, ut metalla in Mercurium resolvantur. p. 170: postquam re ipsa ostendimus metalla ex hydrargyro proxime originem ducere

but one would assume it to be his idea that the super-chemist of a future age, the *Helias artista*, will be able to do with the noblest of metals what at his own time could be accomplished by addition of iron to copper-sulphate. This was the apparent transmutation of iron into copper – well known and widely discussed of old, believed by Nicolaus Cusanus, Paracelsus and Libavius and already contested at the time of Eglin's publication.[29]

For the messianic overtones of his chemical achievements and expectations his authority is Paracelsus. He was the first to mention a certain *Elias artista* to come after him and Basilius Valentinus and Alexander of Suchten left chemical works which will be opened to us through "Helias who is to come". *Helias* thus stands for a future age and the hopes which can be attached to his practical success, *qua* products of his own time as appropriate to the standard of the art which he pursues. The "Helias" of the Latin tongue should thus have emerged at the age of Cicero.[30] Eglin in particular refers[31] to Paracelsus' idea of a *golden age* when man no longer lives like beast and swine, but dedicates himself to the study of the "great secret in nature" *(grosse heimlikeit in der natur)*. Such would yield immediate fruit for the better. Alas, the present is the time when man is all intent on lechery and this will last until one third of the world is slain, another third perishes of its roguery and the third just survives. However it will be returned to its proper "stable" *(in sein rechten stall)*. Also the guilds must perish and be eradicated from the world, otherwise the golden age *(güldin welt)* will not rise, the age when man comes to his senses and to life human and not brutish and not piggish and not spent in the taverns.[32]

But, characteristically he asks: what about *now?* The world is full of alchemical books and fumes – there is hardly a corner not redolent with chemical smoke. Hence already before Helias we are not allowed to "take a holiday" from chemical work. It was Paracelsus himself who raised the question of the *etiam nunc*, of the "also now",[33] conscious as he was of his

---

[29] See above p. 7.

[30] Ibidem, p. 134.

[31] Ibidem, p. 143, on the Theophrastea catastrophe and the Paracelsica temporum distributio, licet nescio quo spiritu ab ipso praedicata et ad akmen Heliae artistae ab ipso relata sit, quando ipsius Theoria cum Praxi florebit et passim, ut ait, in vulgus dispergetur . . .

[32] Paracelsus, Von den natürlichen dingen, I, von terpentin . . . vitriol, cap. 8: vom Vitriol, ed. Sudhoff, II, p. 164–165. Eglin cites: lib. de mineralibus, cap. 8 and for the golden age, ibid. cap. 7: the tempus Helianum Paracelsi, when all will recognise his teaching, will be the 58th year which according to Eglin can only mean: 1658, not 1558. Cheiragogia, p. 132 seq.

[33] Paracelsus, Libellus de tinctura physicorum, Prologus, ed. Sudhoff, XIV, p. 392: jezt folgt in der mittlern welt die monarchei aller künsten an Theophrastum den fürsten langend . . . Ibid., cap. 5, p. 397: sucht, sucht, spricht der höchste spagirus, so werd ir finden . . . wo Du iezt der alchemisten handgriffen geflissen und erfaren bist, als dan so ist nichts so subtils oder scharfs in dingen der natur das dir nicht ofenbar werden.

own position in an intermediate age when he could be of use to the lovers of truth. He calls the adepts of the age *astrales,* that is of angelical nature related to the astral forces which actuate the inner life of metals.[34] It is thus that Eglin finds justification for counting himself among those adepts or *mentales* (as they were called by Suchten) being in no conflict with the task and the laws of Nature and the godly love of the neighbour.[35]

The *Cheiragogia* as well as the *Disquisitio Heliana* are sober technical treatises. They deal with the changes that can be brought about in metals by chemical manipulation. They are alchemical to the extent of subscribing to the idea of the origin of all metals in an "embryonic" metal, namely mercury, and of sulphur lending the second fundamental principle in their development, essence and transmutation. They are, however, free of alchemical symbolism and *arcana.* Accordingly the messianic hope which they have to offer is that of technical perfection in a future age – that of the "Helias of Chemistry". This will be the age of Chemistry – just as the age of Rhetoric was that of Cicero, its *Helias.* Authority for all this is found in the sayings of Paracelsus about the *Helias artista* to come and to show how to convert iron, not into copper (as already demonstrable), but into gold. Indeed this will be in a golden age to follow a world catastrophe in which two thirds of mankind will have perished. And yet there is no time for waiting and vacation after the impact made by the solid Paracelsian progress. This is the raison d'être for the author's own efforts, however short they may fall of the ultimate aim.

No such modesty can be credited to Johann Rudolph Glauber (1604–1670) and his tract: *De Elia Artista or what a man he is and what he will reform in the World or improve and when he cometh.*[36] The answer is: he will extricate from oblivion the true spagyric medicine of the Egyptian philosophers of old which was lost for more than a thousand years; he will renovate and illustrate it by new inventions, he will abolish much useless muck and bring along and show the present erring World a nearer, better, easier and also less costly way towards good medicine. He may come soon after Glauber's own day and at a time of grand changes in several kingdoms such as notably the Roman Empire when ruler wants to vanquish ruler and make himself monarch. Helias' monarchy, however, is different – his name stands *magice* for *salia* into which it converts when read from back to front. Indeed in

[34] Manuale de lapide philosophico medicinali, Vorrede, ed. Sudhoff, XIV, p. 421: etliche menschen als englische naturen. Ibid., p. 427: dan was ich jetzt mit kürze schreib ... damit es die astralischen discipuli vernemen. Eglin, p. 144–145.

[35] Eglin, p. 145 seq.

[36] De Elia artista oder wass Elias Artista für einer sey, und was Er in der Welt reformiren, oder verbessern werde, wann Er kombt? Nemblich die Wahre Spagirische Medicin der alten Aegyptischen Philosophen ... Amsterdam, Joh. Waesberge, 1668, No. 24 in Kurt F. Gugel, Joh. Rud. Glauber. Leben u. Werk. Würzburg 1955, p. 24. – H. M. E. de Jong, Glauber und die Weltanschauung der Rosenkreuzer, in: Janus, 1969, LVI, 278–304, p. 289.

the philosophers' world *Elias Artista* indicates *secret salia – salia artis* – still unknown and destined to achieve "great, nay incredible" things. From salts, then, and in particular his own newly discovered *"Glauber's-salt" (sodium sulphate)*, new alchemical effects and indeed a universal medicine can be expected to develop.[37] His *sal mirabile*, the "universal salt of the philosophers'", will be capable of "exalting" gold to the "highest purple-red" and silver to the "utmost white colour". Glauber himself had already achieved and demonstrated this to friends, but illness prevented him from bringing such experiments to the level of confirmed and sure knowledge – this will surely be accomplished by the chemist of the future whom his work has "awakened".[38]

Eight years before the tract *De Elia Artista* was published Glauber had been even more explicit about the super-chemist to come namely in the second part of his *Miraculum mundi*. This, it says on the title-page, will present the "triumphant entry on horse-back of Elias Artista presaged of old". Also it will show what sort of person Elias Artista is, namely the "*Sal Artis Mirificum*", the "highest medicine of all vegetables, animals and minerals". This will be proved by the growth-promotion of seeds and roots, the miraculous healing of all internal and external diseases of man and beast. To this must be added the real conversion of base metals into silver and gold and also increase of the fire-resisting degree of the latter by four units. Finally what is even more it will make it possible to extract a "natural gold" from all herbs and to bring back a "fixed gold" into any herb whereby its growth will be enhanced. Hence an "Illustrious, Glorious and Triumphant Monarch is

ELIAS AR TISTA, known to few
Et ART IS SALIA, famed by many."[39]

Introducing the treatise Glauber points to the disrepute into which the noble art of alchemy has fallen. He therefore decided to set out to defend those who have written truthfully about it, with the help of the "Philosophers' artful Salt" *(Philosophorum Sal Artis)* or, as Paracelsus called his "Salt of Art", Elias Artista *(Paracelsi Eliam Artistam)*. His followers assumed that with this a person was intended, a super-chemist of the future who will teach the transmutation of metals. However, not a person, but a super-salt, the *sal artis*, was meant by Paracelsus – it occurs where he

[37] Glauber, De Elia artista, loc. cit. 1668, Preface, p. 3 – 6.
[38] Ibidem, p. 12.
[39] Johan Rudolph Glauber, Miraculi mundi ander theyl oder dessen vorlängst geprophezeiten Eliae Artistae triumphirlicher Einritt und auch was der Elias Artista für einer sey? Nemlich der Weisen ihr SAL ARTIS Mirificum, als aller Vegetabilien, Animalien und Mineralium höchste Medicin, wie beweislich . . . dieses alles durch die grosse Gnad und Barmhertzigkeit Gottes erfunden und durch desselben weitere Hülff und Beystandt den Freunden Publice zu demonstriren, und wahr zu machen sich erbietet Johan Rudolph Glauber. Amsterdam 1660.

deals with the transmutation of metals and cuts his text short because he "is not allowed to reveal the right Salt of the sages". Instead he uses *Elias Artista* as anagram for *Et Artis Salia.* Indeed, as Glauber found out for himself, he who "has and knows that *Sal Artis* can accomplish great things and he it is to whom that *Elias Artista* has appeared to teach him marvels." [40] Paracelsus had associated the "Salt of the Art" with vitriol, both secretly and in so many words. Where he wrote of the great virtue of vitriol he could not go farther into detail and reveal that *Elias Artista* or *Salt of the Art* "dwells hidden in vitriol". Instead he had to restrict himself stating that the art of converting base metals into noble ones had been granted to him and that this wisdom will pass away with him until *Elias Artista* "will come and truly teach and make known transmutation in the subsequent century in the fifty-eight year". Alas such keen expectations have never been fulfilled – "no *Elias Artista* was willing to come" *(aber ess hat kein Elias Artista kommen wollen).* [41] Much disappointment could have been saved through a correct interpretation of Paracelsus' intentionally cryptic verdict and the insight that *Elias Artista* had been present all the time, namely in the form of the salt which can achieve medical miracles. "Thus I shall not let Paracelsus rest in his grave, but take him out and turn him towards morn (as he presaged) that is to the light of day so that everyone may see that his prophecy has come true".[42] The same rescue from the grave may be Glauber's own fate when his followers and disciples will undo the work of his ennemies and bring about a great reformation in medicine and alchemy. Not again, as in Paracelsus' days, will the Star of destiny sink and be lost, but *Elias Artista, Et Sal Artis* will have opened the door to all divine and natural secrets, to a better secular age and the Land of Promise. Perhaps not surprisingly Glauber raises claims for his own *Sal mirabile* as the messianic guide into this future – the "*Glauber-salt*" *(sodium sulphate)* of our days. He says he had clearly identified it with *Elias Artista* in his tract *De natura salium* which he published in 1658, the very year envisaged by Paracelsus as the turning point when after a "catastrophe" the light of wisdom and humanity will shine again. [43] He has no doubt that Paracelsus and Basilius Valentinus had produced the marvellous salt from vitriol and that it can achieve naturally what the prophets Elia and Elisa wrought divinely – for their names stand anagrammatically for *Salia.* Indeed there neither is nor can be a single man, beast, plant or mineral in the world to which "our salt" is not the "highest medicine". [44]

Glauber would thus seem to arrogate to himself the claim of being the very *Elias Artista* whom Paracelsus had envisaged, the super-chemist who knows

---

[40] Miraculi mundi ander theyl, 1660, loc. cit., Preface, sig. A3 verso.
[41] Ibidem, A4 recto.
[42] Ibidem, A4 verso – A5 recto.
[43] Ibidem, preface, sig. A4 recto.
[44] Ibidem, preface, sig. A6 recto et verso.

how to convert iron into gold. Glauber still subscribes to alchemical transmutation in strong terms including the conversion of iron into copper that had been discredited already in his early days.[45] Accordingly he says that he has indicated the possibility of the transmutation of iron into gold in several of his treatises in cryptic terms *(obscure)*. The method, however, by which this can be accomplished he has not put to paper, largely because he had not yet mastered it completely, but "I have often seen the possibility and truth that gold is increased from iron, just as copper is increased and amplified from iron".[46] He concludes his treatise with extracts from several Paracelsian treatises, notably the *Tinctura physicorum* and the section on Vitriol from *Von den natürlichen Dingen*,[47] which are related to *Elias Artista* as well as the production of the miracle-salt.

In Glauber's work, then, the *Elias Artista* has assumed a complexion that is at variance with tradition. In this the emphasis lay on messianic hopes for the future. Glauber speaks of the present, his own generation and age to whom he was able to present an almost universal medicine, his "Salt of Art and Miracle". This *is* already the Elias or Elisa – not therefore a figure of the future and indeed not a man at all, but a chemical which had always existed, was known to Paracelsus and had to be newly invented and artificially produced by himself. That it had to be a salt follows from the anagrammatic identity of its name with that of the prophet. It is true, Glauber feels he has not fully relieved alchemy of its main burden – the transmutation of base metal into gold. He sees himself close to this ultimate goal, but not yet in that full mastery which would justify communication of his secret. Perhaps he did expect the coming of the true *Elias Artista* after all who will discover and divulge it in the distant future as tradition had foreseen it.

### *Knorr von Rosenroth and the Purifying Fire of The Kabbala Unveiled*

Knorr von Rosenroth (1636 – 1689), friend and collaborator of the younger Van Helmont (1614 – 1699), Hebrew scholar, poet, translator, philosopher and keen expert in alchemy,[48] promises on the title-page of his kabbalistic encyclopaedia, the *Kabbala denudata* (1677 – 1684), that it will contain the *Compendium* of a "cabbalistico-chymical" book called *Aesch-Mczareph* ("Fire purifying", "Fire smelting") on the "Philosophers' Stone etc". Kopp, the father of chemical and alchemical history, looked in vain for this *compendium* in the two massive quarto-volumes of the work.[49] However, as

[45] Ibidem, p. 33 seq. and 36 – 40. See above p. 7.
[46] Ibidem, p. 35.
[47] As quoted above, p. 12 and note 32/33.
[48] See Friedhelm Kemp in the post-script to the reprint of J. B. Van Helmont's Aufgang der Arzneikunst, translated and annotated by Knorr (1683). München, 1971, p. IX – XVII.
[49] Herm. Kopp, Alchemie, loc. cit., 1886, II, p. 232.

Scholem has shown, its substance is there albeit not as a continuous entity.[50] It has the hallmarks of a translation from a Hebrew original. It treats of individual metals at various disconnected places in the first – *lexicon* – part of the *Apparatus to the Book Sohar* dealing with kabbalistic commonplaces. Thus gold with its numero-mystical and sephirotic associations is found under the topos *Lion (arjeh)*, called as it is in alchemical parlance *Red Lion* and also under *Strength (geburah)*.[51] It ends with iron which appears under *Lance (romach)* – iron mainly occurs under its proper topos – *barsel, ferrum* – revealing a number of connotations mystical and kabbalistical of great interest.[52]

We are not concerned, however, with the position of the individual metals and minerals in their kabbalistic and historical context – this has been examined in depth by Scholem.[53] What is of acute interest here is the Introduction to the alchemical sections of the whole *Apparatus* of *Kabbalistic Commonplaces*. For this introduction emerges under the topos *Elisha*, the follower of *Elia*. He is figured as the "most famed Prophet, an exemplary naturalist sage and disdainful of riches" *(sapientiae naturalis exemplar et divitiarum Contemtor)*.[54] This statement is based on the well known story of Naamani and the punishment of the pupil Gehazi for his greed, as told in II. Kings, 5 v. 6. As the sayings of the Fathers have it: who is rich? He who rejoices in his portion. Thus the true healer of impure metals *(verus impurorum metallorum medicus)* has not riches that appear as such, but has them like the *thohu* of primaeval inane and empty nature – the term sharing with *Elijscha* the same numerical value, namely 411.[55] As the Talmud[56] says: "what creates riches is like riches themselves", and this is naturalist wisdom *(talis est sapienta naturalis)*. The mysteries of this wisdom are by no means alien to the higher mysteries of the *Kabbala*. *Sephirot*, the archetypical divine creative forces, are the same on High *(aziluth)* as those in the lower world *(asiah)* and apply to the mineral Kingdom, however more excellent the former than the latter. A "metallic root" thus

[50] G. Scholem, Alchemie und Kabbala. In: Monschr. f. Gesch. u. Wissensch. d. Judent., 1925, **LXIX**, p. 13–30 and 95–110 (p. 97 seq). Already thirty-seven years after the publication of the first volume of the Kabbala denudata an unknown English author attempted a palingenesis of the Esch m'zareph: A short enquiry concerning the Hermetick Art. Address'd to the Studious therein. By a Lover of Philalethes. To which is annexed a collection from Kabbala denudata, and Translation of the Chymical-Cabbalistical Treatise, Intituled, Aesch mezareph: or, Purifying Fire. 1714. 252 pp. in 12°. Sine loco; no imprint. R. A. Gilbert (Bristol), Cat. XI, item 25, 1976. Briefly quoted by Scholem, p. 105, note (1) after Waite, Doctrine and literature of the Kabalah. 1902, p. 308–314.

[51] Kabbala denudata, I, Sulzbaci 1677, p. 152 and 227. Scholem, p. 102 for the traditional sephirotic and planetary correspondencies of individual metals.

[52] P. 206–208 and 683–684.

[53] Loc. cit., p. 100 and passim, 1925.

[54] Kabb. denud., I, p. 116.

[55] Ibidem, p. 117.

[56] Babah bathra, fol. 25, col. 2.

occupies the *sephirah Crown (kether).* From it and its occult nature all metals take their origin – the nature of their root being just as much of a mystery as the *sephirah Crown,* the occult origin of the other *sephiroth.* What immediately springs from the metallic root is lead, the most primitive metal. It therefore falls under the *sephirah Wisdom (chochmah),* the immediate neighbour of *Kether* on the tree of *sephiroth.* Tin, white like old age and through its creaking symbolising judicial severity and rigour, comes under the following *sephirah, Binah* (reason), white silver under *Chessed* (benignity), red gold under *Geburah* (strength), not only because of its colour, but also its heat and sulphur. *Jesod* (foundation) is mercury, metal-water that is "alive", *argentum vivum,* the whole basis of metallic nature and art.[57] Finally what improves, "heals" and confers nobility on metals, the *medicina metallorum,* belongs to *Malchuth* (kingdom),[58] the opposite pole of the first *sephirah* – it stands for an epitome to the sum total of *sephiroth,* as well as for the lowest manifestation of a creative force; it forms the conjunction of the divine with the elemental world. It probably indicates the Philosophers' Stone, although this term may have been advisedly avoided. Not only metals are thus correlated with the *sephiroth* whereby the key is provided for the opening up of the more intimate sanctuaries of Nature. It is also the three Paracelsian Principles, Salt, Sulphur and Mercury which are included in the collation, for "all tend to the One". Indeed the three highest *sephiroth, Kether, Chochmah* and *Binah,* can be regarded as their source: mercury (water) from Kether, salt from *Chochmah* and sulphur from *Binah.* The remaining seven *sephiroth* would thus be reserved for the metals, *Gedulah* (greatness) and *Geburah* (strength) for silver and gold, *Tiphereth* (glory) for iron, *Nezach* (firmness) and *Hod* (splendour) for tin and copper, *Jesod* (foundation) for lead, whilst *Malchuth* (kingdom) would be the female metallic principle and the Moon of the Wise *(Foemina metallica* and *Luna sapientum),* the field into which the seeds of the secret minerals are to be sown such as the "Water of Gold". "However, heed, my Son, that in these matters there lie such mysteries as no human tongue can utter."[59]

*Elias Artista,* thus, has become the prophet Elisha of old. He, who condemned the riches of the world saw the riches which lie hidden in that chaotic matter which challenges the naturalist and kabbalist. He will gain knowledge and mastery, he will convert it into a kosmos through correlation of

[57] Jesod est argentum vivum ... et aqua haec viva omnino est fundamentum totius naturae et artis metallicae, p. 118 – to be compared with Kether, the highest sephirah with a less concrete Radix metallica, p. 117 and above.

[58] P. 118. To this, Scholem, loc. cit. 1925, p. 98–99, note (4).

[59] Kab. denud., I, p. 118: sed scito, fili mi, in his talia latere mysteria, quae nulla hominum lingua effari poterit: Ego autem ulterius non peccabo lingua mea, sed custodiam os meum clausura ex Psalm 39,2. Esch mezareph, cap. 1 (probably end of the introductory chapter, Scholem, l. c., p. 99).

each component with the archetypal creative forces. This sephirotic differentiation separates and reunites like the fire of the alchemist, the Fire of Purgation *(esch mezareph).*

*In conclusion,* then, *Elias Artista* has gone through a characteristic sequence of changes. Starting as a venerable name to be adopted for the unknown author of mediaeval alchemical manuscripts connected with Franciscan tradition he became the messianic figure of the super-chemist who will reveal the secret of the conversion of iron into gold to a future age. This will follow a cataclysm to which two thirds of mankind fell victim. Then the high ethical standards reclaimed will merit the coming of the chemical "redeemer" of base metal and the truth of Paracelsianism will be commonplace. The technical-chemical overtones thus attached to the figure of a remote past and future helped to concentrate attention to the present – Rosicrucian times when there was hardly a corner free of alchemical smoke. Thus finally *Elias Artista* was depersonalised – he indicated a universal medicine, a product of chemical manipulation. That was already in the grasp of such chemical inventors as Glauber who also felt he possessed the secret of transmutation into gold. At the same time (if not before) a new dimension was added – the mystical and cosmosophic correlation of the minerals and their origin with the ten creative attributes of Divinity, the *sephiroth* of the Kabbala. It was connected with Elisha, the naturalist who preferred the hidden riches which can be earned by those who search for the cosmic order in the chaos before us to the manifest riches that are grasped by the greedy. This cosmic – sephirotic – order comprises not only individual metals and their common "metallic root" (mercury), but also the three Paracelsian principles, salt, sulphur and mercury.

Indeed the kabbalistic version of the *Elias artista* is indebted to Paracelsus. In his main metaphysical work, the *Philosophia sagax,* not Elijah, but Elisha – *Heliseus* – already dominates the scene as a magus who wrought supernatural effects. Figures of his stamp, the *Heliesati,* are related to those who like the Enoch-men acquire long life through union with cosmic forces. In the *Esch m'zareph,* the kabbalistic coordination of minerals with the *Sephiroth,* it is again Elisha and not Elijah who is invoked as the introductory authority, the keeper of unknown treasures of naturalist wisdom.

# INDEX